Advances in the Science of Mating, Love, and Attachment in Romantic Relationships

Advances in the Science of Mating, Love, and Attachment in Romantic Relationships

Guest Editors

Bianca P. Acevedo
Adam Bode

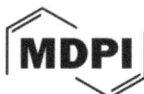

Basel • Beijing • Wuhan • Barcelona • Belgrade • Novi Sad • Cluj • Manchester

Guest Editors

Bianca P. Acevedo
Department of Psychological
and Brain Sciences
University of California
Santa Barbara
United States

Adam Bode
School of Archaeology
and Anthropology
Australian National
University
Canberra
Australia

Editorial Office
MDPI AG
Grosspeteranlage 5
4052 Basel, Switzerland

This is a reprint of the Special Issue, published open access by the journal *Behavioral Sciences* (ISSN 2076-328X), freely accessible at: www.mdpi.com/journal/behavsci/special_issues/L72811IAM8.

For citation purposes, cite each article independently as indicated on the article page online and using the guide below:

Lastname, A.A.; Lastname, B.B. Article Title. *Journal Name* **Year**, *Volume Number*, Page Range.

ISBN 978-3-7258-4034-2 (Hbk)
ISBN 978-3-7258-4033-5 (PDF)
https://doi.org/10.3390/books978-3-7258-4033-5

© 2025 by the authors. Articles in this book are Open Access and distributed under the Creative Commons Attribution (CC BY) license. The book as a whole is distributed by MDPI under the terms and conditions of the Creative Commons Attribution-NonCommercial-NoDerivs (CC BY-NC-ND) license (https://creativecommons.org/licenses/by-nc-nd/4.0/).

Contents

About the Editors vii

Preface ix

Brian N. Chin, Lauryn Kim, Shelby M. Parsons and Brooke C. Feeney
Attachment Orientation and Preferences for Partners' Emotional Responses in Stressful and Positive Situations
Reprinted from: *Behav. Sci.* **2024**, *14*, 77, https://doi.org/10.3390/bs14010077 1

Farnaz Mosannenzadeh, Maartje Luijten, Dominique F. MacIejewski, Grace V. Wiewel and Johan C. Karremans
Adult Attachment and Emotion Regulation Flexibility in Romantic Relationships
Reprinted from: *Behav. Sci.* **2024**, *14*, 758, https://doi.org/10.3390/bs14090758 19

Junnan Tian and Harry Freeman
"All You Need Is Love" a Social Network Approach to Understanding Attachment Networks in Adulthood
Reprinted from: *Behav. Sci.* **2024**, *14*, 647, https://doi.org/10.3390/bs14080647 45

Miriam Jacqueline Muñoz-Aucapiña, Rosa Elvira Muñoz-Aucapiña, Inmaculada García-García, María Adelaida Álvarez-Serrano, Ana María Antolí-Jover and Encarnación Martínez-García
Correction: Muñoz-Aucapiña et al. (2025). Psychometric Validation of the Dating Violence Questionnaire (DVQ-R) in Ecuadorians. *Behavioral Sciences*, 15(1), 68
Reprinted from: *Behav. Sci.* **2025**, *15*, 461, https://doi.org/10.3390/bs15040461 65

Rhonda N. Balzarini, Anya Sharma and Amy Muise
Virtually Connected: Do Shared Novel Activities in Virtual Reality Enhance Self-Expansion and Relationship Quality?
Reprinted from: *Behav. Sci.* **2025**, *15*, 67, https://doi.org/10.3390/bs15010067 67

Cailee M. Nelson, Christian O'Reilly, Mengya Xia and Caitlin M. Hudac
Coupling Up: A Dynamic Investigation of Romantic Partners' Neurobiological States During Nonverbal Connection
Reprinted from: *Behav. Sci.* **2024**, *14*, 1133, https://doi.org/10.3390/bs14121133 92

Adam Bode and Phillip S. Kavanagh
Romantic Love and Behavioral Activation System Sensitivity to a Loved One
Reprinted from: *Behav. Sci.* **2023**, *13*, 921, https://doi.org/10.3390/bs13110921 108

Sara Cloonan, Lara Ault, Karen L. Weihs and Richard D. Lane
Development and Preliminary Validation of the Lovebird Scale
Reprinted from: *Behav. Sci.* **2024**, *14*, 747, https://doi.org/10.3390/bs14090747 126

Seo Jung Shin, Ji Seong Yi and Song Yi Lee
Emerging Love: A Subjective Exploration of Romantic Bonds in Early Adulthood Within the South Korean Context
Reprinted from: *Behav. Sci.* **2024**, *14*, 1135, https://doi.org/10.3390/bs14121135 147

Ana María Fernández, Maria Teresa Barbato, Pamela Barone, Belén Zavalla, Diana Rivera-Ottenberger and Mónica Guzmán-González
What Is the Link of Closeness and Jealousy in Romantic Relationships?
Reprinted from: *Behav. Sci.* **2025**, *15*, 132, https://doi.org/10.3390/bs15020132 169

Thomas B. Sease, Emily K. Sandoz, Leo Yoke, Julie A. Swets and Cathy R. Cox
Loneliness and Relationship Well-Being: Investigating the Mediating Roles of Relationship Awareness and Distraction among Romantic Partners
Reprinted from: *Behav. Sci.* **2024**, *14*, 439, https://doi.org/10.3390/bs14060439 . . . . **182**

Miriam Jacqueline Muñoz-Aucapiña, Rosa Elvira Muñoz-Aucapiña, Inmaculada García-García, María Adelaida Álvarez-Serrano, Ana María Antolí-Jover and Encarnación Martínez-García
Psychometric Validation of the Dating Violence Questionnaire (DVQ-R) in Ecuadorians
Reprinted from: *Behav. Sci.* **2025**, *15*, 68, https://doi.org/10.3390/bs15010068 . . . . **196**

Sandra J. E. Langeslag
Refuting Six Misconceptions about Romantic Love
Reprinted from: *Behav. Sci.* **2024**, *14*, 383, https://doi.org/10.3390/bs14050383 . . . . **210**

About the Editors

Bianca P. Acevedo

Dr. Bianca P. Acevedo (BA, NYU; PhD, Stony Brook University) is a researcher at the University of California, Santa Barbara, and Northwell Health in NYC. She has conducted extensive research on the neural basis of pair bonding, attachment, sensory processing sensitivity, and interventions for healthy aging. She was the recipient of the 2012 International Women in Science Award, and her research has been funded by the National Science Foundation, the National Institute of Health, and the Alzheimer's Association. Her first book, *The Highly Sensitive Brain*, was nominated for the 2021 PROSE Award in Neuroscience, and her second book, *The Science and Art of Sensory Processing Sensitivity* (Elsevier), examines the impact of personality and the environment on the expression of high sensitivity.

Adam Bode

Adam Bode is an interdisciplinary romantic love and human mating researcher who employs an ethological framework in his theory and analysis. He has a Bachelor of Psychology (Honours) and a Bachelor of Laws from the Australian National University. He is currently enrolled in a PhD program in Biological Anthropology at the Australian National University and holds a position as sessional academic at Federation University Australia. Adam's research investigates romantic love using methods and approaches from biological anthropology, human ethology, and psychology.

Preface

In recent decades, researchers have made notable advances in the science of pair bonding, romantic love, and attachment. Access to novel instruments and methods, as well as animal studies, have provided a platform to advance our understanding of the factors and mechanisms that underly the formation and maintenance of pair bonds and attachment relationships.

From short to long-term pair bonds, the great variation in relationship strategies has opened up important areas of research. Thus, this Special Issue, entitled "The Advances in the Science of Love and Attachment", showcases the emerging and evolving field of relationship science, and it includes a collection of studies that represent countries around the globe, various methods, and topics that reveal the complexity of love and attachment. It includes studies using virtual reality, EEG, and Q methodology. Also, it explores themes related to attachment style, as well as other topics that are at the heart of our field, such as closeness, social networks, nonverbal romantic communication, emotion regulation, self-expansion, relationship flourishing, relationship quality, dating violence, jealousy, loneliness, and misconceptions about romantic love. In sum, the works in this Special Issue highlight the complexity, utility, and centrality of attachment, romantic love, and pair bonding in humans. This Special Issue also marks a goal of casting a wide net, resulting in a collection of studies that expand borders and broaden our understanding of human relationships around the globe. Nevertheless, there is still much to be understood in regards to human pair bonding and attachment. These works, while advancing knowledge, also suggest that there are still gaps in the field and important questions of inquiry that require further research.

Bianca P. Acevedo and Adam Bode
Guest Editors

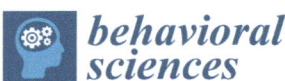

Article

Attachment Orientation and Preferences for Partners' Emotional Responses in Stressful and Positive Situations

Brian N. Chin [1,*], Lauryn Kim [2], Shelby M. Parsons [2] and Brooke C. Feeney [2]

[1] Department of Psychology, Trinity College, Hartford, CT 06106, USA
[2] Department of Psychology, Carnegie Mellon University, Pittsburgh, PA 15213, USA; bfeeney@andrew.cmu.edu (B.C.F.)
* Correspondence: brian.chin@trincoll.edu

Abstract: Attachment theory proposes that close relationships help us to regulate our emotions in stressful and positive situations. However, no previous studies have examined preferences for a partner's emotional response to one's own stressful and positive situations or tested whether these preferences differ based on attachment orientation. This study examines the association of attachment orientation and preferences for partners' emotional responses relative to one's own emotional responses in stressful and positive contexts among 425 United States adults who were currently in a committed relationship of ≥6 months. Data were collected in 2020. Overall, participants preferred their partners to feel and express less distress, less worry, more calm, and more hope than themselves during stressful situations and for their partners to feel and express more excitement, pride, and hope than themselves during positive situations. Higher attachment anxiety predicted preferences for partners to feel and express more distress/worry in stressful situations, whereas higher attachment avoidance predicted preferences for partners to feel and express less hope in stressful situations. Statistical interactions of attachment anxiety × attachment avoidance indicated that the combination of low attachment anxiety and high attachment avoidance (dismissing avoidance) was associated with preferences for partners to feel and express less positive emotions in positive situations, whereas the combination of high attachment anxiety and high attachment avoidance (fearful avoidance) was associated with preferences for partners to feel and express more negative emotions in stressful situations and less positive emotions in positive situations. This investigation provides novel evidence for links between attachment orientation and preferences for partners' emotional responses in two theoretically important contexts, which has implications for the nature and function of emotion regulation in close relationships. Future research is needed to determine the generalizability of these findings to more collectivist cultural contexts.

Keywords: close relationships; relational regulation; emotion regulation; social support; affect

Citation: Chin, B.N.; Kim, L.; Parsons, S.M.; Feeney, B.C. Attachment Orientation and Preferences for Partners' Emotional Responses in Stressful and Positive Situations. *Behav. Sci.* **2024**, *14*, 77. https://doi.org/10.3390/bs14010077

Academic Editors: Bianca P. Acevedo and Adam Bode

Received: 25 November 2023
Revised: 13 January 2024
Accepted: 18 January 2024
Published: 22 January 2024

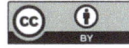

Copyright: © 2024 by the authors. Licensee MDPI, Basel, Switzerland. This article is an open access article distributed under the terms and conditions of the Creative Commons Attribution (CC BY) license (https:// creativecommons.org/licenses/by/ 4.0/).

1. Introduction

We often turn to our close relationships to cope with stressful events or to celebrate good news. Sometimes, relationship partners provide emotional support by expressing the same emotions we are experiencing. Other times, partners provide support by calming us down from intense negative emotions or by helping us enjoy and amplify positive emotions. Although there have been numerous studies demonstrating the benefits of receiving support from one's partner in both stressful and positive contexts [1], there has been no research focused on preferences for partners' emotional responses to one's own stressful and positive situations. Understanding preferences for a partner's emotional responses relative to one's own could provide insight into the ways that individuals regulate (e.g., amplify, maintain, dampen) their emotions with close partners in stressful and positive situations [2]. To address this gap in the literature, we examined attachment-related individual differences in preferences for partners' emotional responses to stressful and positive situations relative to one's own emotional responses.

Attachment Orientation and Emotions

We used attachment theory as a theoretical framework for investigating individual differences in preferences for partners' emotional responses to one's own stressful and positive situations, relative to one's own emotional responses to these situations. According to attachment theory, humans possess an innate propensity to form strong and enduring emotional bonds with close others (i.e., attachment figures) [3]. Experiences with one's attachment figures (i.e., the extent to which needs for security are met), particularly in contexts involving stressors and positive contexts involving novel exploration, underlie the development of individual differences in attachment orientation [3,4]. Individual differences in attachment orientation have been identified across the lifespan and have been shown to influence the way one experiences and regulates one's emotions in the presence of close others [2,5]. In the current investigation, we extended this literature by conducting a novel test of whether individual differences in attachment orientation are associated with preferences for partners' emotional responses in two contexts through which adult attachment relationships facilitate optimal well-being—stressful situations and positive situations involving exploration behavior (e.g., goals, opportunities, accomplishments) [1].

Individual differences in adult attachment orientation are measured in two dimensions—attachment anxiety and attachment avoidance. Attachment anxiety is associated with a preoccupation with close others, hypervigilance to signs of rejection or abandonment by close others, and a worry that close others will be unavailable or unresponsive during times of need. Anxiously attached individuals frequently engage in emotional hyperactivation strategies that are intended to elicit reassurance or affection from close others, such as by heightening their expression of negative emotions during interactions with their partners [6,7]. Attachment avoidance is associated with compulsive self-reliance, mistrust of others, and the belief that close others will be unavailable and unresponsive in times of need. Avoidantly attached individuals prefer to engage in emotional suppression strategies that allow them to avoid relying on others and keep their attachment needs deactivated, such as minimizing their expression of negative emotions during interactions with their partners [2,8].

There is considerable evidence for attachment-related individual differences in one's own emotional responses to stressful events. Past research has generally demonstrated that anxious attachment is associated with hyperactivation of negative emotions in stressful contexts, whereas avoidant attachment is associated with deactivation of negative emotions in stressful contexts [2]. For example, studies of emotional responses to recalled negative memories demonstrate that anxiously attached individuals more readily recall negative memories and report experiencing more intense negative emotions during recall, whereas avoidantly attached individuals less readily recall negative memories and report experiencing less intense negative emotions during recall [9]. Moreover, there is evidence that both trait attachment anxiety and experimentally induced attachment anxiety are associated with a greater propensity for experiencing false memories of relational stimuli [10,11]. Other studies have found attachment-related differences in how individuals attend to negative stimuli, with anxious individuals preferentially attending to negative stimuli [12,13] and avoidant individuals tending to suppress attention to negative stimuli [14]. Earlier investigations have also found that attachment anxiety and attachment avoidance are both associated with lower optimism and more catastrophic appraisals of potential threats [15]. Especially relevant to this investigation, Simpson et al. [16] demonstrated that securely attached individuals were most soothed by their partner's emotional caregiving behaviors during relationship conflict, whereas avoidantly attached individuals responded more favorably to instrumental caregiving behaviors.

There is also evidence for attachment-related individual differences in one's own emotional responses to positive events. Studies of attachment-related differences in emotional response to positive events have generally demonstrated that both anxious attachment and avoidant attachment interfere with the experience and expression of positive emotions [17]. For example, laboratory studies using emotion-induction procedures and facial coding have found that avoidantly attached individuals show less positive facial affect when viewing positive stimuli [18,19], whereas anxiously attached individuals show more negative facial affect when viewing positive stimuli (i.e., happy faces) [20]. Similarly, a daily diary study indicated that anxious attachment and avoidant attachment are both associated with blunted positive emotional responses to positive daily events [21].

2. Current Research

We aimed to build on past research examining attachment and emotional responses by investigating whether attachment orientation predicts individuals' preferences for partners' emotional responses, relative to their own emotional responses, in stressful situations (Aim 1) and positive situations (Aim 2). We conducted an online survey study of individuals who were currently in a committed romantic relationship that had been ongoing for at least six months. Participants reflected on times when they discussed stressful situations and positive situations with their romantic partners and indicated their preferences for their partners' emotional responses (relative to their own responses) in those situations. We assessed participants' preferences about two aspects of partners' emotional responses to each type of situation—their partner's emotional experience (felt emotion) and their partner's emotional expression (expressed emotion). We assessed preferences for specific emotions that were theoretically relevant to stressful situations (distress, worry, calm, hope) and positive situations (excitement, pride, hope, calm). We tested the following specific hypotheses based on the postulates of attachment theory and past research on adult attachment orientation and emotions.

First, we predicted that attachment anxiety would be associated with preferences for partners to respond to one's stressful situations by feeling and expressing more distress, more worry, less calm, and less hope than themselves (Hypothesis 1a). We also predicted that attachment avoidance would be associated with preferences for partners to respond to one's stressful situations by feeling and expressing less distress, less worry, less calm, and less hope than themselves (Hypothesis 1b). We hypothesized that these preferences would help anxious individuals, who tend to hyperactivate their negative emotions in stressful situations, and avoidant individuals, who tend to deactivate their positive and negative emotions in stressful contexts, to accomplish their emotion regulation goals in stressful situations.

Second, we predicted that attachment anxiety would be associated with preferences for partners to respond to one's positive situations by feeling and expressing more excitement, more pride, more hope, and less calm than themselves (Hypothesis 2a). We also predicted that attachment avoidance would be associated with preferences for partners to respond to one's positive situations by feeling and expressing less excitement, less pride, less hope, and more calm than themselves (Hypothesis 2b). We hypothesized that these preferences would help anxious individuals, who desire their partner's approval and validation, and avoidant individuals, who prefer to keep their attachment needs deactivated, to accomplish their emotion regulation goals in positive situations.

3. Method

3.1. Participants and Procedures

Participants were 425 adults recruited through Amazon Mechanical Turk (n = 253) and Volunteer Science (n = 172) for a study of romantic relationships. Participants' ages ranged from 18 to 88 years (M = 41.3, SD = 12.9). In total, 51.5% identified as female, 47.5% as male, and 0.9% as genderqueer or nonbinary. In total, 56.7% of participants identified as White, 32.0% as Asian, 3.5% as Black, 3.5% as multiracial, 2.8% as Hispanic, 0.5% as Native/Indigenous, and 0.7% as another race; 1 participant preferred not to disclose their race. In total, 79.8% of participants were cohabiting with their romantic partner. Sample size was determined based on the desire to maximize power by collecting data from as many participants as possible; data collection was halted when funding was no longer available. Data were collected between March and December 2020. Inclusion criteria were being ≥18 years old, fluent in English, and in a committed romantic relationship of at least six months. All study procedures were approved by a university institutional review board and complied with APA ethical standards for the treatment of human participants.

After providing informed consent, participants completed questionnaires via Qualtrics assessing their demographic information, attachment orientation, and preferences for being supported by romantic partners in stressful and positive situations. Participants were compensated USD 3 for completing the study via Amazon Mechanical Turk; participants did not receive compensation for completing the study via Volunteer Science.

We conducted a post hoc power analysis using G*Power version 3.1.9.7 [22] to compute achieved power for a linear regression with two tested predictors, a significance criterion of $\alpha = 0.05$, and sample size = 425. Achieved power was 1.00 to detect a medium effect ($f^2 = 0.15$) and 0.74 to detect a small effect ($f^2 = 0.02$).

3.2. Measures

3.2.1. Attachment Orientation

We assessed general attachment orientation using a 14-item version of the Experiences in Close Relationships (ECR) scale [23]. Participants rated the extent to which they agreed with statements assessing attachment anxiety (seven items, e.g., "I worry about being abandoned") and attachment avoidance (seven items, e.g., "I try avoiding getting too close to people") in their global attachment relationships (1 = strongly disagree, 7 = strongly agree). Attachment anxiety ($\alpha = 0.92$) and attachment avoidance ($\alpha = 0.88$) composites were computed by averaging the scores of items for each subscale.

3.2.2. Preferences for Partners' Emotional Responses to Stressful Situations

Participants were prompted to reflect on times when they discussed their own stressful situations with their romantic partner and rate how they wanted their partner to respond in these situations:

"Please take a moment to think about times in your life when you have been distressed by significant, major stressors. For example, you might have been worried about a serious health problem that you or a family member was having, you might have performed poorly at something that was very important to you, you might have been treated badly at work, you may be having a hard time finding a job or getting accepted into an academic program, etc. These should be significant personal stressors that were NOT caused by your partner. When discussing these stressors with your partner, to what extent do you typically prefer that your partner respond in the following ways? Some questions below ask about two different aspects of your emotional life. One is your emotional experience, or what you feel inside. The other is your emotional expression, or how you communicate your emotions to others in the way you talk, gesture, or behave."

Participants rated four items assessing the extent to which they preferred their partner to feel distressed, calm, hopeful, and worried about the stressor relative to their own feelings (−3 = much less than me, 0 = as much as me, 3 = much more than me). Participants also rated four items assessing the extent to which they preferred their partner to express distress, calmness, hopefulness, and worry about the stressor relative to their own expressions of each emotion (−3 = much less than me, 0 = as much as me, 3 = much more than me).

3.2.3. Preferences for Partners' Emotional Responses to Positive Situations

Participants were prompted to reflect on times when they discussed their own positive situations or events with their romantic partner and rate how they wanted their partner to respond in these situations:

"Please take a moment to think about times in your life when you have felt excited about something positive. For example, you may have received good news about getting a new job or receiving an award or a promotion, or you may have an exciting new hobby or goal or opportunity to pursue. When discussing these positive experiences with your partner,

to what extent do you typically prefer that your partner respond in the following ways? Some questions below ask about two different aspects of your emotional life. One is your emotional experience, or what you feel inside. The other is your emotional expression, or how you communicate your emotions to others in the way you talk, gesture, or behave."

Participants rated four items assessing the extent to which they preferred their partner to feel excitement, calm, pride, and hope about the positive situation relative to their own feelings (−3 = much less than me, 0 = as much as me, 3 = much more than me). Participants also rated four items assessing the extent to which they preferred their partner to express excitement, calm, pride, and hope about the positive situation relative to their own expressions of each emotion (−3 = much less than me, 0 = as much as me, 3 = much more than me).

4. Data Analysis

Our descriptive analyses included bivariate correlations between predictor and outcome variables and paired samples t-tests evaluating whether participants differed in their preferences for partners to feel vs. express distress, worry, calm, and hope in stressful situations or in their preferences for partners to feel vs. express excitement, pride, calm, and hope in positive situations.

To address our first aim, we used linear regression models to test associations of attachment orientation (attachment anxiety, attachment avoidance, and the interaction of attachment anxiety × attachment avoidance) and preferences for partners' emotional responses to stressful situations (feeling and expressing distress, worry, calm, and hope) relative to their own feelings and expressions.

To address our second aim, we used linear regression models to test associations of attachment orientation and preferences for partners' emotional responses to positive situations (feeling and expressing excitement, calm, pride, and hope) relative to their own feelings and expressions.

To interpret statistically significant interactions of attachment anxiety × attachment avoidance, we conducted planned follow-up analyses of simple slopes of attachment anxiety at one standard deviation above and below the mean value of attachment avoidance.

We conducted these analyses with and without controlling for participants' gender. Because all associations were unaffected by the inclusion of gender as a covariate, we only report the results of the more parsimonious models that did not control for gender.

Transparency and Openness

We report how our sample size was determined and all data exclusions, manipulations, and measures in this study. Data were analyzed using SPSS, version 28.0.1.1, and the PROCESS macro, version 4.2, model 1 [24]. This study was not pre-registered. Data and analysis code are available at https://osf.io/nkmbw/?view_only=bb9aa20a40fc4e26a89866ed7b264efc (accessed on 20 November 2023).

5. Results

Descriptive Analyses

Descriptive statistics for preferred partner emotions in stressful situations and positive situations are shown in Table 1. Bivariate correlations of primary outcome variables are shown in Table 2.

Table 1. Descriptive statistics for study variables.

	M (SD)
Attachment anxiety	3.3 (1.5)
Attachment avoidance	3.6 (1.4)
During stressful situations:	

Table 1. Cont.

	M (SD)
I want my partner to feel:	
Distress	−0.7 (1.6)
Worry	−0.7 (1.5)
Calm	1.0 (1.4)
Hope	1.3 (1.2)
I want my partner to express:	
Distress	−0.6 (1.6)
Worry	−0.7 (1.5)
Calm	1.0 (1.5)
Hope	1.2 (1.4)
During positive situations:	
I want my partner to feel:	
Excitement	0.8 (1.2)
Pride	1.1 (1.2)
Hope	1.0 (1.2)
Calm	0.2 (1.3)
I want my partner to express:	
Excitement	0.8 (1.3)
Pride	0.9 (1.3)
Hope	0.9 (1.3)
Calm	0.1 (1.2)

Table 2. Bivariate correlations of study variables.

	1	2	3	4	5	6	7	8	9	10	11	12	13	14	15	16	17	18
1. Attachment anxiety	--																	
2. Attachment avoidance	0.53	--																
3. Partner feels distress	0.34	0.18	--															
4. Partner feels worry	0.28	0.18	0.55	--														
5. Partner feels calm	−0.07	−0.08	−0.43	−0.28	--													
6. Partner feels hope	−0.11	−0.18	−0.11	−0.19	0.32	--												
7. Partner expresses distress	0.23	0.08	0.74	0.52	−0.43	−0.12	--											
8. Partner expresses worry	0.24	0.18	0.54	0.82	−0.29	−0.17	0.56	--										
9. Partner expresses calm	−0.16	−0.10	−0.47	−0.30	0.76	0.35	−0.44	−0.34	--									
10. Partner expresses hope	−0.06	−0.15	−0.15	−0.16	0.30	0.62	−0.10	−0.13	0.39	--								
11. Partner feels excitement	0.15	−0.02	0.43	0.30	−0.27	0.14	0.38	0.32	−0.27	0.00	--							
12. Partner feels pride	0.18	0.01	0.29	0.21	−0.10	0.22	0.29	0.26	−0.10	0.14	0.65	--						
13. Partner feels hope	0.10	−0.12	0.28	0.23	−0.13	0.19	0.32	0.23	−0.10	0.14	0.57	0.71	--					
14. Partner feels calm	0.13	0.12	0.12	0.15	0.15	−0.01	0.05	0.11	0.05	−0.10	0.11	0.11	0.15	--				
15. Partner expresses excitement	0.06	−0.09	0.30	0.20	−0.18	0.12	0.34	0.23	−0.17	0.06	0.76	0.56	0.57	0.04	--			
16. Partner expresses pride	0.00	−0.14	0.12	0.13	−0.04	0.19	0.23	0.14	0.03	0.22	0.45	0.74	0.60	−0.04	0.55	--		
17. Partner expresses hope	−0.05	−0.18	0.16	0.13	−0.12	0.17	0.28	0.17	−0.03	0.21	0.49	0.62	0.79	0.05	0.51	0.63	--	
18. Partner expresses calm	0.05	0.04	0.04	0.05	0.12	−0.04	0.01	0.07	0.10	−0.08	0.07	0.07	0.15	0.79	0.04	−0.06	0.13	--

Note. Bolded coefficients denote statistical significance at $p < 0.05$.

As shown in Table 1, participants generally preferred their partners to feel and express less distress, less worry, more calm, and more hope relative to themselves during stressful situations and for their partners to feel and express more excitement, pride, and hope relative to themselves during positive situations. Participants also generally preferred their partners to feel more calm, but not express more calm, relative to themselves during positive situations.

Participants reported a stronger preference for partners to feel (vs. express) more hope than themselves in stressful situations (M_{diff} = 0.11, 95CI$_{diff}$ = 0.00, 0.22, paired samples $t(424)$ = 2.01, p = 0.045, d = 0.10). Participants did not differ in their preferences for partners to feel vs. express distress (M_{diff} = −0.08, 95CI$_{diff}$ = −0.19, 0.03, paired samples $t(423)$ = −1.39, p = 0.17, d = −0.07), to feel vs. express worry (M_{diff} = 0.05, 95CI$_{diff}$ = −0.04, 0.14, paired samples $t(424)$ = 1.16, p = 0.25, d = 0.06), or to feel vs. express calm (M_{diff} = 0.00, 95CI$_{diff}$ = −0.09, 0.10, paired samples $t(423)$ = 0.05, p = 0.96, d = 0.00).

Participants reported a stronger preference for partners to feel (vs. express) more pride (M_{diff} = 0.11, 95CI$_{diff}$ = 0.03, 0.20, paired samples $t(424)$ = 2.58, p = 0.010, d = 0.13), more hope (M_{diff} = 0.13, 95CI$_{diff}$ = 0.05, 0.20, paired samples $t(424)$ = 3.28, p = 0.001, d = 0.16), and more calm (M_{diff} = 0.16, 95CI$_{diff}$ = 0.08, 0.24, paired samples $t(424)$ = 4.05, p < 0.001, d = 0.16) than themselves in positive situations. Participants did not differ in their preference for partners to feel vs. express excitement (M_{diff} = 0.06, 95CI$_{diff}$ = −0.03, 0.14, paired samples $t(424)$ = 1.36, p = 0.18, d = 0.07).

Aim 1: Preferences for partners' emotional responses to one's own stressful situations.

We examined whether participants' attachment orientation was associated with their preferences for partners' emotional responses, relative to their own emotional responses, during the participants' stressful situations (Table 3).

Table 3. Main effect and interaction of attachment anxiety and avoidance on preferences for partners' felt and expressed emotions when providing support in stressful situations.

	B	SE	t	p	95CI
Partner Feels Distress					
Step 1					
Intercept	−0.72	0.08	−9.62	<0.001	−0.86, −0.57
Attachment anxiety	0.55	0.09	6.30	<0.001	0.38, 0.73
Attachment avoidance	−0.01	0.09	−0.07	0.95	−0.18, 0.17
Step 2					
Attachment anxiety × attachment avoidance	0.24	0.08	3.07	0.002	0.09, 0.39
Partner Feels Worry					
Step 1					
Intercept	−0.66	0.07	−9.28	<0.001	−0.80, −0.52
Attachment anxiety	0.39	0.08	4.59	<0.001	0.22, 0.55
Attachment avoidance	0.07	0.08	0.83	0.41	−0.10, 0.24
Step 2					
Attachment anxiety × attachment avoidance	0.14	0.07	1.91	0.06	−0.00, 0.29
Partner Feels Calm					
Step 1					
Intercept	1.02	0.07	14.92	<0.001	0.88, 1.15
Attachment anxiety	−0.06	0.08	−0.80	0.43	−0.22, 0.09
Attachment avoidance	−0.08	0.08	−0.93	0.35	−0.23, 0.08
Step 2					
Attachment anxiety × attachment avoidance	0.07	0.07	1.02	0.31	−0.07, 0.21
Partner Feels Hope					
Step 1					
Intercept	1.30	0.06	22.56	<0.001	1.19, 1.42
Attachment anxiety	−0.02	0.07	−0.36	0.72	−0.16, 0.11
Attachment avoidance	−0.20	0.07	−2.90	0.004	−0.33, −0.06
Step 2					
Attachment anxiety × attachment avoidance	0.11	0.06	1.88	0.06	−0.01, 0.23

Table 3. *Cont.*

	B	SE	t	p	95CI
Partner Expresses Distress					
Step 1					
Intercept	−0.64	0.08	−8.53	<0.001	−0.79, −0.49
Attachment anxiety	0.41	0.09	4.69	<0.001	0.24, 0.59
Attachment avoidance	−0.09	0.09	−1.06	0.29	−0.27, 0.08
Step 2					
Attachment anxiety × attachment avoidance	0.02	0.08	0.24	0.81	−0.13, 0.17
Partner Expresses Worry					
Step 1					
Intercept	−0.71	0.07	−9.81	<0.001	−0.85, −0.57
Attachment anxiety	0.32	0.09	3.69	<0.001	0.15, 0.48
Attachment avoidance	0.11	0.09	1.22	0.22	−0.06, 0.27
Step 2					
Attachment anxiety × attachment avoidance	0.17	0.08	2.27	0.02	0.02, 0.32
Partner Expresses Calm					
Step 1					
Intercept	1.01	0.07	14.16	<0.001	0.87, 1.15
Attachment anxiety	−0.21	0.08	−2.52	0.012	−0.38, −0.05
Attachment avoidance	−0.03	0.08	−0.41	0.68	−0.20, 0.13
Step 2					
Attachment anxiety × attachment avoidance	0.08	0.07	1.04	0.30	−0.07, 0.22
Partner Expresses Hope					
Step 1					
Intercept	1.19	0.07	17.51	<0.001	1.06, 1.32
Attachment anxiety	0.03	0.08	0.33	0.74	−0.13, 0.19
Attachment avoidance	−0.22	0.08	−2.76	0.006	−0.38, −0.06
Step 2					
Attachment anxiety × attachment avoidance	0.00	0.07	0.06	0.96	−0.13, 0.14

Consistent with Hypothesis 1a, participants with higher attachment anxiety preferred their partners to feel and express more distress, to feel and express more worry, and to express less calm relative to themselves during the participants' stressful situations. Contrary to Hypothesis 1a, attachment anxiety was not associated with preferences for partners to feel calm, feel hope, or express hope during stressful situations.

Consistent with Hypothesis 1b, participants with higher attachment avoidance preferred their partners to feel and express less hope relative to themselves during the participants' stressful situations. Contrary to Hypothesis 1b, attachment avoidance was not associated with preferences for partners to feel or express distress, worry, or calm during stressful situations.

Next, we tested the interaction of attachment anxiety × attachment avoidance on preferences for partners' emotional responses during the participants' stressful situations. We observed interactions of attachment anxiety × attachment avoidance predicting preferences for partners to feel distress and express worry during the participants' stressful situations. Examination of marginal slopes for attachment anxiety at low and high levels of attachment avoidance in Figure 1 indicated that: (A) attachment anxiety was more strongly associated with the preference for partners to feel more distress (relative to themselves) during stressful situations when participants also had higher levels of attachment avoidance (fearful avoidance) ($b = 0.79$, $SE = 0.12$, $t = 6.82$, $p < 0.001$, 95CI = 0.56, 1.01) than when participants had lower levels of attachment avoidance (preoccupied attachment) ($b = 0.32$, $SE = 0.12$, $t = 2.71$, $p = 0.007$, 95CI = 0.09, 0.55); and (B) attachment anxiety was associated with the preference for partners to express more worry (relative to themselves) during stressful situations when participants also had higher levels of attachment avoidance (fearful avoidance) ($b = 0.48$, $SE = 0.11$, $t = 4.29$, $p < 0.001$, 95CI = 0.26, 0.71) but not when participants had lower levels of attachment avoidance (preoccupied attachment) ($b = 0.14$, $SE = 0.11$, $t = 1.26$, $p = 0.21$, 95CI = $-0.08, 0.37$).

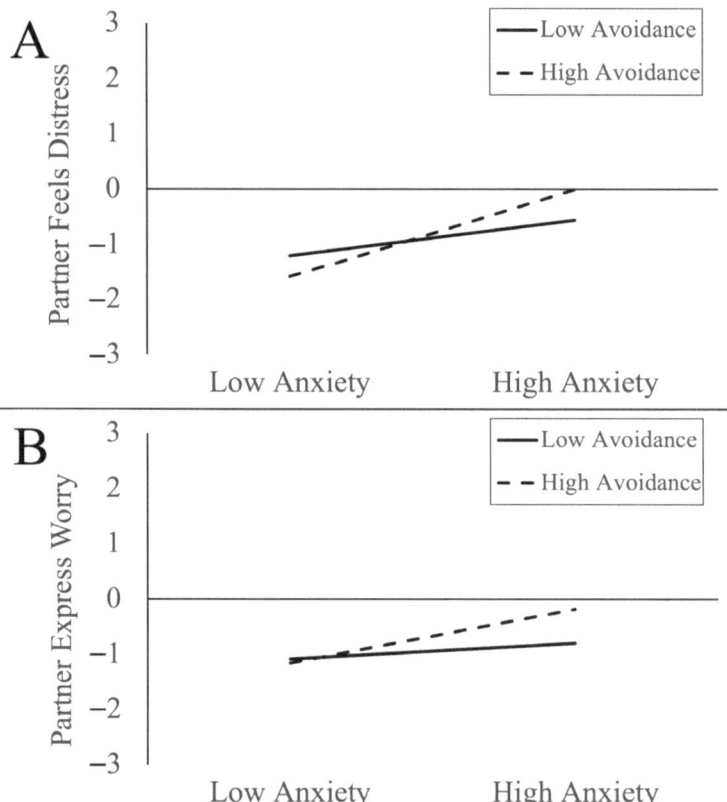

Figure 1. Interaction plots showing preferences for partners to feel distress (**A**) and express worry (**B**) during stressful situations by attachment anxiety and attachment avoidance.

There was no interaction of participants' attachment anxiety × attachment avoidance predicting preferences for partners' other felt or expressed emotions.

Aim 2: Preferences for partners' emotional responses to one's own positive situations.

We examined whether participants' attachment orientation was associated with their preferences for partners' emotional responses, relative to their own emotional responses, during the participants' positive situations (Table 4).

Consistent with Hypothesis 2a, participants with higher attachment anxiety preferred their partners to feel and express more excitement, to feel and express more pride, and to feel more hope than themselves during positive situations. Contrary to Hypothesis 2a, attachment anxiety was not associated with preferences for partners to feel calm, express calm, or express hope during positive situations.

Consistent with Hypothesis 2b, participants with higher attachment avoidance preferred their partners to feel and express less excitement, less pride, and less hope than themselves during the participants' positive situations. Contrary to Hypothesis 2b, attachment avoidance was not associated with preferences for partners to feel calm or express calm during positive situations.

Table 4. Main effect and interaction of attachment anxiety and avoidance on preferences for partners' felt and expressed emotions (relative to one's own emotions) when providing support in positive situations.

	B	SE	t	p	95CI
Partner Feels Excitement					
Step 1					
Intercept	0.81	0.06	13.99	<0.001	0.70, 0.93
Attachment anxiety	0.27	0.07	3.97	<0.001	0.14, 0.41
Attachment avoidance	−0.17	0.07	−2.43	0.016	−0.30, −0.03
Step 2					
Attachment anxiety × attachment avoidance	0.15	0.06	2.55	0.011	0.04, 0.27
Partner Feels Proud					
Step 1					
Intercept	1.05	0.06	18.40	<0.001	0.94, 1.16
Attachment anxiety	0.30	0.07	4.41	<0.001	0.17, 0.43
Attachment avoidance	−0.15	0.07	−2.25	0.025	−0.28, −0.02
Step 2					
Attachment anxiety × attachment avoidance	0.17	0.06	2.86	0.004	0.05, 0.28
Partner Feels Hope					
Step 1					
Intercept	0.98	0.06	17.32	<0.001	0.87, 1.09
Attachment anxiety	0.28	0.07	4.13	<0.001	0.14, 0.41
Attachment avoidance	−0.29	0.07	−4.35	<0.001	−0.42, −0.16
Step 2					
Attachment anxiety × attachment avoidance	0.09	0.06	1.53	0.13	−0.03, 0.20
Partner Feels Calm					
Step 1					
Intercept	0.21	0.06	3.39	<0.001	0.09, 0.33
Attachment anxiety	0.12	0.07	1.67	0.10	−0.02, 0.27
Attachment avoidance	0.09	0.07	1.26	0.21	−0.05, 0.24
Step 2					
Attachment anxiety × attachment avoidance	0.21	0.06	3.35	<0.001	0.09, 0.34
Partner Expresses Excitement					
Step 1					
Intercept	0.76	0.06	12.34	<0.001	0.64, 0.88
Attachment anxiety	0.19	0.07	2.63	0.009	0.05, 0.33
Attachment avoidance	−0.21	0.07	−2.94	0.004	−0.36, −0.07
Step 2					
Attachment anxiety × attachment avoidance	0.14	0.06	2.25	0.025	0.02, 0.27
Partner Expresses Pride					
Step 1					
Intercept	0.94	0.06	15.28	<0.001	0.82, 1.06
Attachment anxiety	0.15	0.07	2.01	0.046	0.00, 0.29
Attachment avoidance	−0.26	0.07	−3.62	<0.001	−0.41, −0.12
Step 2					
Attachment anxiety × attachment avoidance	0.03	0.06	.41	0.68	−0.10, 0.15
Partner Expresses Hope					
Step 1					
Intercept	0.85	0.06	14.14	<0.001	0.73, 0.97
Attachment anxiety	0.08	0.07	1.13	0.26	−0.06, 0.22
Attachment avoidance	−0.27	0.07	−3.78	<0.001	−0.41, −0.13
Step 2					
Attachment anxiety × attachment avoidance	0.09	0.06	1.50	0.13	−0.03, 0.22
Partner Expresses Calm					
Step 1					
Intercept	0.05	0.06	0.85	0.40	−0.07, 0.16
Attachment anxiety	0.05	0.07	0.73	0.47	−0.09, 0.19
Attachment avoidance	0.02	0.07	0.23	0.82	−0.12, 0.15
Step 2					
Attachment anxiety × attachment avoidance	0.17	0.06	2.91	0.004	0.06, 0.29

Next, we tested the interaction of attachment anxiety × attachment avoidance on preferences for partners' emotional responses during the participants' positive situations. We observed interactions of attachment anxiety × attachment avoidance predicting preferences for partners to feel and express excitement, to feel and express calm, and to feel pride. Examination of marginal slopes for attachment anxiety at low and high levels of attachment avoidance in Figure 2 indicated that each of these interactions followed a similar pattern.

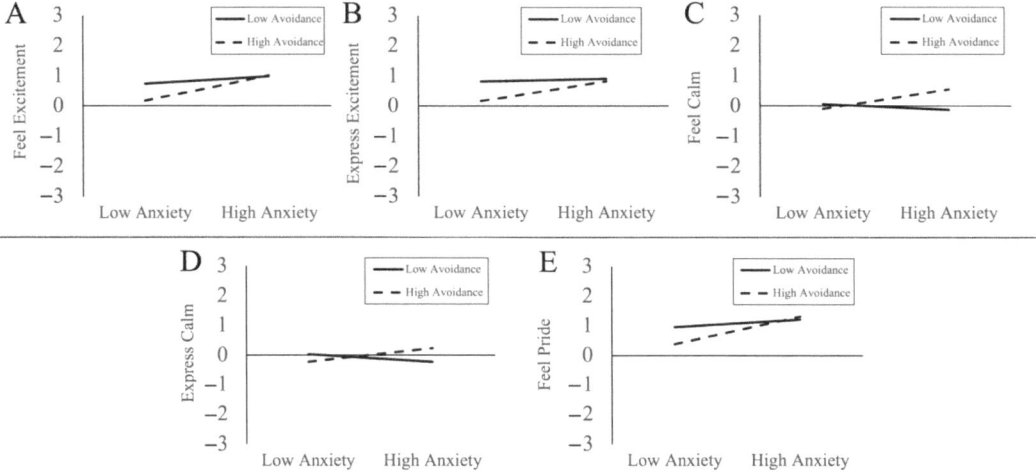

Figure 2. Interaction plots showing preferences for partners to feel excitement (**A**), express excitement (**B**), feel calm (**C**), express calm (**D**), and feel pride (**E**) during positive situations by attachment anxiety and attachment avoidance.

When participants had high attachment avoidance, higher attachment anxiety was associated with the preference for partners to feel more excitement ($b = 0.42$, $SE = 0.09$, $p < 0.001$, $95CI = 0.25, 0.60$), express more excitement ($b = 0.33$, $SE = 0.10$, $p = 0.001$, $95CI = 0.14, 0.52$), feel more calm ($b = 0.33$, $SE = 0.10$, $p = 0.001$, $95CI = 0.14, 0.52$), express more calm ($b = 0.22$, $SE = 0.09$, $p = 0.014$, $95CI = 0.05, 0.40$), and feel more pride than themselves during the participants' positive situations ($b = 0.33$, $SE = 0.10$, $p = 0.001$, $95CI = 0.14, 0.52$).

When participants had low attachment avoidance, higher attachment anxiety was not associated with the preference for partners to feel excitement ($b = 0.12$, $SE = 0.09$, $p = 0.20$, $95CI = -0.06, 0.30$), express excitement ($b = 0.05$, $SE = 0.10$, $p = 0.63$, $95CI = -0.14, 0.24$), feel calm ($b = -0.09$, $SE = 0.10$, $p = 0.34$, $95CI = -0.28, 0.10$), express calm ($b = -0.13$, $SE = 0.09$, $p = 0.17$, $95CI = -30, 0.05$), or feel pride (relative to themselves) during the participants' positive situations ($b = 0.13$, $SE = 0.09$, $p = 0.15$, $95CI = -0.05, 0.30$).

There was no interaction of participants' attachment anxiety × attachment avoidance predicting preferences for partners to express pride, feel hope, or express hope.

6. Discussion

To our knowledge, this study was the first to investigate preferences for partners' emotional responses to one's own stressful and positive situations relative to one's own emotional responses in these situations. This design facilitated interpretation of these preferences in terms of whether they reflected a desire for partners' emotional responses to amplify, dampen, or maintain individuals' own emotions in each context. Overall, we found that participants preferred for their partners to dampen their negative emotions in stressful contexts and to amplify their positive emotions in both stressful and positive contexts. We found evidence for most hypothesized associations of attachment orientation and preferences for partners' emotional responses in each context. Compared to securely attached individuals, anxiously attached individuals preferred their partners to feel and express more negative emotions in stressful situations and more positive emotions in positive situations, while avoidantly attached individuals preferred their partners to feel and express less positive emotions in both stressful situations and positive situations. We also found that individuals with high anxiety and high avoidance (i.e., fearful avoidance) preferred their partners to feel and express more negative emotions in stressful situations and fewer positive emotions in positive situations, whereas individuals with high avoidance and low anxiety (i.e., avoidant dismissing) preferred their partners to feel and express less positive emotions in positive situations. These findings provide a greater understanding of the emotion regulation strategies that individuals prefer to use in their close relationships and how these preferences are shaped by our general attachment working models.

6.1. Preferences about Partners' Emotional Responses to Stressful Situations

Overall, participants preferred their partners to feel and express less distress, less worry, more calm, and more hope than themselves during stressful situations. This suggests that individuals generally wanted their partners to serve as a safe haven that helped them to dampen their negative emotions and amplify their positive emotions in stressful contexts.

Hypothesis 1a was supported. Anxiously attached individuals preferred their partners to feel and express more distress, more worry, and less hope during their own stressful situations. These observations are consistent with attachment theory's description of anxiously attached individuals as strongly desiring their partner's validation and approval. Because anxiously attached individuals tend to experience hyperactivation of their own negative emotions in stressful contexts [2], it is possible that these preferences reflect a desire for partners to respond in a way that validates their hyperactivated negative affect and confirms their negative mental representations of themselves and others [25].

Hypothesis 1b was partially supported. Avoidantly attached individuals preferred for their partners to feel and express less hope during their own stressful situations. These preferences are consistent with earlier studies suggesting that attachment avoidance is associated with lower optimism and more catastrophic appraisals of potential threats [15]. Contrary to our initial hypothesis, attachment avoidance was not associated with preferences for partners to feel or express distress or worry during stressful situations. This was surprising given attachment theory's description of avoidantly attached individuals as being motivated to deactivate their emotions and attachment needs during stressful situations [2]. One possible reason that this hypothesis was not supported is because we observed an interaction of attachment avoidance and attachment anxiety indicating that it was the combination of high attachment avoidance and high attachment anxiety (i.e., fearful avoidance) that was associated with a stronger preference for partners to feel more distress and express more worry during one's own stressful situations. This observation is consistent with theoretical descriptions of individuals with a fearful-avoidant attachment orientation as engaging in "incoherent" coping strategies that tend to reflect their extreme dysregulation during stressful situations [26]. It is also consistent with theoretical descriptions of fearful-avoidant individuals as being worried about potential signs of rejection from close others [27].

6.2. Preferences about Partners' Emotional Responses to Positive Situations

Overall, participants preferred their partners to feel and express more excitement, pride, and hope than themselves during positive situations. This suggests that individuals generally wanted their partners to serve as a catalyst or secure base for exploration, encouraging their embracing of opportunities and challenges [28]. These preferences are also consistent with the broad literature demonstrating the benefits of interpersonal capitalization in romantic relationships [29].

Hypotheses 2a and 2b were supported. During their own positive situations, anxiously attached individuals preferred their partners to feel and express more excitement, pride, and hope, while avoidantly attached individuals preferred their partners to feel and express less excitement, pride, and hope. These preferences are consistent with earlier theoretical descriptions of anxiously attached individuals as desiring their partner's validation and approval and of avoidantly attached individuals as wanting to deactivate their emotions and attachment needs [3,27]. They are also consistent with earlier research showing that partners' capitalization attempts elicit less favorable responses from avoidantly attached individuals and ambivalent responses (i.e., involving feelings of both appreciation and indebtedness) from anxiously attached individuals [29]. Findings for avoidantly attached individuals support earlier work suggesting that attachment avoidance may interfere with the experience of pride in response to a partner's positive events. Specifically, Mikulincer and Shaver [30] posited that avoidantly attached individuals may experience hubris or hostile envy in response to a partner's positive events instead of the normative experience of pride.

We also observed interactions of attachment anxiety and attachment avoidance. The combination of high anxiety and high avoidance (i.e., fearful avoidance) was associated with preferences for partners to feel and express more calm in positive situations, while the combination of low anxiety and high avoidance (i.e., avoidant dismissing) was associated with preferences for partners to feel less pride and to feel and express less excitement in positive situations. These observations are consistent with theoretical descriptions of fearful-avoidant individuals and avoidant-dismissing individuals as engaging in coping strategies that are focused on deactivating their emotions and their attachment needs. In theory, these preferences may serve the respective interpersonal and emotion regulation goals of avoidant-dismissing individuals, who are primarily motivated to maintain their autonomy and independence, and fearful-avoidant individuals, who desire closeness with their partners but also fear their potential rejection [27].

6.3. Broader Theoretical Contributions

This study provides insight into the types of emotional support that are most desired by different individuals. Our results suggest several novel hypotheses about the effectiveness of different emotional support strategies in stressful and positive situations and how this may differ by general attachment orientation. First, they suggest that individuals will feel most supported in stressful situations when partners dampen their negative emotions; however, this strategy will be less effective for individuals with higher attachment anxiety. Second, they suggest that individuals will feel most supported in positive situations when partners amplify their positive emotions; this strategy will be more effective for individuals with higher attachment anxiety but less effective for individuals with higher attachment avoidance.

Our findings are consistent with Collins and Allard's [25] assertion that a core function of our attachment working models is to guide our emotional response patterns and how we think about ourselves and others. These findings also raise additional theoretical questions about whether individuals will feel more supported when there is a match between their stated preferences and their partners' actual emotional responses to stressful and positive situations. Indeed, it is possible that individuals' preferences accurately reflect the emotional responses that would help them to feel most supported in each context. However, it is equally plausible that these preferences are not necessarily adaptive and instead a reflection of an individual's general working models of the self and others that developed based on their earlier experiences in close relationships—regardless of whether these models are accurate or adaptive in their current relationship. Consistent with the latter possibility, we found that the emotional responses that anxiously and avoidantly attached individuals preferred from their partners tended to mirror the ways that these individuals respond themselves in stressful and positive situations. For example, anxiously attached individuals, who tend to experience hyperactivation of their own negative emotions during their stressful situations, also preferred for partners to feel and express more distress/worry in these situations. Future observational and experimental studies are needed to disentangle these possibilities by testing whether the individual or dyad benefits when there is a match between individuals' preferred and received partner emotional responses in each context. Insecure individuals, in particular, may benefit from partners who assist them in regulating their emotions by dampening negative emotions in stressful contexts and by amplifying positive emotions in positive contexts.

Finally, our questionnaire asked participants to differentiate between their preferences for their partners to feel and express emotions. Although the experience and expression of emotions are distinct from a theoretical perspective [31], we did not observe a strong empirical distinction between preferences for partners to feel and express emotions in our study. We measured these preferences separately to account for the possibility that some participants might prefer for their partners to regulate their emotional expressions (i.e., to outwardly exaggerate or downplay their inner feelings) or that dimensions of attachment insecurity would have different associations with preferences for felt and expressed emotions. However, we observed strong correlations between preferences for partners to feel and express specific emotions in each context and found similar associations between attachment orientation and preferences for partners to feel and express specific emotions in each context. One possible reason why we did not observe a stronger distinction between felt and expressed emotions is because our self-report assessment approach was suboptimal for distinguishing between these preferences. As suggested by the strong correlations of felt and expressed emotions and their similar associations with attachment orientation, it is possible that our participants had trouble distinguishing between preferences for their partners' outward emotional expressions and internal emotional experiences. Future observational studies that assess felt and expressed emotions in both relationship partners could help to distinguish between the impact of partners' emotional expressions and emotional experiences in these support contexts. Studies assessing relationship partners' physiological reactivity and physiological synchrony during specific support interactions may also be helpful for addressing these questions [32]. Studies that assess partners' emotional expressions using observer ratings could also help to distinguish between the impact of felt and expressed emotions on perceived supportiveness and relationship outcomes.

6.4. Strengths, Limitations, and Conclusions

Strengths of our study include its investigation of a novel theoretical question based on the predictions of attachment theory in a relatively large and diverse sample of adults in the United States. However, there are also several limitations of this work that represent opportunities for future investigation. First, participants were asked to report how they preferred their partners to respond emotionally in stressful and positive situations. Although self-report methods are important for assessing preferences, the extent to which participants are willing or able to accurately report these preferences is unknown and should be investigated. For example, a future study could aim to replicate these associations by experimentally manipulating how partners respond to disclosures about stressful and positive events in a laboratory discussion. Future research in this area could also examine whether manipulating felt attachment security, such as by using attachment security priming, impacts preferences for partners' felt or expressed emotions in these contexts. Other future work could comprehensively assess felt and expressed emotions and preferences regarding own and partner emotions from both the disclosing and responding partners, as well as observer ratings of both partners' emotional expressions, during real-time interactions in the laboratory. Second, our measures asked participants how they preferred their partners to feel and express emotions relative to their own feelings and expressions of emotions. However, it is likely that attachment orientation also influences one's own emotional responses to stressful and positive events [21]. For example, people with higher attachment avoidance may express lower amounts of hope during positive situations and also prefer that their partners express even less hope than that. Future studies could disentangle this by measuring preferences for partners' emotions on an absolute measurement scale that is not relative to one's own emotional feelings and expressions (e.g., assessing preferences for partners' expressed hope using anchors of not at all and extremely). Third, we prompted participants to reflect on times when they have discussed stressful and positive events with their romantic partner. However, it is unknown whether the types or intensity of events recalled by participants was impacted by their attachment orientation. For example, future studies are needed to test the alternative possibility that anxiously attached individuals preferred their partners to feel more distress because they recalled more intense stressful events than securely attached individuals [10,21]. Future studies could also address this limitation by including measures to assess the type and intensity of events recalled by each participant and statistically controlling for these characteristics.

Overall, these findings contribute to research on attachment theory and interpersonal emotion regulation by demonstrating that attachment insecurity shapes how individuals prefer to regulate their emotions in close relationships in two theoretically important contexts. In general, we observed that anxiously attached individuals' preferences were consistent with a desire for their partners' validation and approval, whereas avoidantly attached individuals' preferences were consistent with a desire to deactivate their emotions and attachment needs. Future research is needed to establish the types of partner emotional responses that will most benefit individuals during their stressful and positive life contexts and over time. Moreover, there is a general need for continued research on preferences for how partners listen and respond to different types of self-disclosures in close relationships [33].

6.5. Constraints on Generality

The main boundary condition of this research is its examination of adults from the United States who mostly identified as White or Asian. It is unknown whether similar associations of attachment orientation and preferences for partners' emotional responses would be observed among adults of other nationalities, cultures, or racial/ethnic backgrounds. Because an earlier review found significant evidence for variation in social support processes (e.g., perceptions of various behaviors as supportive) between individualist and collectivist cultures [34], it will be especially important for future research to evaluate the generalizability of our findings to individuals from more collectivist cultures than the United States. A second potential boundary condition of this research is that our data were collected online in 2020 during the COVID-19 pandemic. Given the impacts of the COVID-19 pandemic on mental health and close relationships, the historical specificity of our observed effects is also unknown. A final potential boundary condition of this research is that our outcome was assessed using newly developed prompts and questionnaires. Certain aspects of these prompts and questionnaires may influence the generalizability of our findings. For example, it is possible that we might have observed more varied associations between attachment orientation and preferences for partners to feel vs. express emotions if this distinction had been made clearer in our prompt. In addition, we assessed individuals' preferences for their partners to feel and express theoretically relevant positive and negative emotions in each context; it is unknown whether the observed associations would generalize to other types of positive and negative emotions that were not assessed in this study.

Author Contributions: Conceptualization, B.N.C., L.K., S.M.P. and B.C.F.; formal analysis, B.N.C.; methodology, B.N.C., L.K., S.M.P. and B.C.F.; writing—original draft, B.N.C.; writing—review and editing, L.K., S.M.P. and B.C.F. All authors have read and agreed to the published version of the manuscript.

Funding: This research was partially supported by a small undergraduate research grant for a senior honors thesis project conducted at Carnegie Mellon University, and by a faculty completion grant from the dean of faculty office at Trinity College awarded to the first author.

Institutional Review Board Statement: This study was conducted according to the guidelines of the Declaration of Helsinki and approved by the Institutional Review Board of Carnegie Mellon University in 2019 with protocol code STUDY2019_00000486.

Informed Consent Statement: Informed consent was obtained from all participants involved in this study.

Data Availability Statement: The data and analysis code for this study are available at: https://osf.io/nkmbw/?view_only=bb9aa20a40fc4e26a89866ed7b264efc.

Conflicts of Interest: All authors declare no conflicts of interest.

References

1. Feeney, B.C.; Collins, N.L. A New Look at Social Support. *Pers. Soc. Psychol. Rev.* **2015**, *19*, 113–147. [CrossRef] [PubMed]
2. Mikulincer, M.; Shaver, P.R. Attachment orientations and emotion regulation. *Curr. Opin. Psychol.* **2019**, *25*, 6–10. [CrossRef] [PubMed]
3. Bowlby, J. *Attachment and Loss: Vol. 1 Attachment*, 2nd ed.; Basic Books: New York, NY, USA, 1982.
4. Ainsworth, M.S. Infant–mother attachment. *Am. Psychol.* **1979**, *34*, 932–937. [CrossRef] [PubMed]
5. Cassidy, J. Emotion Regulation: Influences of Attachment Relationships. *Monogr. Soc. Res. Child Dev.* **1994**, *59*, 228–249. [CrossRef] [PubMed]
6. Cassidy, J.; Berlin, L.J. The Insecure/Ambivalent Pattern of Attachment: Theory and Research. *Child Dev.* **1994**, *65*, 971. [CrossRef] [PubMed]
7. Collins, N.L.; Read, S.J. Adult attachment, working models, and relationship quality in dating couples. *J. Pers. Soc. Psychol.* **1990**, *58*, 644–663. [CrossRef] [PubMed]
8. Cassidy, J.; Kobak, R.R. Avoidance and its relation to other defensive processes. In *Clinical Implications of Attachment*; Lawrence Erlbaum Associates, Inc.: Mahwah, NJ, USA, 1988; pp. 300–323.
9. Mikulincer, M.; Orbach, I. Attachment styles and repressive defensiveness: The accessibility and architecture of affective memories. *J. Pers. Soc. Psychol.* **1995**, *68*, 917–925. [CrossRef]
10. Hudson, N.W.; Chopik, W.J. Seeing you reminds me of things that never happened: Attachment anxiety predicts false memories when people can see the communicator. *J. Pers. Soc. Psychol.* **2023**, *124*, 396–412. [CrossRef]
11. Hudson, N.W.; Fraley, R.C. Does attachment anxiety promote the encoding of false memories? An investigation of the processes linking adult attachment to memory errors. *J. Pers. Soc. Psychol.* **2018**, *115*, 688–715. [CrossRef]
12. Reynolds, S.; Searight, R.; Ratwik, S. Adult attachment styles and rumination in the context of intimate relationships. *N. Am. J. Psychol.* **2014**, *16*, 495–506.
13. Silva, C.; Soares, I.; Esteves, F. Attachment insecurity and strategies for regulation: When emotion triggers attention. *Scand. J. Psychol.* **2012**, *53*, 9–16. [CrossRef] [PubMed]
14. Fraley, R.C.; Shaver, P.R. Adult attachment and the suppression of unwanted thoughts. *J. Pers. Soc. Psychol.* **1997**, *73*, 1080–1091. [CrossRef]
15. Mikulincer, M.; Shaver, P.R. *Attachment in Adulthood: Structure, Dynamics, and Change*, 2nd ed.; Guilford Press: New York, NY, USA, 2016.
16. Simpson, J.A.; Winterheld, H.A.; Rholes, W.S.; Oriña, M.M. Working models of attachment and reactions to different forms of caregiving from romantic partners. *J. Pers. Soc. Psychol.* **2007**, *93*, 466–477. [CrossRef] [PubMed]
17. Mikulincer, M.; Shaver, P.R. *Adult Attachment and Happiness: Individual Differences in the Experience and Consequences of Positive Emotions*; Oxford University Press: Oxford, UK, 2013. [CrossRef]
18. Magai, C.; Hunziker, J.; Mesias, W.; Culver, L.C. Adult attachment styles and emotional biases. *Int. J. Behav. Dev.* **2000**, *24*, 301–309. [CrossRef]
19. Spangler, G.; Zimmermann, P. Attachment representation and emotion regulation in adolescents: A psychobiological perspective on internal working models. *Attach. Hum. Dev.* **1999**, *1*, 270–290. [CrossRef]
20. Sonnby-Borgstrom, M.; Jonsson, P. Models-of-self and models-of-others as related to facial muscle reactions at different levels of cognitive control. *Scand. J. Psychol.* **2003**, *44*, 141–151. [CrossRef] [PubMed]
21. Gentzler, A.; Kerns, K. Adult attachment and memory of emotional reactions to negative and positive events. *Cogn. Emot.* **2006**, *20*, 20–42. [CrossRef]
22. Faul, F.; Erdfelder, E.; Lang, A.-G.; Buchner, A. G*Power 3: A flexible statistical power analysis program for the social, behavioral, and biomedical sciences. *Behav. Res. Methods* **2007**, *39*, 175–191. [CrossRef]
23. Brennan, K.A.; Clark, C.L.; Shaver, P.R. Self-report measurement of adult attachment: An integrative overview. In *Attachment Theory and Close Relationships*; The Guilford Press: New York, NY, USA, 1998; pp. 46–76.
24. Hayes, A.F. *Introduction to Mediation, Moderation, and Conditional Process Analysis: A Regression-Based Approach*, 2nd ed.; Guilford Press: New York, NY, USA, 2018.
25. Collins, N.L.; Allard, L.M. Cognitive representations of attachment: The content and function of working models. In *Blackwell Handbook of Social Psychology: Interpersonal Processes*; Blackwell Publishers Ltd.: Hoboken, NJ, USA, 2001; Volume 2, pp. 60–85.
26. Simpson, J.A.; Rholes, W.S. Fearful-avoidance, disorganization, and multiple working models: Some directions for future theory and research. *Attach. Hum. Dev.* **2002**, *4*, 223–229. [CrossRef]
27. Collins, N.L. Working models of attachment: Implications for explanation, emotion, and behavior. *J. Pers. Soc. Psychol.* **1996**, *71*, 810–832. [CrossRef]
28. Feeney, B.C.; Van Vleet, M.; Jakubiak, B.K.; Tomlinson, J.M. Predicting the Pursuit and Support of Challenging Life Opportunities. *Pers. Soc. Psychol. Bull.* **2017**, *43*, 1171–1187. [CrossRef] [PubMed]

29. Peters, B.J.; Reis, H.T.; Gable, S.L. Making the good even better: A review and theoretical model of interpersonal capitalization. *Soc. Pers. Psychol. Compass* **2018**, *12*, e12407. [CrossRef]
30. Mikulincer, M.; Shaver, P.R. Attachment theory and emotions in close relationships: Exploring the attachment-related dynamics of emotional reactions to relational events. *Pers. Relatsh.* **2005**, *12*, 149–168. [CrossRef]
31. Simpson, J.A.; Collins, W.A.; Tran, S.; Haydon, K.C. Attachment and the experience and expression of emotions in romantic relationships: A developmental perspective. *J. Pers. Soc. Psychol.* **2007**, *92*, 355–367. [CrossRef] [PubMed]
32. Butler, E.A.; Randall, A.K. Emotional Coregulation in Close Relationships. *Emot. Rev.* **2013**, *5*, 202–210. [CrossRef]
33. Itzchakov, G.; Reis, H.T. Listening and perceived responsiveness: Unveiling the significance and exploring crucial research endeavors. *Curr. Opin. Psychol.* **2023**, *53*, 101662. [CrossRef]
34. Wu, D.C.; Kim, H.S.; Collins, N.L. Perceived responsiveness across cultures: The role of cultural fit in social support use. *Soc. Pers. Psychol. Compass* **2021**, *15*, e12634. [CrossRef]

Disclaimer/Publisher's Note: The statements, opinions and data contained in all publications are solely those of the individual author(s) and contributor(s) and not of MDPI and/or the editor(s). MDPI and/or the editor(s) disclaim responsibility for any injury to people or property resulting from any ideas, methods, instructions or products referred to in the content.

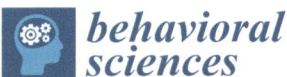
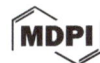

Article

Adult Attachment and Emotion Regulation Flexibility in Romantic Relationships

Farnaz Mosannenzadeh [1], Maartje Luijten [1], Dominique F. MacIejewski [2], Grace V. Wiewel [1] and Johan C. Karremans [1,*]

[1] Behavioural Science Institute, Radboud University, 6525 XZ Nijmegen, The Netherlands; farnaz.mosannenzadeh@ru.nl (F.M.); maartje.luijten2@ru.nl (M.L.); grace.wiewel@ru.nl (G.V.W.)
[2] Tilburg School of Social and Behavioral Sciences, Tilburg University, 5037 AB Tilburg, The Netherlands; d.f.maciejewski@tilburguniversity.edu
* Correspondence: johan.karremans@ru.nl

Abstract: Adults with attachment insecurity often struggle in romantic relationships due to difficulties in emotion regulation (ER). One potentially influential yet understudied factor is the inflexible over-reliance on either intrapersonal (self-directed, e.g., suppression) or interpersonal (involving others, e.g., sharing) ER. This study investigates the association between attachment insecurity and flexibility in using interpersonal versus intrapersonal ER in response to daily stressors in romantic relationships. We hypothesized that higher attachment avoidance and anxiety are associated with (H1) higher reliance on either intrapersonal or interpersonal ER over the other, respectively; (H2) less variable use of interpersonal compared to intrapersonal ER over time; and (H3) less flexible use of interpersonal compared to intrapersonal ER depending on the availability of a romantic partner. Study 1 ($N = 174$; 133 females, $M_{age} = 23.79$, $SD_{age} = 7.63$) used an online cross-sectional survey to measure average inter/intrapersonal ER, addressing H1. Study 2 ($N = 124$; 104 females, $M_{age} = 22.45$, $SD_{age} = 6.39$), combined a baseline survey with experience sampling (7 days, 8 notifications/day), addressing H1, H2, and H3. Results showed that higher attachment avoidance was associated with lower interpersonal compared to intrapersonal ER. Higher attachment anxiety was associated with less variable use of interpersonal compared to intrapersonal ER and less flexible use of interpersonal ER depending on partner availability. These findings suggest distinct associations between attachment orientations and ER flexibility, explaining ER difficulties in individuals with high attachment insecurity.

Keywords: adult attachment; emotion regulation; flexibility; romantic relationships; ESM

Citation: Mosannenzadeh, F.; Luijten, M.; MacIejewski, D.F.; Wiewel, G.V.; Karremans, J.C. Adult Attachment and Emotion Regulation Flexibility in Romantic Relationships. *Behav. Sci.* **2024**, *14*, 758. https://doi.org/10.3390/bs14090758

Academic Editors: Bianca P. Acevedo and Adam Bode

Received: 6 June 2024
Revised: 19 August 2024
Accepted: 20 August 2024
Published: 27 August 2024

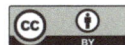

Copyright: © 2024 by the authors. Licensee MDPI, Basel, Switzerland. This article is an open access article distributed under the terms and conditions of the Creative Commons Attribution (CC BY) license (https://creativecommons.org/licenses/by/4.0/).

1. Introduction

Most people seek a fulfilling romantic relationship, which is known to enhance health and longevity [1]. However, adults with higher attachment insecurity have difficulties in the formation and maintenance of satisfying romantic relationships partially due to difficulties in regulating their emotions [2–5]. Understanding how attachment insecurity is associated with difficulties in the regulation of emotions is a key step to enhancing individual well-being and nurturing more satisfying relationships for people with higher attachment insecurity.

Emotion regulation (ER) refers to all processes through which individuals change their emotions; for example, reducing negative emotions [6]. Strategies for ER range from distracting oneself to seeking support from others [6,7]. While extensive research has examined the general effectiveness of various ER strategies [8], the more recent literature has recognized that successful ER is not necessarily about using *particular* ER strategies, but depends on the ability to flexibly use *a variety of different* ER strategies that suit specific personal and situational demands [9,10]. This ability is termed emotion regulation flexibility (ER flexibility) [9–11].

Higher attachment insecurity has been linked to lower cognitive and psychological flexibility [12–14], raising the question whether it may also be related to limited ER flexibility. As we will explain in more detail, individuals with higher attachment insecurity may struggle with seeking support from others for emotion regulation, resulting in either excessive self-reliance or dependency on others [5,15,16]. This over- or under-dependence on support from others may suggest a limited ER flexibility. This is important because limited ER flexibility may at least to some extent explain and thus provide a better understanding of ER difficulties of adults with higher attachment insecurity. However, previous research has not directly investigated the association between adult attachment and ER flexibility. The present research aims to investigate if and to what extent attachment insecurity is associated with ER flexibility in the context of romantic relationships.

1.1. Adult Attachment and Emotion Regulation in Romantic Relationships

According to attachment theory [17–19], attachment is an innate behavioral system designed to ensure a person's safety through proximity to a caregiver, known as the attachment figure [3]. Individuals with a more secure attachment hold positive views of themselves as worthy of love and view close others as being reliable in times of need [3,20]. In contrast, insecure attachment is marked by self-doubt and skepticism towards other's reliability in times of need [3]. In adulthood, attachment-related dynamics extend into romantic relationships, with romantic partners serving as attachment figures [21,22]. Individual differences in attachment behavior in adulthood are measured by two continuous dimensions (called attachment orientations): attachment anxiety and attachment avoidance [23]. In the context of romantic relationships, higher attachment anxiety is characterized by an exaggerated fear of being abandoned by romantic partners. *Higher attachment avoidance* is characterized by a high reluctance to shape interdependence with romantic partners [3].

Adult attachment orientations play a pivotal role in how individuals regulate their emotions in the context of romantic relationships. In times of stress, the primary attachment-related ER strategy, associated with a secure attachment, is seeking proximity to a romantic partner [5,15,16,22]. For example, John who is having a stressful conflict at work, reaches out to his romantic partner Mary by phone, seeking her support and proximity to deal with his stress. Notably, this primary strategy is a form of interpersonal ER, which refers to the processes in which "a person's emotions are regulated by others" [24] (p. 342). Interpersonal ER can be contrasted to intrapersonal ER, which refers to regulation of emotions without the help of others [6]. For example, John suppresses his negative emotions or brings his attention to the positive aspects of his work to feel better [25]. In attachment terms, effective interpersonal ER occurs when the attachment figure is available and responsive to one's needs and requests for support [5,26]; for example, when Mary picks up the phone and assures John that he can well-handle the conflict, making John feel less stressed.

However, if the attachment figure appears unavailable, for example, if Mary does not respond to John's phone call, individuals may use secondary emotion regulation strategies. These secondary strategies, called hyperactivating and deactivating strategies, are associated with attachment insecurity [5,15,16] and may indicate an over-reliance on either interpersonal or intrapersonal ER over the other.

Hyperactivation occurs when the attachment figure appears unavailable but proximity seeking is still perceived viable [5]. It involves intensification of attachment related emotions (e.g., stress) and behaviors (e.g., proximity seeking) [5,15]. For instance, John becomes angry when Mary does not pick up the phone and keeps calling her. Hyperactivating strategies are typically used by individuals with higher attachment anxiety [5,27,28]. For example, empirical research has found links between higher attachment anxiety and higher rumination on negative feelings [29], self-blame [30], and catastrophizing [30], all leading to more intense negative emotions. Higher attachment anxiety is also linked to high or excessive reassurance seeking [4,31,32] and more interpersonal ER strategies in general [4]. Notably, the underlying drive for hyperactivating strategies seems to be an exaggeration of self-helplessness [33] in order to elicit the attention, proximity, and support of the romantic partner. This suggests that hyperactivating strategies may reflect difficulties in self- or intrapersonal ER and an insistence on interpersonal ER; in other words, an over-reliance on interpersonal compared to intrapersonal ER, particularly when the romantic partner's availability is under question.

By contrast, the use of deactivation strategies occurs when proximity seeking is perceived inviable [5]. Deactivation includes suppression of attachment-related emotions and inhibition of proximity-seeking behaviors [5]. For example, John, assuming that Mary is incapable or unwilling to be of help, will not seek contact with Mary but instead withdraws and experientially suppresses stressful feelings. People with higher attachment avoidance more often use deactivating strategies [5,28]. For example, empirical research has shown an association between higher attachment avoidance and higher denial or suppression of emotions [5,34,35], as well as less reassurance seeking [4,31], and lower care-seeking in response to a threatening stimuli [36], all indicating more intrapersonal and less interpersonal ER. Notably, the underlying drive for deactivating strategies seems to be dampening interdependence to protect oneself from rejection-related stress and vulnerability [37]. Deactivating strategies are thus characterized by avoiding reliance on others, and "compulsive self-reliance" or autonomy [5,17–19]. This suggests that deactivating strategies may reflect an over-reliance on intrapersonal compared to interpersonal ER.

Considering individuals frequently employ multiple ER strategies concurrently [9], simultaneous investigation of how individuals use interpersonal compared to intrapersonal ER would provide a holistic and realistic perspective on individuals' ER. It would also capture the relative emphasis an individual places on interpersonal compared to intrapersonal ER across different contexts. However, while previous research has investigated the association between adult attachment and interpersonal or intrapersonal ER [4,30,31,34,38,39], a direct examination of the association between adult attachment and the use of interpersonal compared to intrapersonal ER is lacking. Investigating the association between adult attachment and the *relative* use of interpersonal compared to intrapersonal ER is particularly important as it may indicate that those with higher attachment insecurity may have a limited ER flexibility.

1.2. Adult Attachment and Emotion Regulation Flexibility in Romantic Relationships

Recent developments in ER research underscore that successful ER depends on ER flexibility: the extent to which one can use a variety of different ER strategies with respect to specific personal and situational demands across time [9,40,41]. Bonanno and Burton [42] proposed that a flexible ER is one that is sensitive to the contextual demands, uses a wide repertoire of ER strategies and is responsive to feedback. Aldao et al. [9] expanded on the work of Bonanno and Burton [42] and stated that a necessary but not sufficient condition for ER flexibility is ER variability, defined as "the variation in the use of one or more ER strategies across a number of situations" [9] (p. 268). In the previous paragraphs, we explained how adult attachment orientations might be associated with the use of interpersonal compared to intrapersonal ER. In the following paragraphs, we explain how that association may suggest a link between attachment and ER variability and ER flexibility.

1.2.1. Emotion Regulation Variability

People can use ER strategies variably. For example, they can use various ER strategies in response to one specific occasion (e.g., John tries to suppress his stress, but if that does not work, he resorts to asking support from Mary), termed between-strategy variability in the ER flexibility literature [9,11]. Using both interpersonal and intrapersonal ER to a similar extent represents high variability, while a preference for one strategy over the other is an indicator of low variability [43]. Additionally, the preference for ER strategies may vary across different occasions over time (e.g., John asks Mary for support when stressed on one occasion, and on the next occasion John tries coping with stress himself) [9,43]. Variations in the use of an ER strategy across situations over time is termed within-strategy variability in the ER flexibility literature [9,11]. We expect that those with higher attachment insecurity show lower variability in the use of interpersonal compared to intrapersonal ER. Specifically, as we discussed above, we hypothesize that attachment anxiety is linked to a strong preference for and use of interpersonal over intrapersonal ER; and attachment avoidance is linked to a strong preference for and use of intrapersonal over interpersonal ER. Since the ER preferences of individuals with attachment insecurity seem to be compulsive, we also expect these preferences not to vary much across different occasions over time.

1.2.2. Emotion Regulation Flexibility

Emotion regulation flexibility indicates the extent to which the variability in the use of ER strategies covaries with changes in the environment or the situational context [9]. In the context of attachment-related ER in romantic relationships, a crucial contextual factor is the availability of the romantic partner [5,21]. In this sense, a flexible ER would indicate varying interpersonal and intrapersonal ER according to changes in partner availability. More specifically, it would indicate using interpersonal ER (e.g., seeking company and support of the partner) when the romantic partner is available, and being able to resort to intrapersonal ER (i.e., dealing with the emotions by oneself, through for example relaxation, distraction, suppression, and so on), when the romantic partner is absent. By contrast, insisting on either interpersonal or intrapersonal ER irrespective of partner availability would indicate limited ER flexibility. As discussed above, people with higher attachment anxiety use hyperactivating ER strategies, relying on interpersonal over intrapersonal ER, even if their partner is unavailable (e.g., John keeps calling Mary for support even when she apparently is not available, and he does not resort to intrapersonal ER instead). In contrast, people with higher attachment avoidance tend to perceive that their romantic partner is unwilling or incapable of being responsive to their needs, and therefore, even if their partner is available, they may tend to use deactivating strategies, relying on intrapersonal over interpersonal ER (e.g., John tries solving his stress about work using intrapersonal ER, irrespective of whether Mary is available to support him). Thus, variation in the relative use of interpersonal compared to intrapersonal ER for people with higher attachment insecurity should be less dependent on the availability of their partner, indicating a limited ER flexibility.1.3. The Current Research

In the current research, we aim to investigate if and to what extent romantic attachment insecurity is associated with ER flexibility in the use of interpersonal compared to intrapersonal ER when regulating one's own negative emotions in times of stress. To address this aim, we first investigated the basic question whether individuals with higher romantic attachment insecurity have a tendency to consistently rely on either inter- or intrapersonal ER, relative to the other, as an indicator of ER variability (Research Question 1; RQ1). We used two strategies to examine this research question: Firstly, we investigated the relative use of interpersonal ER compared to intrapersonal ER, with a strong preference for either one of them indicating low variability. Secondly, we investigated the extent to which the relative use of interpersonal compared to intrapersonal ER varies across multiple occasions over time, with less variation indicating low variability.

To measure the relative use of interpersonal compared to intrapersonal ER, in both Studies 1 and 2, in an online cross-sectional survey, after assessing their level of attachment anxiety and avoidance, participants reported their general tendency to use interpersonal ER and intrapersonal ER in response to stressful life events. In addition, in Study 2, we measured the relative use of interpersonal ER compared to intrapersonal ER in multiple occasions per day in a 7-day period, using an experience sampling method (ESM). ESM allows participants to momentarily and repeatedly report on their actual life experiences and behaviors. A meta-analysis comparing global self-reports and daily measures [44] revealed that global self-report measures of a given ER strategy often do not strongly or specifically match the actual use of that strategy in daily life. This finding highlights the advantage of using ESM to capture more accurate and context-specific data on ER. We hypothesized that higher scores on romantic attachment anxiety and avoidance are associated with lower variability, with attachment anxiety being linked to a higher preference for interpersonal over intrapersonal ER (H1.1); attachment avoidance being linked to a higher preference for intrapersonal over interpersonal ER (H1.2); and both attachment anxiety and avoidance being linked to lower variation in the relative use of interpersonal compared to intrapersonal ER across multiple occasions in a given time period (H2.1, H2.2, respectively).

As the second research question (RQ2), we investigated whether the relative use of interpersonal compared to intrapersonal ER varies depending on the availability of the romantic partner, indicating ER flexibility. In general, we hypothesized that the relative use of interpersonal compared to intrapersonal ER would increase when the partner is available compared to when they are absent (H3.1). We then hypothesized that individuals with higher attachment anxiety and/or avoidance will show less ER flexibility, indicated by a weaker association between partner availability and the relative use of interpersonal compared to intrapersonal ER (H3.2; H3.3, respectively).

While our primary focus was on the relative use of interpersonal compared to intrapersonal ER, for each hypothesis, we additionally investigated the unique associations between attachment orientations and these two types of ER separately. This approach allowed us to discern how attachment orientations influence the use of each ER strategy individually, providing more clarity on the origins of ER variability and flexibility.

2. Study 1

In this study, we investigated the association between romantic attachment and the general tendency to use interpersonal compared to intrapersonal ER in times of stress using a cross-sectional online survey. We computed a variability index to measure the relative use of interpersonal compared to intrapersonal ER, called inter-vs-intrapersonal ER, by subtracting participants' self-reported general tendency to use intrapersonal ER from their tendency to use interpersonal ER. The scores closer to 0 indicate more similarity in the use of interpersonal and intrapersonal ER and thus a higher variability. Larger positive or negative scores indicate lower variability; with positive scores indicating a preference for interpersonal ER, and negative scores indicating a preference for intrapersonal ER. The advantage of employing the subtraction method to calculate variability over the often-used standard deviation (SD) method [9,43] is its capability to not only quantify the extent but also the direction of variability. In other words, it not only shows the extent to which one strategy was preferred over the other, but also allows us to understand which ER strategy (interpersonal or intrapersonal) was preferred. This approach offers clear interpretability and is particularly relevant to our research question and hypothesis. Based on our hypotheses, we expected a positive association between attachment anxiety and inter-vs-intrapersonal ER (H1.1) and a negative association between attachment avoidance and inter-vs-intrapersonal ER (H1.2). For a visualization of hypotheses, see Figure 1. This study was pre-registered on the Open Science Framework (OSF; see https://osf.io/m2t9g, accessed on 1 February 2021; see Table S9 for deviations from pre-registration).

In order to limit the influence of confounding and other extraneous variables, we controlled for other potential variables that might influence inter-vs-intrapersonal ER. More specifically, we controlled for participants' gender, relationship duration and relationship quality as they are shown to influence interpersonal processes in romantic relationships, particularly support seeking; for example, to regulate emotions [45]. Furthermore, the personality trait neuroticism is shown to be strongly associated with intrapersonal ER strategies such as suppressing and avoiding emotions, rumination on negative emotions, and isolating oneself [46]. Additionally, the personality trait extraversion is shown to be associated with support seeking from others [47]. Therefore, we also controlled for neuroticism and extraversion. Since the study was conducted during the spread of the COVID-19 pandemic, we also controlled for the extent to which participants' responses were influenced by the COVID situation.

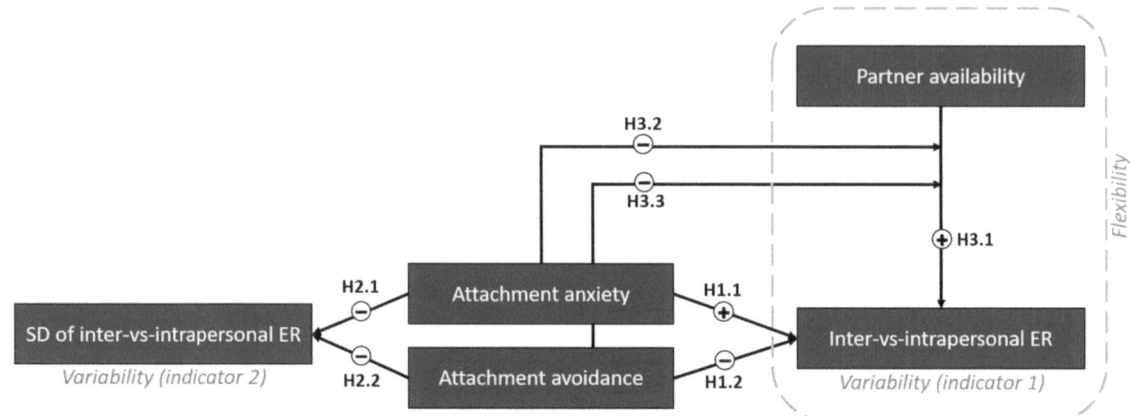

Figure 1. Research hypotheses of Study 1 and Study 2. Note. Study 1 investigated H1.1 and H1.2 in an online cross-sectional survey. Study 2 investigated all hypotheses in an online survey combined with experience sampling method. Inter-vs-intrapersonal ER is interpersonal ER minus intrapersonal ER at a given period of time. SD is standard deviation. The signs in the circles indicate the direction of the hypothesized effect.

3. Materials and Methods of Study 1

3.1. Participants

The participants were included in the study if they were at least 18 years old, involved in a monogamous romantic relationship for at least six months, and in possession of a smartphone. To ensure independent data, only one partner of a couple could participate. Participants were not excluded based on physical or mental illness. Participants were recruited from April to October 2020, via the Radboud University participant recruitment system (SONA), and online advertisement on social media (e.g., Facebook, Instagram, WhatsApp). Based on a prior power analysis using G*Power 3.1.9.2 [48], for a multiple linear regression analysis, the sample should consist of at least 73 participants when using an estimated effect size of 0.15, significance level of 0.05, and a power of 0.90. Initially, 203 persons signed up for the study. The participants were excluded if they did not consent to participate ($n = 3$), did not complete the questionnaire ($n = 23$), reported that they did not answer the questionnaire seriously ($n = 2$), and did not meet the inclusion criteria concerning relationship length ($n = 1$). The final sample included 174 adults (133 female), aged between 18 and 58 ($M = 23.79$, $SD = 7.63$) with a relationship length between 6 months and 41 years ($M = 3.5$ years, $SD = 6.1$ years). The majority of participants were White/Caucasian (87%), unmarried (93%), not cohabiting with their partner (62%), and without children (95%). For details of the demographic characteristics of the participants, see Table S1. The participants were compensated via study credit points (if applicable) and/or entering a lottery of 50 Euros.

3.2. Procedure

The study included an online survey (on Qualtrics) with a battery of questionnaires. Before proceeding with the questionnaires, participants received information about the study and were asked to give their consent. The survey took an average of 25 min to complete.

3.3. Measures

3.3.1. Adult Attachment

The independent variables, adult attachment anxiety and avoidance, were measured using Experiences in Close Relationships-Revised (ECR-R) [49]. This scale consists of two subscales, attachment anxiety (18 items; $\alpha = 0.88$) and attachment avoidance (18 items;

$\alpha = 0.90$). Participants indicated their level of agreement with each item on a Likert-type scale from 1 = strongly disagree to 7 = strongly agree. Attachment anxiety and attachment avoidance scores were computed by calculating the mean of participants' responses on the corresponding items. Higher means indicate higher attachment anxiety or avoidance.

3.3.2. Inter-vs-Intrapersonal Emotion Regulation

The dependent variable inter-vs-intrapersonal ER was defined as an index of variability, indicating the relative use of interpersonal compared to intrapersonal ER. Inter-vs-intrapersonal ER was measured using a 2-item self-constructed scale that asked participants about their general ER tendency when experiencing negative or distressing emotions (i.e., My general tendency is to: 1 item for interpersonal emotion regulation, "seek out the company or support of my romantic partner or other people close to me"; 1 item for intrapersonal emotion regulation: "try to handle the situation by myself"). The participants responded to the items on a Likert-type scale from 1 = almost never to 5 = almost always. To compute inter-vs-intrapersonal ER score, the interpersonal score minus intrapersonal score was calculated. The scores closer to 0 indicate more similarity in the use of interpersonal and intrapersonal ER and thus a higher variability between strategies. Larger positive or negative scores indicate lower variability. Positive scores indicate more use of interpersonal compared to intrapersonal ER. Negative scores indicate less use of interpersonal compared to intrapersonal ER.

3.3.3. Relationship Quality

The control variable relationship quality was measured using a 18-item Perceived Relationship Quality Component (PRQC) [50]. An example item is "How satisfied are you with your relationship?". Participants responded to each item on a Likert-type scale, from 1 = not at all to 7 = extremely. The relationship quality score was computed by calculating the mean of the participants' responses on all items ($\alpha = 0.93$).

3.3.4. Personality Types

The control variables neuroticism and extraversion were measured using the 10-item Personality Inventory (TIPI) scale [51]. The TIPI scale comprises two items for each of five personality traits. Participants indicated their agreement with each item on a Likert-type scale from 1 = strongly disagree to 7 = strongly agree. Extraversion ($\alpha = 0.79$) and neuroticism ($\alpha = 0.75$) were computed by calculating the mean of the participants' responses on the corresponding items.

3.3.5. COVID

At the final stage of the survey, we asked participants to respond to a 1-item question "To what extent do you think your answers are different from a normal time when there was no Corona?" on a sliding bar ranging from 0 = not at all to 100 = very much. This self-developed variable was called COVID and was controlled for in the analysis.

3.4. Data Preparation and Analysis

All data preparation and analysis were performed in R version 4.0.3 [52]. Since all survey questions were forced response, we had no missing values. In participants' responses to relationship length, some entries did not specify whether the indicated number referred to years or months. For these cases, we coded the entries as "NA" to denote missing information. To analyze the data, we ran a multiple linear regression using the function lmer [53] with attachment anxiety, attachment avoidance and their interaction term as independent variables and inter-vs-intrapersonal ER as the outcome variable. We also controlled for relationship length (in months), gender (dummy coded: 1 = female, 0 = male; named female), relationship quality, extraversion, neuroticism, and COVID. All continuous variables were centered around the sample mean scores before entering in the analysis. Notably, the interaction between attachment anxiety and avoidance was included in the analysis following Fraley's [54] advice. Additionally, the initial model included age as a control variable; however, due to collinearity between age and relationship length, and since the model with relationship length (and not with age) could better capture the variance in the dependent variable than the model with age (and not relationship length), age was excluded from the final model.

4. Results of Study 1

4.1. Preliminary Analysis of Data

Descriptive statistics are presented in Table 1. Notably, the mean score for inter-vs-intrapersonal ER ($M = -0.01$) indicates that, on average, individuals exhibited an equal inclination toward using interpersonal and intrapersonal ER, with a slightly higher tendency toward intrapersonal ER. Participants reported varying levels of attachment insecurity, with mean levels falling in the lower to mid-range of the scale. On average, participants reported little influence of COVID on their responses.

Table 1. Descriptive statistics across studies and analyses.

Variable	Study 1			Study 2 Baseline			Study 2 Baseline + ESM			
	n	M (SD)	Range	n	M (SD)	Range	n	M (SD)	Range	ICC
Baseline measurements										
Inter-vs-intrapersonal ER	174	−0.01 (1.85)	−4 to 4	287	0.24 (1.90)	−4 to 4	124	0.31 (2.07)	−4 to 4	-
Interpersonal ER	174	3.55 (1.08)	1 to 5	287	3.63 (1.08)	1 to 5	124	3.68 (1.13)	1 to 5	-
Intrapersonal ER	174	3.56 (1.11)	1 to 5	287	3.39 (1.07)	1 to 5	124	3.36 (1.13)	1 to 5	-
Attachment anxiety	174	2.53 (0.88)	1 to 5.06	287	2.60 (1.06)	1 to 6.5	124	2.49 (0.99)	1 to 5.6	-
Attachment avoidance	174	2.40 (0.83)	1 to 5.39	287	2.56 (0.80)	1 to 5	124	2.55 (0.78)	1 to 4.6	-
Age (years)	174	23.79 (7.63)	18 to 58	287	22.13 (5.04)	18 to 58	124	22.45 (6.39)	18 to 58	-
Relationship length (months)	169	42.07 (72.74)	6 to 492	286	30.66 (30.02)	3 to 249	123	33.74 (36.68)	3 to 249	-
Relationship quality	174	5.94 (0.80)	3.17 to 7	282	6.10 (0.79)	2.3 to 7	124	6.18 (0.68)	3.1 to 7	-
Neuroticism	174	4.15 (1.52)	1 to 7	287	4.28 (1.43)	1 to 7	124	4.36 (1.45)	1 to 7	-
Extraversion	174	4.30 (1.73)	1 to 7	287	4.49 (1.47)	1 to 7	124	4.44 (1.51)	1 to 7	-
COVID	174	23.44 (23.67)	0 to 100	287	30.02 (24.49)	0 to 100	124	31.39 (25.18)	0 to 92	-
Momentary measurements										
Participant-centered values										
Inter-vs-intrapersonal ER							124	−2.93 (3.05)	−10 to 5.4	-
Interpersonal ER							124	3.58 (1.93)	0 to 9	-
Intrapersonal ER							124	6.51 (1.66)	0.7 to 10	-
Stressfulness of event							124	5.12 (1.56)	1.6 to 8.4	-
Partner availability							124	0.32 (0.23)	0 to 0.9	-
Others availability							124	0.42 (0.21)	0 to 0.9	-
Grand values										
Inter-vs-intrapersonal ER							2654	−3.1 (5.62)	−10 to 10	0.22
Interpersonal ER							2663	3.5 (3.66)	0 to 10	0.21
Intrapersonal ER							2654	6.61 (2.96)	0 to 10	0.25
Stressfulness of event							2666	5.12 (2.52)	0 to 10	0.35
Partner availability							2672	0.31 (0.46)	0 to 1	0.20
Others availability							2672	0.41 (0.49)	0 to 1	0.14

Correlations between variables are presented in Supplemental Materials (Table S2). Attachment anxiety and avoidance were positively correlated ($r = 0.41$, $p < 0.001$). Inter-vs-intrapersonal ER was significantly negatively correlated with attachment avoidance ($r = -0.39$, $p < 0.001$) but not significantly with attachment anxiety ($r = -0.13$, $p = 0.071$). Furthermore, higher inter-vs-intrapersonal ER was reported by females ($r = 0.29$, $p < 0.001$), participants with higher relationship quality ($r = 0.19$, $p = 0.013$), and those with lower neuroticism ($r = -0.27$, $p < 0.001$). Age and relationship length were highly correlated ($r = 0.80$, $p < 0.001$).

4.2. Main Analysis

The model explained 21.8% of the variance in inter-vs-intrapersonal ER ($F(9, 159) = 6.204$, $p < 0.001$). As can be seen in Table 2, the effect of attachment anxiety was not significant, meaning that unlike H1.1, the relative use of interpersonal compared to intrapersonal ER did not depend on one's level of attachment anxiety. Attachment avoidance was significantly negatively associated with inter-vs-intrapersonal ER (H1.2), meaning that individuals with higher attachment avoidance reported a lower reliance on interpersonal compared to intrapersonal ER when dealing with their negative emotions when stressed. The results also indicated that the variability between strategies decreased at higher scores of attachment avoidance with an increased preference for intrapersonal compared to interpersonal ER (see Figure 2). Attachment anxiety and attachment avoidance did not significantly interact in influencing inter-vs-intrapersonal ER, suggesting that the effect of attachment avoidance on the relative use of interpersonal compared to intrapersonal ER did not depend on different levels of attachment anxiety.

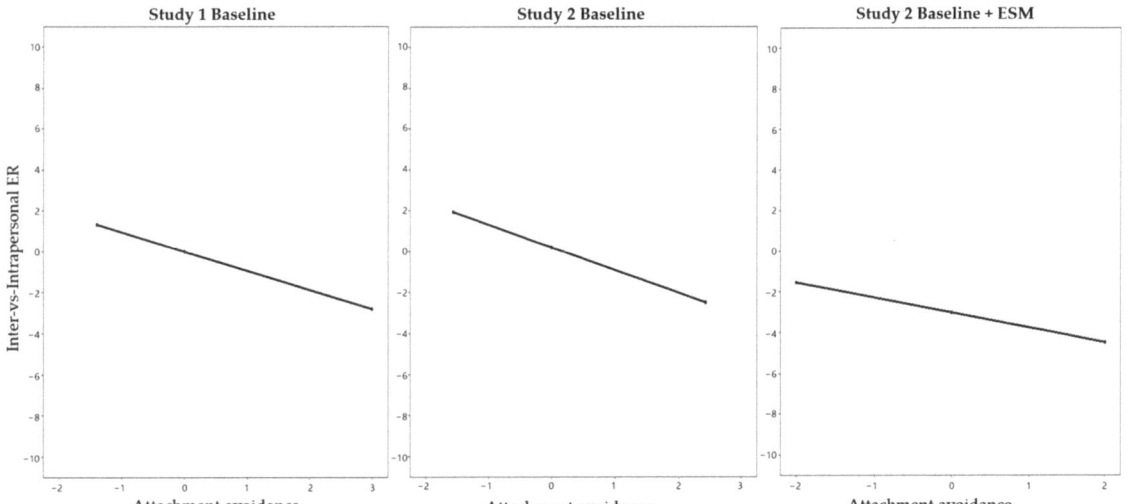

Figure 2. The effect of attachment avoidance on inter-vs-intrapersonal emotion regulation across studies and analyses. Note: the inter-vs-intrapersonal scores closer to 0 indicate more similarity in the use of interpersonal and intrapersonal ER and thus a higher variability. Larger positive or negative scores indicate lower variability.

Table 2. The effect of attachment on the use of interpersonal compared to intrapersonal emotion regulation across studies and analyses.

	Study 1 Baseline (N = 174)				Study 2 Baseline (N = 287)				Study 2 ESM (N = 124)				
	b	SE	t	p	b	SE	t	p	b	SE	DF	t	p
(Intercept)	−0.69	0.28	−2.45	**0.016**	−0.41	0.28	−1.48	0.139	**−5.67**	**0.55**	**2483**	**−10.38**	**<0.001**
Attachment anxiety	−0.13	0.18	−0.73	0.464	0.02	0.12	0.14	0.885	0.03	0.26	113	0.10	0.922
Attachment avoidance	**−0.94**	**0.21**	**−4.37**	**<0.001**	**−1.11**	**0.14**	**−7.78**	**<0.001**	**−0.77**	**0.32**	**113**	**−2.45**	**0.016**
Attachment anxiety × Attachment avoidance	−0.02	0.17	−0.13	0.900	0.15	0.11	1.395	0.164	**0.50**	**0.23**	**113**	**2.13**	**0.035**
Relationship length	−0.01	0.01	−0.34	0.732	0.00	0.00	0.17	0.869	−0.01	0.01	113	−1.57	0.120
Female	**0.92**	**0.33**	**2.81**	**0.006**	**0.74**	**0.30**	**2.46**	**0.015**	0.41	0.57	113	0.72	0.471
Others					−0.86	1.02	−0.85	0.399					
Relationship quality	−0.38	0.23	−1.71	0.090	−0.27	0.15	−1.71	0.088	0.05	0.36	113	0.13	0.899
Neuroticism	**−0.23**	**0.09**	**−2.47**	**0.015**	−0.14	0.08	−1.73	0.084	0.28	0.16	113	1.76	0.081
Extraversion	−0.03	0.08	−0.44	0.661	**0.15**	**0.07**	**2.13**	**0.034**	0.13	0.14	113	0.96	0.339
COVID	−0.01	0.01	−0.79	0.432	−0.01	0.00	−1.38	0.169	0.02	0.01	113	1.83	0.070
Stressfulness of event									**0.15**	**0.06**	**2483**	**2.45**	**0.014**
Partner availability									**5.89**	**0.36**	**2483**	**16.48**	**<0.001**
Others availability									**1.10**	**0.24**	**2483**	**4.56**	**<0.001**
Time									−0.01	0.01	2483	−1.39	0.166

Note: the significant results are presented in bold.

4.3. Exploratory Analysis

To attain further insight into the association between attachment and the measure of interpersonal relative to intrapersonal ER, we performed two other exploratory regression analyses with interpersonal ER and intrapersonal ER separately. The results (see Table S3) showed that attachment anxiety was not significantly associated with interpersonal ER ($b = -0.06$, $SE = 0.10$, $p = 0.542$) or intrapersonal ER ($b = 0.07$, $SE = 0.12$, $p = 0.559$). In contrast, higher attachment avoidance was associated with both a lower tendency to use interpersonal ER ($b = -0.61$, $SE = 0.12$, $p < 0.001$) and a higher tendency to use intrapersonal ER ($b = 0.33$, $SE = 0.14$, $p = 0.023$). That is, individuals with higher attachment avoidance reported less proximity and support seeking and more self-regulation compared to those with lower attachment avoidance. We did not find significant interactions between the two attachment orientations for interpersonal ($b = -0.05$, $SE = 0.09$, $p = 0.577$), nor for intrapersonal ($b = -0.03$, $SE = 0.11$, $p = 0.774$).

5. Discussion of Study 1

As a brief discussion of results of the Study 1, attachment anxiety had no influence on the amount of using interpersonal versus intrapersonal ER, providing no support for our first hypothesis that people with higher attachment anxiety have lower ER variability with an over-reliance on interpersonal versus intrapersonal ER (H1.1). However, the results supported our second hypothesis (H1.2), as higher attachment avoidance was associated with lower interpersonal compared to intrapersonal ER, indicating a lower variability in higher levels of attachment avoidance. In other terms, individuals with higher (compared to lower) attachment avoidance had a higher tendency to rely on intrapersonal ER strategies over seeking proximity and support from close others. These findings provide support for overreliance on one particular ER strategy for avoidantly attached individuals, but not for anxiously attached individuals.

6. Study 2

In this study, we combined a baseline online survey with an ESM study for a period of one week. This study was pre-registered on the OSF (see https://osf.io/et5a2, accessed on 1 February 2021; see Table S9 for deviations from pre-registration). Our first aim was to replicate the results of the first study regarding the association between attachment and the relative use of interpersonal compared to intrapersonal ER in both baseline data and ESM data. In the baseline survey, similar to Study 1, we calculated an index of ER variability, indicating the relative use of interpersonal compared to intrapersonal ER, called inter-vs-intrapersonal ER. This index was calculated as a self-report on the extent to which people generally tend to use interpersonal ER minus the extent to which they generally tend to use intrapersonal ER when they experience stress.

Similarly, in ESM, we calculated momentary inter-vs-intrapersonal ER as momentary self-report on the extent to which individuals used interpersonal ER minus the extent to which they used intrapersonal ER when they experienced stressful events in daily life. We particularly asked for stressful life events since it is the focus of our research. Based on our hypotheses outlined in the Introduction, in both baseline and ESM data, we tested for a positive association between attachment anxiety and inter-vs-intrapersonal ER (H1.1) and a negative association between attachment avoidance and inter-vs-intrapersonal ER (H1.2).

In addition, as a second indicator of variability, we calculated the extent to which inter-vs-intrapersonal ER varied over time. Following Aldao et al.'s [9] advice and similar to Blanke et al. [43], we calculated the standard deviation of all momentary assessments of inter-vs-intrapersonal ER for each participant. In concrete terms, a higher standard deviation reflects higher variation in the relative use of interpersonal compared to intrapersonal ER. We expected that people with higher attachment anxiety or avoidance will show lower standard deviations (H2.1, H2.2), indicating lower variability in inter-vs-intrapersonal ER.

Finally, we investigated the association between attachment and ER flexibility; that is, the variable use of ER strategies depending on the specific context, and in this case, partner availability. We used Aldao et al.'s [9] suggestion to calculate a coefficient that measures the extent to which ER variability and changes in the context/environment covary together, where larger coefficients represent higher ER flexibility. We performed a regression analysis to compute the extent to which inter-vs-intrapersonal ER (as an index of ER strategy variability) depends on changes in partner availability. Overall, we expected that individuals would use more interpersonal compared to intrapersonal ER when their romantic partner is available compared to when the partner is unavailable (H3.1). More importantly, we tested whether attachment anxiety and avoidance moderated the association between partner availability and inter-vs-intrapersonal ER. Specifically, we expected the association between partner availability and use of inter-vs-intrapersonal ER to be weaker for those with higher (compared to lower) attachment anxiety and avoidance (H3.2, and H3.3). For a visualization of hypotheses, see Figure 1.

7. Materials and Methods of Study 2

7.1. Participants

As stated before, the study included a baseline survey followed by a 1-week ESM procedure. In our baseline data analysis, we aimed to gather information from a minimum of 110 participants. This decision was guided by an a priori power analysis, considering an estimated effect size (f^2) of 0.07 (the smallest expected effect size based on the results of the Study 1), a significance level of 0.05, and a power of 0.80, calculated using G*Power 3.1.9.2 [48]. For the ESM data, where we collected multiple observations per participant and employed a multi-level model with enhanced power, we expected to have sufficient statistical power with a minimum of 110 participants. The inclusion criteria were being over 18 years old, involved in a monogamous, romantic relationship for at least three months, and in possession of a smartphone. To ensure independent data, only one partner of a couple could participate. Participants were not excluded based on physical or mental illness. Participants were recruited from April 2021 to March 2022, via the Radboud University participant recruitment system (SONA), and online advertisement on social media (e.g., Facebook, Instagram, WhatsApp). A portion (but not all) of participants who completed the baseline survey also completed the ESM procedure. The participants were compensated via study credit points (if applicable) for completing either the baseline or both the baseline and ESM procedures. Furthermore, all participants who completed the baseline questionnaire and the ESM procedure with at least a 75% compliance rate entered a lottery ($4 \times 50€$ cash prizes).

7.1.1. Baseline

In total, 435 persons signed up for the study. We excluded participants who did not consent to participate (n = 74), did not complete the questionnaire (n = 65), reported that they did not answer the questionnaire seriously (n = 4), and did not meet the inclusion criteria concerning minimum relationship length (n = 5). The final sample included 287 adults (244 female, 3 other), aged between 18 and 58 (M = 22.13, SD = 5.04) with a relationship length between 3 months and 21 years (M = 2.5 years, SD = 2.5 years). Compared to Study 1, Study 2 baseline participants were younger ($t(265.84)$ = $-2.56, p$ = 0.011). Similar to Study 1, the majority of participants were White/Caucasian (87%), unmarried (96%), not cohabiting with their partner (72%), and without children (96%). For details of the demographic characteristics of the participants, see Table S1.

7.1.2. Experience Sampling Method

Initially, 136 eligible participants signed up for the ESM part of the study. We excluded data of those who dropped out during the ESM part (n = 9) and did not meet the commonly applied pre-defined 33% compliance rate (n = 3). The final ESM analyses included 124 participants (104 female) aged between 18 and 58 years old (M = 22.45, SD = 6.39 years) with a relationship duration between 3 months and 21 years (M = 2.81 years, SD = 3.5 years) in the ESM analysis. Other demographic characteristics were similar to those of Study 1 and Study 2 baseline participants (for details, see Table S1).

7.2. Procedure

The study included two main parts: (1) an online baseline survey (on Qualtrics) and (2) an ESM procedure, using the SEMA^3 app SEMA3: Smartphone Ecological Momentary Assessment, version 1.4.2(48) [55]. In the baseline survey (first part), participants responded to a battery of questionnaires. Before proceeding with the questionnaires, participants received information about the study and were asked to give their consent. The survey took an average of 25 min to complete. Upon completion of the baseline survey, participants were instructed to schedule an individual online meeting (i.e., briefing session) with the researchers. During the briefing session, participants were guided through the installation and usage of the SEMA3 app on their smartphones and the ESM procedure using a pre-established protocol and an informative PowerPoint presentation.

For each participant, a 7-day ESM procedure started on the next day after their briefing session. Each day, on their smartphones, participants received seven semi-randomly timed prompts throughout the day (one prompt randomly programmed within each 2 h interval within 14 awake hours) and one evening prompt in the evening. The schedule of prompts was adjusted individually to each participant's usual daily schedule so that the prompts would occur when the participant was usually awake.

The daily prompts had to be responded within 30 min; otherwise, the questionnaire would be missed. The daily prompts contained momentary questionnaires which took around two to three minutes to complete. In each questionnaire, participants first reported their momentary emotions. Then, they were instructed to think of a situation when they felt bad/stressed since the last notification. This was followed by questions about the context of the event and the emotion regulation strategies that the participant used to deal with their stress since the last notification. Note that in the briefing session, the participants were instructed to report any major or minor stressful events (e.g., missing a bus). Nevertheless, participants had the option to report that no stressful events occurred since the last prompt, which resulted in receiving a set of filler questions that were very similar to the actual questions in content and number but were not of interest to the current study. Furthermore, participants received a 4 min evening questionnaire on their average ER during each day which was not included in the data analysis of the current study. By the end of the seventh day, upon the request of participants, up to two extra days of ESM procedure were provided to increase the compliance rate. Eleven participants used this opportunity to increase their compliance rate, aiming to qualify for full study credits and/or gaining entry into the lottery. Upon completion, participants received a debriefing via e-mail and access to their data summary provided by the SEMA3 app.

7.3. Measures

The baseline measures were the same as in Study 1, with two differences: Firstly, to measure adult attachment, we used a shorter version of ECR-R (ECR-R-General Short Form) [56] with 10 items for attachment anxiety ($\alpha = 0.87$) and 10 items for attachment avoidance ($\alpha = 0.84$). Additionally, to measure relationship quality, we used only three subscales (trust, commitment, and satisfaction) from the PRQC [50] including 9 items ($\alpha = 0.90$). Notably, the Cronbach's alpha for personality traits neuroticism and extraversion were $\alpha = 0.63$ and $\alpha = 0.73$, respectively. In the ESM part, if the participant indicated that they experienced a bad/stressful event, they were asked to respond to a series of questions about that event, including in the presented order:

7.3.1. Partner Availability

The participants responded to a multi-select multiple choice question "When I felt bad/stressed, I was in contact with ...", with 10 response items (i.e., Nobody, Romantic partner, Housemates, Family, Family (living elsewhere), Colleagues/Classmates, Friend, Acquaintances, Strangers, Other). The participants were previously informed that being in contact means, for example, face-to-face, via phone call, or online contact. The variable partner availability was dummy coded as 1 if the participant indicated that they were in contact with their partner and as 0 if otherwise. The variable others availability was dummy coded as 1 if the participant indicated that they were with anyone else than their romantic partner and 0 as otherwise.

7.3.2. Stressfulness of the Event

The participants responded to a 1-item question "To what extent did you feel bad/stressed?" on a sliding bar ranging from 0 = not at all to 10 = very much.

7.3.3. Momentary Inter-vs-Intrapersonal Emotion Regulation

The participants responded to "What did you do to deal with your negative feelings/stress" on 3 items (1 item for interpersonal: "I reached out for the company and support of my partner." 1 item for intrapersonal: "I tried to handle my negative feelings/stress by myself." 1 item "I reached out for the company and support of others") on a visual sliding bar from 0 = not at all to 10 = very much. As the first indicator of variability, indicating the relative use of interpersonal compared to intrapersonal ER in each moment, momentary inter-vs-intrapersonal ER was calculated as the interpersonal score minus intrapersonal score for each notification (we left out the scores on the third item, measuring interpersonal ER using others than romantic partner). A score of 0 indicates equal use of interpersonal compared to intrapersonal ER, with scores closer to 0 indicating higher variability and larger positive or negative scores indicating lower variability. Positive scores indicate more use of interpersonal compared to intrapersonal ER. Negative scores indicate less use of interpersonal compared to intrapersonal ER. As the second indicator of ER variability, the variation in the relative use of interpersonal compared to intrapersonal ER over time, the SD of momentary inter-vs-intrapersonal ER was calculated across all momentary assessments for each participant based on previous research [9,43].

All ESM measures were developed based on items found in the ESM Item Repository [57].

7.4. Data Preparation and Analysis

All data preparation and analysis were performed in R, version 4.0.3 [52]. The baseline measures from Qualtrics and ESM measures from SEMA3 were downloaded as separate csv files, and then imported in R, where data were preprocessed, and variable scores were calculated (for details of pre-processing steps, see Supplementary Materials). The analysis of the baseline data was equivalent to the one reported in Study 1. In all analysis, in order to limit the influence of confounding and other extraneous variables, and since we aimed to replicate the results of Study 1, we used the same control variables as Study 1, namely, relationship length, gender, relationship quality, extraversion, neuroticism, and the effect of COVID. Furthermore, in ESM analyses, we controlled for momentary stressfulness of the event, availability of the partner, and availability of others than partner. Notably, since individuals can use interpersonal ER not only with their romantic partner but also with others, we considered controlling for the variable interpersonal ER with others than partner. However, this variable is correlated with and affected by our control variable availability of others than partner and, it is challenging to determine the sequence of events—whether interpersonal ER occurred with the partner or others first. Therefore, for the sake of model parsimony and to avoid potential issues related to reverse causality and multicollinearity, we opted not to include interpersonal ER with others.

7.4.1. Main Analyses

For the analysis of the ESM data to answer RQ1 part 1 (concerning the relative use of interpersonal compared to intrapersonal ER) and RQ2, we performed two multilevel models using the lme function from R package nlme [58] and with momentary inter-vs-intrapersonal ER as an outcome variable and attachment anxiety, attachment avoidance, and their interaction term as independent variables. For both models, time-invariant control variables—including relationship length, gender (female), relationship quality, extraversion, neuroticism, and COVID—as well as time-variant control variable time were included as fixed effects. Furthermore, time-variant control variables such as stressfulness of event, partner availability, and others availability were added as both fixed and random effects. Additionally, for RQ2, the two-way and three-way interactions of partner availability with attachment anxiety and attachment avoidance were entered as fixed effects. Following Bolger and Laurenceau's [59] advice, all continuous independent time-invariant variables were grand-mean centered around the population mean. All continuous independent time-variant variables were person-mean centered around participant means.

To answer RQ2 part 2 (the variation in the relative use of interpersonal compared to intrapersonal ER over time), a multiple linear regression analysis was performed with SD of momentary inter-vs-intrapersonal ER as the outcome variable, and attachment anxiety, attachment avoidance, and their interaction term as independent variables. In the initial phase of data analysis, a set of control variables, namely relationship length, female, relationship quality, extraversion, neuroticism, and COVID, were included in the model. However, the model did not significantly explain the variance in the dependent variable. To refine the model, control variables were systematically removed one by one, starting with those exhibiting the lowest correlation with the outcome variable. Following the sequential removal of extraversion and female, the model achieved statistical significance. Therefore, the final model included centered values of relationship length, relationship quality, neuroticism, and COVID as control variables. Notably, the patterns of effect size and significance did not change with removal of extraversion and female. Additionally, we computed mean levels of stressfulness of events, partner availability, and others availability for each participant and added it to the model as control variables.

7.4.2. Exploratory Analysis

For each model in the main analyses, two additional exploratory analyses were performed, maintaining the main analysis model's independent variables but using different outcome variables: one with interpersonal ER as the outcome and another with intrapersonal ER.

8. Results of Study 2
8.1. Preliminary Analyses

Participants completed a total of 6052 ESM notifications with an average 38 out of 49 responses, yielding a mean compliance rate of 78.50% ($SD = 14$). Participants reported experiencing a stressful event in 2677 notifications, averaging 22 notifications per participant, meaning a mean 57.90% ($SD = 24$) of responded notifications. Participants reported their partner was available in a mean 32% ($SD = 23$) of the stressful events. Descriptive statistics are presented in Table 1. Notably, compared to Study 1, Study 2 baseline had a higher relationship quality, $t(363.08) = 2.08$, $p = 0.038$, reported an average higher attachment avoidance, $t(352.92) = 2.12$, $p = 0.035$, and indicated a higher influence of COVID on their responses $t(374.85) = 2.86$, $p = 0.005$. Participants of Study 2 baseline did not differ from Study 1 participants in their average attachment anxiety, $t(416.64) = 0.78$, $p = 0.439$, and inter-vs-intrapersonal ER, $t(372.57) = 1.37$, $p = 0.172$. Study 2 ESM did not differ from the larger sample of Study 2 baseline in average scores of baseline variables (e.g., attachment anxiety; see Table S5).

Correlations between Study 2 baseline variables are presented in the Supplementary Materials (Table S2). Attachment anxiety and avoidance were positively correlated ($r = 0.30$, $p < 0.001$). Similar to Study 1, inter-vs-intrapersonal ER was negatively correlated with attachment avoidance ($r = -0.42$, $p < 0.001$) but not correlated with attachment anxiety ($r = -0.05$, $p = 0.467$). That is, individuals with higher attachment avoidance had a lower tendency to use inter-vs-intrapersonal ER.

Correlations between Study 2 ESM variables are presented in the Supplementary Materials (Table S4). Notably, baseline and ESM measures of inter-vs-intrapersonal ER were only moderately positively correlated ($r = 0.31$, $p < 0.001$). Nevertheless, similar to the baseline measure, ESM measure of inter-vs-intrapersonal ER was negatively correlated with attachment avoidance ($r = -0.29$, $p < 0.001$) but not with attachment anxiety ($r = -0.09$, $p = 0.283$). Inter-vs-intrapersonal ER was also positively correlated with relationship quality ($r = 0.19$, $p = 0.019$).

8.2. Emotion Regulation Variability

8.2.1. Inter-vs-Intrapersonal Emotion Regulation: Baseline Cross-Sectional Data

Main Analysis

The model explained 21.8% of the variance in inter-vs-intrapersonal ER ($F(10, 271) = 8.812$, $p < 0.001$), as an index of ER strategy variability, indicating the relative use of interpersonal compared to intrapersonal ER. The results are presented in Table 2. As in Study 1, the effect of attachment anxiety was not significant, meaning that the relative use of interpersonal compared to intrapersonal ER did not depend on one's level of attachment anxiety, not supporting H1.1. Replicating the findings of Study 1, the association with attachment avoidance was negative and significant, supporting H1.2; that is, on average, the higher one's level of attachment avoidance, the less they reported to use interpersonal compared to intrapersonal ER—or put differently, the more they relied on intrapersonal compared to interpersonal ER. The results indicated a lower ER strategy variability for people with high levels of attachment avoidance (see Figure 2). Attachment anxiety and attachment avoidance did not significantly interact in influencing inter-vs-intrapersonal ER, suggesting that the effect of attachment avoidance on inter-vs-intrapersonal ER did not depend on different levels of attachment anxiety.

Exploratory Analysis

The results (see Table S3) replicated the findings of Study 1. Attachment anxiety was not significantly associated with neither interpersonal ER ($b = 0.07$, $SE = 0.07$, $p = 0.290$) nor intrapersonal ER ($b = 0.06$, $SE = 0.07$, $p = 0.438$). In contrast, on average, an increase in attachment avoidance was associated with both a lower tendency to use interpersonal ER ($b = -0.62$, $SE = 0.08$, $p < 0.001$) and a higher tendency to use intrapersonal ER ($b = 0.48$, $SE = 0.08$, $p < 0.001$). The association between attachment avoidance and interpersonal or intrapersonal ER did not depend on the levels of attachment anxiety, as indicated by the insignificant interactions between the two attachment orientations (for interpersonal $b = 0.09$, $SE = 0.06$, $p = 0.151$; for intrapersonal $b = -0.06$, $SE = 0.07$, $p = 0.331$).

8.2.2. Inter-vs-Intrapersonal Emotion Regulation: Experience Sampling Method Data
Main Analysis

The results are reported in Table 2. The results replicated our previous results of the Study1 and Study 2 baseline analyses. Using our first indicator of variability (the relative use of interpersonal vs. intrapersonal ER), the effect of attachment anxiety was not significant, providing no support for H1.1; that is, the momentary relative use of interpersonal compared to intrapersonal ER did not depend on one's level of attachment anxiety. The effect of attachment avoidance was significant, supporting H1.2; that is, on average, higher levels of attachment avoidance were associated with less use of interpersonal compared to intrapersonal ER on average across all momentary assessments. The results indicated a lower ER strategy variability for those with higher attachment avoidance (see Figure 2). In contrast to the baseline data, the ESM results showed a significant interaction effect of attachment anxiety and avoidance in predicting momentary inter-vs-intrapersonal ER. Plotting the interaction effect showed that the effect of attachment avoidance on the relative use of interpersonal compared to intrapersonal ER decreased as the level of attachment anxiety increased (see Figure 3). The analysis of the simple slopes showed that on average, higher attachment avoidance was associated with less use of interpersonal compared to intrapersonal ER when attachment anxiety was low ($-1SD$; $b = -1.26$, $p = 0.002$) or average ($b = -0.77$, $p = 0.015$). When attachment anxiety was high ($+1SD$), more avoidance was not significantly associated with momentary relative use of interpersonal compared to intrapersonal ER ($b = -0.28$, $p = 0.453$). Thus, participants higher in avoidance showed a lower use of interpersonal compared to intrapersonal ER only when their attachment anxiety was low or medium.

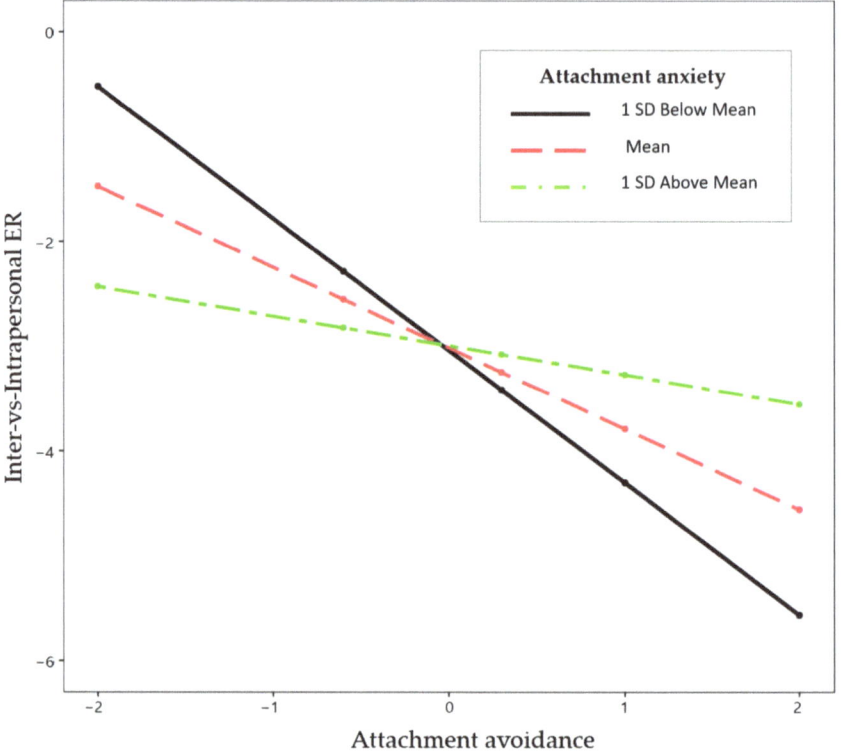

Figure 3. The interaction between attachment anxiety and avoidance affecting inter-vs-intrapersonal emotion regulation.

Exploratory Analysis

The results (see Table S3) replicated the findings of the Study 1 and Study 2 baseline, showing no effect of attachment anxiety on neither interpersonal ER ($b = 0.12$, $SE = 0.16$, $p = 0.496$) nor intrapersonal ER ($b = 0.12$, $SE = 0.16$, $p = 0.465$). In contrast to attachment anxiety, on average, an increase in attachment avoidance was associated with a lower momentary use of interpersonal ER ($b = -0.66$, $SE = 0.20$, $p = 0.001$), replicating our earlier findings; this association did not depend on the levels of attachment anxiety, as indicated by the insignificant interactions between the two attachment orientations ($b = 0.15$, $SE = 0.15$, $p = 0.311$). Different from our earlier findings, attachment avoidance was not associated with the momentary use of intrapersonal ER ($b = 0.17$, $SE = 0.20$, $p = 0.408$). However, there was a significant interaction between the two attachment orientations ($b = -0.31$, $SE = 0.15$, $p = 0.035$). Exploring the interaction effect showed that the association between attachment avoidance and intrapersonal ER was positive when attachment anxiety was low ($b = 0.48$, $z = 1.81$, $p = 0.070$) or average ($b = 0.17$, $z = 0.83$, $p = 0.404$), and negative when attachment anxiety was high ($b = -0.14$, $z = -0.60$, $p = 0.548$). None of these associations were, however, significant.

8.2.3. Standard Deviation of Inter-vs-Intrapersonal Emotion Regulation

Main Analysis

The results are presented in Table 3. The model explained 7.2% of the variance in SD of inter-vs-intrapersonal ER ($F(10, 112) = 1.944$, $p = 0.046$). Supporting H2.1, higher attachment anxiety was significantly associated with a lower SD in the relative use of interpersonal compared to intrapersonal ER among people high in attachment anxiety, indicating lower variability. Providing no support for H2.2, the effect of attachment avoidance on SD was not significant, indicating that the variability in the relative use of interpersonal compared to intrapersonal ER did not depend on one's level of attachment avoidance. Furthermore, attachment anxiety and attachment avoidance did not significantly interact in influencing SD; that is the association between attachment anxiety and the variation in the relative use of interpersonal compared to intrapersonal ER did not differ across different levels of attachment avoidance.

Table 3. Analysis of attachment insecurities affecting variability in the use of inter-vs-intrapersonal emotion regulation across momentary assessments.

Independent Variable	b	SE	t	p
(Intercept)	4.41	0.62	7.70	<0.001
Attachment anxiety	−0.46	0.18	−2.56	0.012
Attachment avoidance	0.09	0.23	0.39	0.699
Attachment anxiety × Attachment avoidance	0.25	0.17	1.50	0.137
Relationship length	−0.01	0.00	−1.48	0.143
Relationship quality	0.12	0.27	0.44	0.660
Neuroticism	−0.11	0.12	−0.97	0.336
COVID	0.01	0.01	0.94	0.351
Participant level mean stressfulness of events	−0.08	0.10	−0.85	0.397
Participant level mean partner availability	1.62	0.70	2.36	0.020
Participant level mean others availability	0.50	0.72	0.69	0.490

Note. The significant results are presented in bold.

Exploratory Analysis

The variance in the SD of *interpersonal* ER was not significantly explained by neither the model (R^2 adjusted $= 0.004$, $F(10, 112) = 1.055$, $p = 0.403$), nor attachment anxiety ($b = -0.13$, $SE = 0.11$, $p = 0.222$), attachment avoidance ($b = 0.04$, $SE = 0.14$, $p = 0.756$), or the interaction between them ($b = 0.04$, $SE = 0.10$, $p = 0.718$). However, 9.1 percent of variance in SD of *intrapersonal* ER was explained by the model ($F(10, 112) = 2.222$, $p = 0.021$). Higher attachment anxiety was associated with lower SD of intrapersonal ER ($b = -0.23$, $SE = 0.10$, $p = 0.022$). That is, on average, people with higher attachment anxiety showed less variability in the amount of self-regulation they used during a week. For details of the results, see Table S6. Attachment avoidance was not associated with SD of intrapersonal ER ($b = 0.07$, $SE = 0.13$, $p = 0.613$). The association between attachment anxiety and SD of intrapersonal ER was moderated by attachment avoidance ($b = 0.24$, $SE = 0.09$, $p = 0.012$), as it was larger when attachment avoidance was low ($b = -0.42$, $z = -1.04$, $p = 0.300$) compared to when it was high ($b = -0.05$, $z = -0.12$, $p = 0.905$). None of the simple slopes were, however, significant.

8.3. Emotion Regulation Flexibility

8.3.1. Main Analysis

The results are presented in Table 4. Partner availability (versus partner absence) predicted higher inter-vs-intrapersonal ER as a main effect; that is, when their partner was available, people used more interpersonal compared to intrapersonal ER than when their partner was not available (H3.1). This indicates a general flexibility in the use of interpersonal compared to intrapersonal ER with respect to the contextual factor of partner availability. The results, however, showed no significant interaction between partner availability and neither attachment anxiety (H3.2) nor attachment avoidance (H3.3), indicating that the level of flexibility was not influenced by attachment orientations.

Table 4. Moderation effect of attachment on the association between partner availability and inter-vs-intrapersonal emotion regulation.

Independent Variable	Inter-vs-Intrapersonal ER				
	b	SE	DF	t	p
(Intercept)	−5.70	0.55	2480	−10.44	**<0.001**
Attachment anxiety	0.19	0.28	113	0.67	0.505
Attachment avoidance	**−0.87**	**0.35**	**113**	**−2.51**	**0.013**
Partner availability	**5.98**	**0.36**	**2480**	**16.43**	**<0.001**
Attachment anxiety: Attachment avoidance	**0.58**	**0.26**	**113**	**2.26**	**0.026**
Attachment anxiety: Partner availability	−0.55	0.37	2480	−1.50	0.133
Attachment avoidance: Partner availability	0.29	0.46	2480	0.63	0.527
Attachment anxiety: Attachment avoidance: Partner availability	−0.38	0.41	2480	−0.92	0.357
Relationship length	−0.01	0.01	113	−1.57	0.119
Female	0.42	0.57	113	0.74	0.462
Relationship quality	0.04	0.36	113	0.12	0.904
Neuroticism	0.28	0.16	113	1.73	0.087
Extraversion	0.14	0.14	113	1.00	0.320
COVID	0.02	0.01	113	1.87	0.065
Stressfulness of event	**0.15**	**0.06**	**2480**	**2.44**	**0.015**
Others availability	**1.11**	**0.24**	**2480**	**4.58**	**<0.001**
Time	−0.01	0.01	2480	−1.41	0.159

Note: the significant results are presented in bold.

8.3.2. Exploratory Analysis

The results (see Table S7) revealed that participants used higher interpersonal ER when their partner was available (versus absent; $b = 4.03$, $SE = 0.23$, $p = <0.001$). This association was moderated by attachment anxiety ($b = -0.51$, $SE = 0.23$, $p = 0.030$). That is, as expected, the association between partner availability and interpersonal ER was weaker for those with high attachment anxiety ($b = 3.53$, $t = 10.67$, $p < 0.001$) than for those with low anxiety ($b = 4.54$, $t = 13.95$, $p < 0.001$; see Figure 4). This suggests lower flexibility in the use of interpersonal ER for people with higher attachment anxiety. Partner availability was negatively associated with intrapersonal ER ($b = -1.92$, $SE = 0.18$, $p < 0.001$). That is, when their partner was available (compared to absent), participants used less self-regulation. This association was, however, not moderated by neither attachment anxiety ($b = 0.10$,

$SE = 0.18$, $p = 0.573$) nor attachment avoidance ($b = 0.02$, $SE = 0.23$, $p = 0.943$). That is, neither attachment anxiety nor avoidance were associated with lower flexibility in self-regulation.

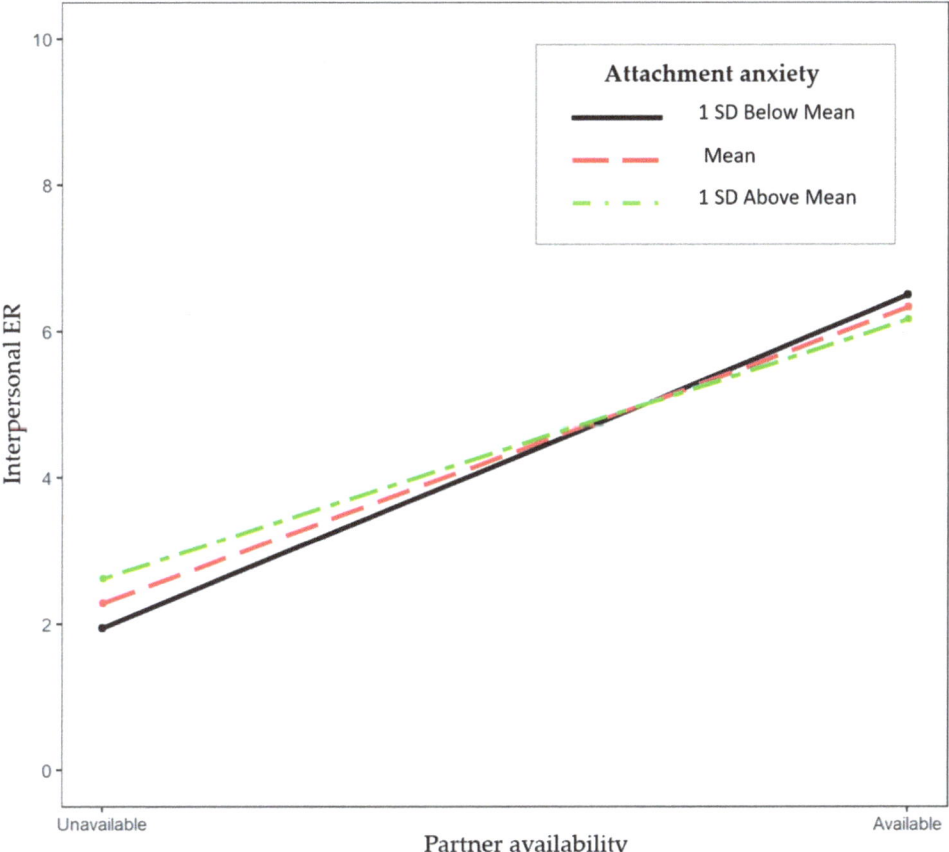

Figure 4. The interaction between attachment anxiety and partner availability affecting interpersonal emotion regulation.

9. General Discussion

We investigated the association between adult attachment to a romantic partner and the extent to which one flexibly uses interpersonal compared to intrapersonal ER when regulating their own emotional response to daily life stressful situations. Specifically, we measured the extent to which one (1) variably uses different ER strategies, and (2) flexibly varies the use of ER strategies depending on the context (in this case: whether the partner was available or not). Before discussing the implications, we summarize the various results of our studies and clarify their conceptual meaning.

Across two studies and three different types of analyses (based on two cross-sectional data and one ESM data), our results consistently suggested that in contrast to what we hypothesized (H1.1), individuals higher (compared to lower) in attachment anxiety did not show a stronger preference for interpersonal compared to intrapersonal ER. However, as hypothesized (H2.1), they showed a lower variability (SD) in the relative use of interpersonal compared to intrapersonal ER across different occasions over time. Therefore, their relative use of interpersonal compared to intrapersonal ER did not vary from individuals with lower attachment anxiety on average; however, it did vary or fluctuate significantly less across different occasions. As hypothesized (H1.2), participants higher (compared to lower) in attachment avoidance reported a stronger preference for self-regulation (intrapersonal ER) compared to relying on others (interpersonal ER), indicating lower variability in ER. However, we found no support that higher attachment avoidance was associated with lower variability when looking at the standard deviations of using inter- vs. intrapersonal ER strategies (H2.2). This indicates that, while high (versus low) avoidant people across situations, on average, tend to have a strong preference for intra- over interpersonal ER, high avoidant people are 'variable' in the sense that they range from either having a slight to having a strong preference for intra- over interpersonal ER across occasions.

Finally, as expected (H3.1), in general, individuals' relative use of interpersonal compared to intrapersonal ER increased when the partner was available compared to when they were absent, indicating ER flexibility. We found partial (only in our exploratory analysis) support for our hypothesis that people with higher attachment anxiety show lower flexibility (H3.2). That is, while individuals used higher levels of interpersonal ER when their partner was available (compared to absent), this association between partner availability and interpersonal ER was weaker for those with higher (compared to lower) attachment anxiety. Specifically, when their partner was available, they used slightly less interpersonal ER; and when their partner was not available, they used more interpersonal ER compared to those with lower attachment anxiety. We found no support for our hypothesis that people with higher attachment avoidance show lower flexibility (H3.3); that is, similar to secure people, their relative use of interpersonal compared to intrapersonal ER increased when the partner was available compared to when they were absent. Together, the present findings make a novel contribution to the current literature on attachment and ER by providing initial insights into the role of attachment anxiety and avoidance in the ER flexibility.

9.1. Attachment Anxiety and Emotion Regulation Flexibility

Our results showed, both in the cross-sectional data as well as in the ESM in daily life, that individuals high (compared to low) in attachment anxiety did not show a stronger, or weaker, preference for interpersonal compared to intrapersonal ER. This was surprising as previous theorizing has often considered both emotional distress-amplification as well as heightened behavioral proximity and support seeking as indicators of hyper-activation that is typical of anxiously attached individuals [5,29,31,33,60]. Our findings raise the interesting theoretical question whether attachment anxiety may be characterized mainly by emotional and cognitive hyper-activation in response to threat (e.g., stress, rumination), but that anxious attachment is not typically characterized by interpersonal proximity and support seeking in terms of emotional regulation strategy.

The fact that people high in anxiety displayed a relatively low variability as indicated by lower standard deviations across occasions (and particularly low variability in the use of intrapersonal ER as the result of the exploratory analysis showed), may indicate less flexibility in their ER in response to changes in the environment (in this case, partner availability). Indeed, our exploratory results showed that individuals with higher attachment anxiety showed lower ER flexibility when considering interpersonal ER. That is, their amount of proximity and support seeking was less dependent on their partner availability compared to those with lower attachment anxiety. In John's example, his support-seeking behavior was less covarying with Mary's availability compared to a person who is less anxiously attached to their partner.

One explanation for our results on variability and flexibility can be the heightened sensitivity of highly anxious people to signs of threat [3,60], which perhaps makes it difficult to accurately perceive and respond to social cues. The ability to accurately evaluate a situation and perceive its contextual demands and opportunities is indeed a first step in having higher ER flexibility [11,42]. Less sensitivity to situational circumstances could lead individuals to gravitate toward certain emotion regulation strategies, regardless of the specific demands of a situation [9]. In John's example, if his perception of Mary's ability to be available is not accurate, he might engage in hyperactivating behavior by exaggerating his support seeking when Mary does not respond to his phone call. Another related explanation could be that the partner's unavailability in times of stress may be appraised as particularly stressful by anxiously attached individuals [3,5,60,61], resulting in more support-seeking behaviors (i.e., more interpersonal ER). For example, if Mary does not respond to John's phone call, his stress levels may rise, resulting in higher support seeking.

9.2. Attachment Avoidance and Emotion Regulation Flexibility

Individuals with higher attachment avoidance showed low variability between strategies in that, on average, they displayed a higher preference for the use of intra- over interpersonal ER. This aligns with previous research indicating that higher attachment avoidance correlates with deactivating strategies [5] such as increased autonomy [60,62], decreased interdependence with close others [63], and less support seeking from them [31,36,45]. Our study extends previous findings by simultaneously examining interpersonal and intrapersonal ER in individuals' actual daily lives, with the ESM study providing real-life momentary evidence that highly avoidant individuals indeed tend to prioritize intrapersonal ER strategies over interpersonal ER when coping with daily life stressors.

While, on average, individuals with higher attachment avoidance showed a higher preference for intrapersonal compared to interpersonal ER, they did show variability as the strength of their preference varied largely across situations. That is, they showed a relatively large fluctuation across situations from having only a slightly to a strongly preferred use of intrapersonal ER over interpersonal ER. This finding seems consistent in that they flexibly used different amounts of interpersonal compared to intrapersonal ER depending on their partner's availability. A possible theoretical implication of these observed patterns in our study is that the general lower tendency to use interpersonal compared to intrapersonal ER in avoidant individuals is not a matter of limited repertoire or capability; instead, it is likely that motivational factors and avoidant individuals' perception of the usefulness of relying on others play a role. While they may be capable of using both inter- as well as intrapersonal ER strategies, they simply have a strong preference for intrapersonal ER. Indeed, in our study, similar to previous research [64], participants with higher attachment avoidance rated interpersonal ER as less helpful than those with lower avoidance (see exploratory correlations in Table S8). This also aligns with other previous research where avoidant individuals reported a lower need for support from a romantic partner [65] and a preference for independent problem-solving and avoiding social interaction during distress [66,67].

Finally, analyses of our momentary data revealed that individuals with higher attachment avoidance, across occasions, relied more on intrapersonal compared to interpersonal ER particularly when their attachment anxiety levels were low or average. These results align with prior research, where individuals exhibiting both high avoidance and anxiety are classified as fearful avoidant [20], demonstrating inconsistent behaviors [68]. Our exploratory analyses (Table S7) suggest that higher attachment anxiety may moderate the effect of attachment avoidance on intrapersonal ER. That is, similar to the explanation of Simpson and Rholes [68], the desire of fearful individuals for self-reliance might be buffered by a simultaneous inclination towards interdependence, resulting in ER patterns comparable to those of securely attached individuals in our data. This result shows the importance of looking at interpersonal and intrapersonal ER both individually and simultaneously.

9.3. Implications for Research and Practice

Our results indicate that both attachment anxiety and attachment avoidance are distinctively associated with indicators of limited ER flexibility, implying that lower ER flexibility may partly explain the ER difficulties of individuals with higher attachment insecurity. Specifically, attachment anxiety was associated with less variable and adaptive ER behavior in response to environmental changes, implying less accurate evaluation of situational demands. In contrast, our results imply that individuals with higher attachment avoidance are able to accurately detect environmental changes but exhibit inflexibility due to a general reluctance to rely on others, likely rooted in a predetermined expectation that others are unreliable for ER. This underscores the need for future research to explore the distinct mechanisms linking attachment insecurities with ER (flexibility).

On a more general and theoretical note, our findings reinforce the distinction between attachment anxiety and avoidance, confirming that they are distinct subsystems within the attachment system, rather than two sides of the same dimension. This distinction is crucial for developing targeted interventions and furthering theoretical frameworks in attachment and emotion regulation research.

Our results can also have important applied implications. Our findings imply that interventions for those with attachment insecurity should focus on increasing ER flexibility. For individuals with higher attachment anxiety, interventions could aim to enhance the ability to accurately recognize the situational demands and to use a variety of strategies accordingly. For those with higher attachment avoidance, interventions might focus on enhancing their willingness to rely on others, thereby improving their ability to use interpersonal ER.

9.4. Limitations and Directions for Future Research

Our findings should be interpreted in light of several limitations. First, our study focused on examining attachment-related ER during periods of stress, but our approach lacks insight into participants' ER in positive life situations. Future research could explore attachment-related ER differences between positive and negative life events by incorporating both types of events concurrently in data collection and analysis. Second, in the ESM data, there was an uneven distribution of responses, with some individuals reporting only a few instances of stressful events, while others reported more frequent occurrences. This pattern weakly ($r = 0.21$, $p < 0.05$) correlated with attachment avoidance (see Table S8), indicating that individuals with higher attachment avoidance reported more stressful events on average. This suggests a potential bias as avoidant individuals contributed slightly more data compared to their anxious or securely attached counterparts.

Third, in the absence of a validated scale that measures the relative use of interpersonal and intrapersonal ER simultaneously, we introduced a new measure to capture these dimensions. While our measure exhibits face validity as it directly assesses participants' interpersonal and intrapersonal ER, we recommend developing more validated measures that simultaneously capture interpersonal and intrapersonal ER in both cross-sectional and ESM study designs, similar to a recently developed questionnaire that captured some intrapersonal ER strategies [69].

Fourth, we acknowledge that apart from attachment orientations, other individual, relational, situational, and cultural factors could influence an individual's use of interpersonal compared to intrapersonal ER strategies. While we controlled for key individual factors (gender, age, and personality traits such as neuroticism and extraversion), as well as relational factors (relationship length and relationship quality) and situational factors (such as availability of others), we recognize that other factors could also have impacted ER behavior. For example, individuals with a more collectivistic cultural background might have used higher levels of interpersonal compared to intrapersonal ER [70]. Additionally, past traumatic relational experiences such as intimate partner violence, emotional abuse, and infidelity might influence the use of interpersonal compared to intrapersonal ER. Such additional influences should be considered in future research. Future investigations could also explore other attachment-related contextual factors such as fatigue, event type (relationship related or not), and the amount of stressfulness of the event [17,40].

Fifth, our study was primarily composed of females, students, and Western participants. Therefore, our findings may not generalize to male populations, individuals with diverse gender identities, and the general population, particularly those of non-Western cultures. Additionally, our sample was predominantly young, in relatively new relationships (with a mean relationship length of 2.5 years in Study 2), unmarried, and without children. These demographic factors could influence attachment-related ER behaviors, meaning our results may not fully apply to older adults, those in longer-term relationships, married individuals, or parents. Future research should aim to include more diverse samples to better understand how these factors interact with attachment orientations and ER. Furthermore, our sample did not include participants with very high levels of attachment insecurity (scores above 5.5 on a scale of 1 = highest security to 7 = highest insecurity). This could limit the generalizability of our findings as in populations with higher levels of attachment insecurity, the dynamics of ER may differ. Future research could explore ER flexibility in populations with very high levels of attachment insecurity.

Notably, future research can further explore alternative ways of measuring variability [71] and alternative conceptualizations and measurements of regulatory flexibility. While our study followed Aldao et al.'s [9] conceptualization of ER flexibility, another significant approach is offered by Bonanno et al. [42], conceptualizing ER flexibility within three inter-related components of context-sensitivity, repertoire, and feedback. Incorporating both frameworks could provide a more comprehensive understanding of ER flexibility [72]. Future research should advance this research by examining the relationship between attachment insecurity and ER flexibility using Bonanno's conceptualization. Additionally, examining attachment's association with flexibility in use of specific ER strategies like rumination, suppression, or sharing would be beneficial.

Additionally, another important factor influencing the use of interpersonal versus intrapersonal ER is the responsiveness of the partner to one's attempts at interpersonal ER. Future research should advance the knowledge on the effects of partner responsiveness—both enacted and perceived—on interpersonal ER. Dyadic designs involving both partners may be particularly effective in exploring these dynamics. Furthermore, while previous research suggests that in general greater ER flexibility signifies more effective ER [9,40,41], actual investigation into the adaptiveness of higher ER variability and flexibility is recommended [9,73]. Future research could investigate whether the associations we found between attachment insecurities and regulatory behavior translate into adverse ER outcomes, such as heightened experiences of negative emotions. This exploration could elucidate whether the ER difficulties experienced by insecurely attached individuals stem from lower ER flexibility.

10. Conclusions

To the best of our knowledge, our study was the first to explore the association between adult attachment and ER flexibility in romantic relationships. To do so, we looked at responses of people in daily life and across different contexts. We found that both attachment anxiety and attachment avoidance are significantly but distinctively associated with different indicators of ER flexibility. Our findings suggest that limited ER flexibility is probably a contributing factor to ER difficulties of individuals with higher attachment insecurity, deepening our understanding of how attachment insecurities affect emotion regulation. For practice, our findings imply that interventions designed to help individuals with attachment insecurity should focus on increasing their ER flexibility. To conclude, our research offers valuable insights into overcoming emotion regulation challenges of insecurely attached people. Ultimately, addressing these difficulties could greatly benefit the well-being of individuals with insecure attachment styles and their close relationships.

Supplementary Materials: The following supporting information can be downloaded at: https://www.mdpi.com/article/10.3390/bs14090758/s1, Table S1: Demographic Information of Studies; Table S2: Between-Person Correlations of Variables In Study 1 and Study 2 Baseline; Table S3: Analysis of Attachment Influencing Emotion Regulation Across Studies; Table S4: Between-Person and Within-Person Correlations of Variables in Study 2 Baseline + ESM; Table S5: Comparing Variable Scores Between Studies; Table S6: Analysis of Attachment Influencing Within-Strategy Variability; Table S7: Moderation Effect of Attachment on the Association Between Partner Availability and Inter-Vs-Intrapersonal ER; Table S8: Exploratory Correlations between Study Variables and Other Related Variables Measured During Data Collection of Study 2 [74]; Table S9: Deviations of the Studies from Pre-Registration.

Author Contributions: Conceptualization, F.M., M.L. and J.C.K.; Methodology, F.M., M.L., D.F.M. and J.C.K.; Formal analysis, F.M.; Data curation, F.M. and G.V.W.; Writing—original draft, F.M.; Writing—review & editing, F.M., M.L., D.F.M., G.V.W. and J.C.K.; Visualization, F.M.; Supervision, M.L. and J.C.K. All authors have read and agreed to the published version of the manuscript.

Funding: This research received no external funding.

Institutional Review Board Statement: The study was conducted in accordance with the Declaration of Helsinki, and approved by the Ethics Committee Social Sciences (ECSS) of Radboud University (Nijmegen, The Netherlands) (protocol code ECSW-LT-2022-1-14-45591 and 14 January 2022).

Informed Consent Statement: Informed consent was obtained from all subjects involved in the study.

Data Availability Statement: The data presented in this study as well as analytical codes will be openly available in the Open Science Framework (https://osf.io/et5a2) (accessed on 18 August 2024).

Acknowledgments: We would like to thank San Y. Albers, Marie A. Bogena, Guido F. Knipmeijer, Elena K. Thönnessen, and Stela Zhisheva for their solid work in data collection for Study 1. Special thanks to Bregje A.M. Vosbeek for her valuable assistance, particularly with the SEMA3 app for the ESM study, as well as her contributions to data collection for Study 2. We also appreciate the good collaborative work of Eva T.M. Hafkamp, Leon H. Sickenberg, and Jade Matton in data collection for Study 2. Lastly, we extend our gratitude to Elise Kalokerinos for her insightful advice during the initial stages of the ESM project, particularly regarding the study design and the measurement of ER flexibility.

Conflicts of Interest: The authors declare no conflict of interest.

References

1. Markey, C.N.; Markey, P.M. Leaving Room for Complexity in Attempts to Understand Associations between Romantic Relationships and Health: Commentary on Wanic and Kulik. *Sex Roles* **2011**, *65*, 313–319. [CrossRef]
2. Cassidy, J.; Shaver, P.R. *Handbook of Attachment: Theory, Research, and Clinical Applications*; Rough Guides: New York, NY, USA, 2002.
3. Gillath, O.; Karantzas, G.C.; Fraley, R.C. *Adult Attachment: A Concise Introduction to Theory and Research*; Academic Press: Cambridge, MA, USA, 2016.
4. Messina, I.; Maniglio, R.; Spataro, P. Attachment Insecurity and Depression: The Mediating Role of Interpersonal Emotion Regulation. *Cogn. Ther. Res.* **2023**, *47*, 637–647. [CrossRef]
5. Mikulincer, M.; Shaver, P.R. Attachment orientations and emotion regulation. *Curr. Opin. Psychol.* **2019**, *25*, 6–10. [CrossRef] [PubMed]
6. Gross, J.J. Emotion Regulation: Current Status and Future Prospects. *Psychol. Inq.* **2015**, *26*, 1–26. [CrossRef]
7. Naragon-Gainey, K.; McMahon, T.P.; Chacko, T.P. The structure of common emotion regulation strategies: A meta-analytic examination. *Psychol. Bull.* **2017**, *143*, 384–427. [CrossRef] [PubMed]
8. Aldao, A.; Nolen-Hoeksema, S.; Schweizer, S. Emotion-regulation strategies across psychopathology: A meta-analytic review. *Clin. Psychol. Rev.* **2010**, *30*, 217–237. [CrossRef]
9. Aldao, A.; Sheppes, G.; Gross, J.J. Emotion Regulation Flexibility. *Cogn. Ther. Res.* **2015**, *39*, 263–278. [CrossRef]
10. English, T.; Eldesouky, L. Emotion regulation flexibility. *Eur. J. Psychol. Assess.* **2020**, *36*. [CrossRef]
11. Kalokerinos, E.K.; Koval, P. Emotion regulation flexibility. In *Handbook of Emotion Regulation*, 3rd ed.; The Guilford Press: New York, NY, USA, 2024; pp. 265–273.
12. Dağ, İ.; Gülüm, İ.V. The Mediator Role of Cognitive Features in the Relationship Between Adult Attachment Patterns and Psychopathology Symptoms: Cognitive Flexibility. *Turk. J. Psychiatr.* **2013**, *24*, 1–15.
13. Hadžić, A.; Kantar, D. The Relationships between attachment dimensions and affect in adulthood: The mediating effects of psychological flexibility. *Primenj. Psihol.* **2021**, *14*, 173–188. [CrossRef]
14. Salande, J.D.; Hawkins, R.C., II. Psychological flexibility, attachment style, and personality organization: Correlations between constructs of differing approaches. *J. Psychother. Integr.* **2017**, *27*, 365–380. [CrossRef]
15. Mikulincer, M.; Shaver, P.R. The attachment behavioral system in adulthood: Activation, psychodynamics, and interpersonal processes. *Adv. Exp. Soc. Psychol.* **2003**, *35*, 56–152.
16. Shaver, P.R.; Mikulincer, M. Attachment-related psychodynamics. *Attach. Hum. Dev.* **2002**, *4*, 133–161. [CrossRef] [PubMed]
17. Bowlby, J. *Attachment and Loss*; New York Basic: New York, NY, USA, 1969.
18. Bowlby, J. *Attachment and Loss. Volume 2, Separation, Anxiety and Anger*; Pimlico: London, UK, 1973.
19. Bowlby, J. *Attachment and Loss: Sadness and Depression*; Pimlico: London, UK, 1998.
20. Bartholomew, K.; Horowitz, L.M. Attachment styles among young adults: A test of a four-category model. *J. Personal. Soc. Psychol.* **1991**, *61*, 226. [CrossRef] [PubMed]
21. Hazan, C. Adult romantic attachment: Theory and evidence. *Adv. Pers. Relatsh.* **1993**, *4*, 29–70.

22. Hazan, C.; Shaver, P. Romantic love conceptualized as an attachment process. *J. Personal. Soc. Psychol.* **1993**, *52*, 511–524. [CrossRef]
23. Brennan, K.A.; Clark, C.L.; Shaver, P.R. *Self-Report Measurement of Adult Attachment: An Integrative Overview*; Guilford Press: New York, NY, USA, 1998.
24. Hofmann, S.G.; Carpenter, J.K.; Curtiss, J. Interpersonal Emotion Regulation Questionnaire (IERQ): Scale Development and Psychometric Characteristics. *Cogn. Ther. Res.* **2016**, *40*, 341–356. [CrossRef]
25. Gross, J.J. *Handbook of Emotion Regulation*, 1st ed.; Guilford Press: New York, NY, USA, 2011.
26. Overall, N.C.; Simpson, J.A. Attachment and Dyadic Regulation Processes. *Curr. Opin. Psychol.* **2015**, *1*, 61–666. [CrossRef]
27. Fraley, R.C.; Niedenthal, P.M.; Marks, M.; Brumbaugh, C.; Vicary, A. Adult Attachment and the Perception of Emotional Expressions: Probing the Hyperactivating Strategies Underlying Anxious Attachment. *J. Personal.* **2006**, *74*, 1163–1190. [CrossRef]
28. Eilert, D.W.; Buchheim, A. Attachment-Related Differences in Emotion Regulation in Adults: A Systematic Review on Attachment Representations. *Brain Sci.* **2023**, *13*, 884. [CrossRef]
29. Mikulincer, M.; Florian, V. The relationship between adult attachment styles and emotional and cognitive reactions to stressful events. In *Attachment Theory and Close Relationships*; Simpson, J.A., Rholes, W.S., Eds.; The Guilford Press: New York, NY, USA, 1998; pp. 143–165.
30. Pascuzzo, K.; Cyr, C.; Moss, E. Longitudinal association between adolescent attachment, adult romantic attachment, and emotion regulation strategies. *Attach. Hum. Dev.* **2013**, *15*, 83–103. [CrossRef] [PubMed]
31. Messina, I.; Calvo, V.; Grecucci, A. Attachment orientations and emotion regulation: New insights from the study of interpersonal emotion regulation strategies. *Res. Psychother. Psychopathol. Process Outcome* **2024**, *26*, 703. [CrossRef] [PubMed]
32. Shaver, P.R.; Schachner, D.A.; Mikulincer, M. Attachment style, excessive reassurance seeking, relationship processes, and depression. *Personal. Soc. Psychol. Bull.* **2005**, *31*, 343–359. [CrossRef] [PubMed]
33. Mikulincer, M.; Shaver, P.R.; Pereg, D. Attachment Theory and Affect Regulation: The Dynamics, Development, and Cognitive Consequences of Attachment-Related Strategies. *Motiv. Emot.* **2003**, *27*, 77–102. [CrossRef]
34. Brodie, Z.P.; Goodall, K.; Darling, S.; McVittie, C. Attachment insecurity and dispositional aggression: The mediating role of maladaptive anger regulation. *J. Soc. Pers. Relatsh.* **2019**, *36*, 1831–1852. [CrossRef]
35. Feeney, J.A.; Karantzas, G.C. Couple conflict: Insights from an attachment perspective. *Curr. Opin. Psychol.* **2017**, *13*, 60–64. [CrossRef]
36. Uccula, A.; Mercante, B.; Barone, L.; Enrico, P. Adult Avoidant Attachment, Attention Bias, and Emotional Regulation Patterns: An Eye-Tracking Study. *Behav. Sci.* **2023**, *13*, 1. [CrossRef] [PubMed]
37. Nielsen, S.K.K.; Lønfeldt, N.; Wolitzky-Taylor, K.B.; Hageman, I.; Vangkilde, S.; Daniel, S.I.F. Adult attachment style and anxiety–The mediating role of emotion regulation. *J. Affect. Disord.* **2017**, *218*, 253–259. [CrossRef] [PubMed]
38. Karreman, A.; Vingerhoets, A.J.J.M. Attachment and well-being: The mediating role of emotion regulation and resilience. *Personal. Individ. Differ.* **2012**, *53*, 821–826. [CrossRef]
39. Read, D.L.; Clark, G.I.; Rock, A.J.; Coventry, W.L. Adult attachment and social anxiety: The mediating role of emotion regulation strategies. *PLoS ONE* **2018**, *13*, e0207514. [CrossRef]
40. Aldao, A. The Future of Emotion Regulation Research: Capturing Context. *Perspect. Psychol. Sci.* **2013**, *8*, 155–172. [CrossRef] [PubMed]
41. Levy-Gigi, E.; Bonanno, G.A.; Shapiro, A.R.; Richter-Levin, G.; Kéri, S.; Sheppes, G. Emotion Regulatory Flexibility Sheds Light on the Elusive Relationship Between Repeated Traumatic Exposure and Posttraumatic Stress Disorder Symptoms. *Clin. Psychol. Sci.* **2016**, *4*, 28–39. [CrossRef]
42. Bonanno, G.A.; Burton, C.L. Regulatory Flexibility: An Individual Differences Perspective on Coping and Emotion Regulation. *Perspect. Psychol. Sci.* **2013**, *8*, 591–612. [CrossRef] [PubMed]
43. Blanke, E.S.; Brose, A.; Kalokerinos, E.K.; Erbas, Y.; Riediger, M.; Kuppens, P. Mix it to fix it: Emotion regulation variability in daily life. *Emotion* **2019**, *20*, 473. [CrossRef]
44. Koval, P.; Kalokerinos, E.K.; Greenaway, K.H.; Medland, H.; Kuppens, P.; Nezlek, J.B.; Hinton, J.D.X.; Gross, J.J. Emotion regulation in everyday life: Mapping global self-reports to daily processes. *Emotion* **2023**, *23*, 357–374. [CrossRef] [PubMed]
45. McLeod, S.; Berry, K.; Hodgson, C.; Wearden, A. Attachment and social support in romantic dyads: A systematic review. *J. Clin. Psychol.* **2020**, *76*, 59–101. [CrossRef]
46. Zhu, Z.; Qin, S.; Dodd, A.; Conti, M. Understanding the relationships between emotion regulation strategies and Big Five personality traits for supporting effective emotion regulation tools/interventions design. *Adv. Des. Res.* **2023**, *1*, 38–49. [CrossRef]
47. Amirkhan, J.H.; Risinger, R.T.; Swickert, R.J. Extraversion: A "Hidden" Personality Factor in Coping? *J. Personal.* **1995**, *63*, 189–212. [CrossRef]
48. Faul, F.; Erdfelder, E.; Buchner, A.; Lang, A.-G. Statistical power analyses using G* Power 3.1: Tests for correlation and regression analyses. *Behav. Res. Methods* **2009**, *41*, 1149–1160. [CrossRef]
49. Fraley, R.C.; Waller, N.G.; Brennan, K.A. An item response theory analysis of self-report measures of adult attachment. *J. Personal. Soc. Psychol.* **2000**, *78*, 350–365. [CrossRef]
50. Fletcher, G.J.; Simpson, J.A.; Thomas, G. The measurement of perceived relationship quality components: A confirmatory factor analytic approach. *Personal. Soc. Psychol. Bull.* **2000**, *26*, 340–354. [CrossRef]

51. Gosling, S.D.; Rentfrow, P.J.; Swann, W.B., Jr. A very brief measure of the Big-Five personality domains. *J. Res. Personal.* **2003**, *37*, 504–528. [CrossRef]
52. R Core Team. R: A Language and Environment for Statistical Computing. R Foundation for Statistical Computing (Computer Software). 2020. Available online: https://www.R-project.org/ (accessed on 21 April 2023).
53. Bates, D.; Mächler, M.; Bolker, B.; Walker, S. Fitting Linear Mixed-Effects Models Using lme4. *J. Stat. Softw.* **2015**, *67*, 1–48. [CrossRef]
54. Fraley, R.C. Information on the Experiences in Close Relationships-Revised (ECR-R) Adult Attachment Questionnaire. University of Illinois Psychology Department Labs. November 2012. Available online: http://labs.psychology.illinois.edu/~rcfraley/measures/ecrr.htm (accessed on 1 February 2020).
55. Koval, P.; Hinton, J.; Dozo, N.; Gleeson, J.; Alvarez, M.; Harrison, A.; Vu, D.; Susanto, R.; Jayaputera, G.; Sinnott, R. SEMA3: Smartphone Ecological Momentary Assessment, Version 3. 2019. Computer Software. Available online: http://www.sema3.com (accessed on 1 February 2021).
56. Wilkinson, R.B. Measuring attachment dimensions in adolescents: Development and validation of the Experiences in Close Relationships—Revised—General short form. *J. Relatsh. Res.* **2011**, *2*, 53–62. [CrossRef]
57. Kirtley, O.J.; Hiekkaranta, A.P.; Kunkels, Y.K.; Verhoeven, D.; Van Nierop, M.; Myin-Germeys, I. The Experience Sampling Method (ESM) Item Repository. 2 April 2019. Available online: https://osf.io/kg376/ (accessed on 1 February 2021).
58. Pinheiro, J.; Bates, D.; R Core Team. Nlme: Linear and Nonlinear Mixed Effects Models. R Package Version 3.1-162. Computer Software. 2023. Available online: https://CRAN.R-project.org/package=nlme (accessed on 21 April 2023).
59. Bolger, N.; Laurenceau, J.-P. *Intensive Longitudinal Methods: An Introduction to Diary and Experience Sampling Research*; Guilford Press: New York, NY, USA, 2013.
60. Mikulincer, M.; Shaver, P.R. *Attachment in Adulthood: Structure, Dynamics, and Change*; Guilford Press: New York, NY, USA, 2007; p. 578.
61. Silva, C.; Soares, I.; Esteves, F. Attachment insecurity and strategies for regulation: When emotion triggers attention. *Scand. J. Psychol.* **2012**, *53*, 9–16. [CrossRef]
62. Ren, D.; Arriaga, X.B.; Mahan, E.R. Attachment insecurity and perceived importance of relational features. *J. Soc. Pers. Relatsh.* **2017**, *34*, 446–466. [CrossRef]
63. Simpson, J.A. Influence of attachment styles on romantic relationships. *J. Personal. Soc. Psychol.* **1990**, *59*, 971. [CrossRef]
64. George-Levi, S.; Laslo-Roth, R.; Schmidt-Barad, T. Feeling you, when you feel me: Attachment, empathic concern, and interpersonal emotion regulation. *J. Soc. Psychol.* **2022**, *162*, 655–669. [CrossRef]
65. McLeod, S.; Berry, K.; Taylor, P.; Wearden, A. Romantic attachment and support preferences in new mothers: The moderating role of stress. *J. Soc. Pers. Relatsh.* **2021**, *38*, 1535–1552. [CrossRef]
66. Collins, N.L.; Feeney, B.C. A safe haven: An attachment theory perspective on support seeking and caregiving in intimate relationships. *J. Personal. Soc. Psychol.* **2000**, *78*, 1053. [CrossRef] [PubMed]
67. Davila, J.; Kashy, D.A. Secure base processes in couples: Daily associations between support experiences and attachment security. *J. Fam. Psychol.* **2009**, *23*, 76. [CrossRef]
68. Simpson, J.A.; Rholes, W.S. Fearful-avoidance, disorganization, and multiple working models: Some directions for future theory and research. *Attach. Hum. Dev.* **2002**, *4*, 223–229. [CrossRef] [PubMed]
69. Medland, H.; De France, K.; Hollenstein, T.; Mussoff, D.; Koval, P. Regulating emotion systems in everyday life: Reliability and validity of the RESS-EMA scale. *Eur. J. Psychol. Assess.* **2020**, *36*, 437–446. [CrossRef]
70. Liddell, B.J.; Williams, E.N. Cultural Differences in Interpersonal Emotion Regulation. *Front. Psychol.* **2019**, *10*, 999. [CrossRef] [PubMed]
71. Lo, T.T.; Van Lissa, C.J.; Verhagen, M.; Hoemann, K.; Erbaş, Y.; Maciejewski, D.F. A theory-informed emotion regulation variability index: Bray-Curtis dissimilarity. *Emotion* **2024**, *24*, 1273–1285. [CrossRef] [PubMed]
72. Battaglini, A.M.; Rnic, K.; Jameson, T.; Jopling, E.; LeMoult, J. Interpersonal emotion regulation flexibility: Effects on affect in daily life. *Emotion* **2023**, *23*, 1048–1060. [CrossRef]
73. Lo, T.T.; Verhagen, M.; Pouwels, J.L.; van Roekel, E.; O'Brien, S.T.; Debra, G.; Braet, J.; Vink, J.; Maciejewski, D. Naming before Taming? Emotion Differentiation and Emotion Regulation Variability Hinder Each Other within Adolescents. *PsyArXiv* **2024**. [CrossRef]
74. Williams, W.C.; Morelli, S.A.; Ong, D.C.; Zaki, J. Interpersonal emotion regulation: Implications for affiliation, perceived support, relationships, and well-being. *J. Personal. Soc. Psychol.* **2018**, *115*, 224. [CrossRef] [PubMed]

Disclaimer/Publisher's Note: The statements, opinions and data contained in all publications are solely those of the individual author(s) and contributor(s) and not of MDPI and/or the editor(s). MDPI and/or the editor(s) disclaim responsibility for any injury to people or property resulting from any ideas, methods, instructions or products referred to in the content.

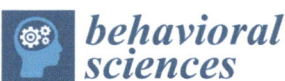
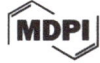

Article

"All You Need Is Love" a Social Network Approach to Understanding Attachment Networks in Adulthood

Junnan Tian [1] and Harry Freeman [2,*]

[1] Department of Psychology, Wuhan University, Wuhan 430072, China; tianjn@whu.edu.cn
[2] Division of Counseling and Psychology in Education, University of South Dakota, Vermillion, SD 57069, USA
* Correspondence: harry.freeman@usd.edu

Abstract: This study examined five dimensions of attachment network structure in a large sample of adults (n = 930, 57% female) between 24 to 80 years of age. We employed a newly validated diagrammatic measure, the web-based hierarchical mapping technique (WHMT), to measure the attachment strength to participants' five closest relationships and the physical distance to and between network members. Our first aim was to replicate existing research on the composition of adult attachment networks, exploring variations in network patterns by age, romantic status, and parental status. Our second aim was to explore four new network dimensions, including physical distance to network members, hierarchical patterns, centrality, and density. The results replicated previous work on network composition, highlighting the pivotal role of romantic partners as primary attachment figures through adulthood. The analysis of the new network dimensions revealed a clear divide between adults in romantic relationships and those who are not. Compared to the single adults, the adults in romantic relationships were more hierarchical in their attachment preferences, reported lower emotional connection to friends and parents, and lived farther from their network, which was also more geographically dispersed. In other words, romantically involved adults put more of their attachment eggs in one basket. The results also showed that the older adults tended to live further away from their attachment network and had a more geographically dispersed network compared to the younger adults.

Keywords: social networks; attachment bonds; social network analysis; romantic relationships; measuring attachment

Citation: Tian, J.; Freeman, H. "All You Need Is Love" a Social Network Approach to Understanding Attachment Networks in Adulthood. *Behav. Sci.* **2024**, *14*, 647. https://doi.org/10.3390/bs14080647

Academic Editors: Bianca P. Acevedo and Adam Bode

Received: 30 May 2024
Revised: 11 July 2024
Accepted: 17 July 2024
Published: 26 July 2024

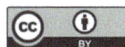

Copyright: © 2024 by the authors. Licensee MDPI, Basel, Switzerland. This article is an open access article distributed under the terms and conditions of the Creative Commons Attribution (CC BY) license (https://creativecommons.org/licenses/by/4.0/).

1. Introduction

Attachment bonds describe a limited number of relationships across the lifespan that are biologically based, durable across time and physical distance, and critical to felt security [1,2]. Infants and young children develop their first attachment bonds to parents and potentially to other adult caregivers, but beyond childhood, the composition of a person's attachment network expands to include close peer relationships [3–8]. Beginning in the 1980s, researchers began studying the normative development of attachment networks beyond childhood, examining how friends and romantic partners become increasingly important targets for attachment support in adolescence and young adulthood [5,9–12]. More recently, this work has expanded to the study of attachment networks through the adult years [8,13–17]. One aim in the current study is to replicate existing research on the composition of adult attachment networks using a newly validated diagrammatic measure called the web-based hierarchical mapping technique (the WHMT) [18]. The second aim is to move beyond the current focus on network composition to study whole network dimensions, including centrality, density, and hierarchical patterns, an aim that is made possible by the new analytics of the WHMT.

Attachment network research has been limited to studying composition due to a reliance on Likert-scaled measures that use ordinal scoring, such as the WHO-TO [7], the Attachment Network Questionnaire (ANQ) [19], and the Important People Interview (IPI) [20]. These measures are well suited to assessing who in a person's social network meets the criteria of an attachment figure and the relative strength to each network member. The ordinal scoring, however, results in non-independent ratings of attachment figures, which constrain whole network metrics that describe the shape or what we call network morphology. Network morphology dimensions include the centrality, density, and degree of hierarchical preference [18,21]. To accurately assess network centrality and hierarchy requires independent ratings of attachment strength to each network figure, and measuring network density requires independent ratings between network figures. The WHMT provides this analytic capability. In the current study, we employ the WHMT to replicate previous findings on adult attachment network composition and extend this work by studying normative patterns of network morphology from emerging adulthood to late adulthood.

1.1. The Study of Adult Attachment Network Composition

In discussing the ontogeny of attachment beyond infancy, Bowlby speculated that "Other adults may come to assume an importance equal to or greater than that of the parents, and sexual attraction to age-mates begins to extend the picture [1]. Theory on adult relationships as attachment bonds gradually took shape during the latter half of the 20th century, beginning with Hazan and Shaver's seminal paper (1987) [22] "Romantic love conceptualized as an attachment process". In this paper, the authors focused on how styles of infant attachment (i.e., infancy-secure, avoidant, and anxious/ambivalent) can be applied to understanding individual differences in adult attachment to romantic partners. Later work by Hazan and others expanded this view to explain why and under what normative conditions romantic partners and other adults can take up attachment functions and become primary targets for attachment behaviors [9–11], culminating in a normative model of parent-to-peer attachment transfer [10]. Based on their findings, Hazan and colleagues indicate that clear-cut adult attachment formation typically occurs around the second anniversary of romantic relationships [5,10]. In addition to romantic attachment, most adults continue to rely on parents as important sources of attachment support, and often forge one or two additional attachments to friends or others. Attachment network research has focused on understanding variations in who adults turn to for attachment support and the relative strength of attachment to each network figure.

Network composition research examines who and how many people are in a person's attachment network, and the relative strength of attachment to each network member. Determining who in a person's social network is a legitimate attachment figure, network members are evaluated against three cognitive/behavioral attachment provisions, including safe haven, proximity maintenance/separation protest, and secure base exploration [7]. When a network member meets all three cognitive/behavioral criteria, they are said to be a "clear-cut" attachment figure [23]. The number of clear-cut attachment figures is limited, typically ranging between one and three individuals at any point in a person's lifespan [10,21,23–25]. On the other hand, this determination may be partly owed to a reliance on ordinal rating scale methods that constrain the number of attachment figures that can be nominated for any single relationship provision [21]. In the current study, we revisit this question on attachment network size using a method that provides independent scoring.

The majority of attachment network research has focused on who adolescents and adults prefer as their primary source of attachment support, called the primary attachment figure. Beyond childhood, three factors have emerged as the most potent indicators of who adolescents and adults view as their primary attachment figure. These include romantic relationship status [5,10,26–29], parental status [16,30,31], and the transition into late adulthood [15,16]. From early to late adolescence, youth form more intimate friendships and enter into their first romantic relationships, a period recognized as the parent-to-peer transfer in attachment preference [10,26,27]. During this time, romantic partners and friends gradually take up attachment provisions from parents; however, a primary preference for a peer is typically delayed until two years into a romantic relationship [5], albeit a rapid transfer to a peer, friend, or romantic partner, is more likely for youth with insecure parental attachments [6]. From early adulthood and beyond, however, being in a committed romantic relationship is typically associated with lower attachment to mothers, fathers, and friends, independent of romantic relationship duration [14,16,32].

The transition to parenthood marks another developmental shift in network composition. In separate studies yielding somewhat contradictory findings, Feeney and colleagues investigated how becoming a parent is associated with differences in the attachment preference to parents and romantic partners [16,31]. In her first study, new parents indicated a stronger preference for parents and lower romantic attachment compared to their childless counterparts [31]. In a second and larger study with parents of older children, being a parent was associated with weaker attachments to parents. The authors interpreted conflicting findings as a matter of new versus experienced parents and parenting infants versus older children, respectively [16]. That is, most experienced parents of older children have come to rely on their spouses, relinquishing parents as primary confidants.

The transition to late adulthood brings additional changes due to network attrition, resulting from parents' death or incapacity, romantic dissolution, or the death of other family members and friends. Adult children become increasing targets for attachment support, and friends and siblings are commonly identified as primary attachment figures among single adults [15–17]. In the current study, we explore these same factors as predictors of network composition through the adult years, using a new measure.

1.2. The Measure of Attachment Networks

Traditional approaches to measuring attachment networks have relied on six- to nine-item ranking scales that capture the relative strength of attachment to significant others, based on safe haven, separation protest/proximity maintenance, and secure base exploration behaviors and cognitions [7]. The first published attachment network measure, the WHO-TO [7], was initially developed as a single forced-choice scale and was later modified by Fraley and Davis [5] for Likert scaling. Similar measures followed, including the Attachment Networks Questionnaire (ANQ) [19], and the Important People Interview (IPI) [20], which used six- and nine-item ranking scales, respectively, to assess the same three dimensions of attachment support.

All three scales—the WHO-TO, ANQ, and IPI—provide ordinal scoring of attachment strength to each rated figure, identifying who in the network meets the criteria for "clear-cut" attachment and who is the primary attachment figure. For a social network member to be considered a clear-cut or "full-blown" attachment figure, they must be ranked first or second on at least one item on each of the three dimensions [16], with the primary attachment figure receiving the highest sum-score. Network figures that do not meet this cut-off score may still be considered a subsidiary attachment figure if they are identified on one or more attachment provisions. The ordinal scoring, however, constrains accurate within-subject comparisons between network figures, given the lack of independence between ratings [18,21].

Moving beyond the measure of network composition. An alternative approach to ordinal scoring came in 2005 with the Bull's Eye diagrammatic measure [33], a modification of Antonucci's [34] hierarchical mapping technique requiring participants to place self-selected support figures on a diagram relative to a "core-self", marked in the center, with three concentric circles. This new approach provides independent and continuous rating scores for each network figure, thereby providing more analytic capability for accurate comparisons between network figures [18]. The Bull's Eye also came with some limitations, including manual delivery and scoring and low discriminate validity [18]. It was originally designed for paper delivery, using self-adhesive dots for support figures and requiring a ruler to score distances. More importantly, when participants evaluate their social network for closeness to "core-self", intimacy and companionship are sometimes evaluated more strongly than attachment support functions, resulting in elevated peer relationship scores [18].

In response to these limitations, the Bull's Eye was modified for online delivery and the middle "core-self" was replaced with "vulnerable-self". Participants were instructed to think about how close they want each network figure when they are feeling insecure and vulnerable. These significant changes resulted in a new measure, which we called the web-based hierarchical mapping technique (WHMT) [18,21]. A psychometric examination of the WHMT captures has shown accurate and reliable capture of safe haven, separation protest, and secure base provisions in adult relationships with parents and romantic partners. The measure is also sensitive to micro-level changes in felt security following interventions [18]. Similar to the Bull's Eye, the WHMT provides independent ratio-scaled scores of emotional closeness and physical proximity to each network figure, as well as between network figures. Compared to traditional ordinal formats, the independent scoring provides a more accurate assessment of each figure's role as an attachment figure. In a qualitative evaluation of the WHMT, the authors found that support figures placed inside the first concentric circle met the definition of clear-cut attachments, indicated by separation protest, safe haven, and secure base themes [18].

In addition to a more accurate assessment of network composition, the WHMT provides whole network analytics, including network density, centrality, and hierarchical shape. The concept of attachment hierarchies is central to Bowlby's assumption that all infants and children are innately predisposed to orient toward a preferred or primary attachment figure, a concept he termed monotropy [1]. Monotropy is difficult to test using ordinal scales, given the dependency of scores between figures. Studies using ordinal scales assume hierarchical order by assigning a primary attachment figure status to the figure with the highest sum score [5,16,19]. One exception is a recent study by Freeman and Simon [21], who applied a significance test to the difference score between the three highest rated figures. They found that 10% of their young adult sample did not significantly differentiate between their top three rated figures, and an additional 25% viewed their top two figures equally, a condition Schaffer and Emerson [35] referred to as "shared primary attachment" in their 18-month-old sample. In the current study, we examine if a clear order of attachment preference exists (i.e., monotropy), compared to having two primary attachment figures (i.e., shared primary), or if all three are undifferentiated, a condition we call distributed attachment based on Freeman and Simon's [21] classification scheme.

In addition to testing hierarchical shape, we explore two additional social network dimensions, including centrality and density. Centrality and density are the most common outcomes assessed in social network analysis (SNA); however, they have yet to be applied to the study of adult attachment networks [36]. In SNA vernacular, attachment networks can be regarded as egocentric networks, also called personal networks, as they are comprised of an ego (the attached), alters (attachment relationships connected to the ego), ties between the ego and alters, and ties between alters [37]. Centrality is the strength of the ties connecting the ego to all the alters, and density is the strength of the ties between alters. Centrality is evaluated in terms of attachment strength to each member of the network based on how close each figure is placed to the ego. Given that participants are not asked to place alters in relation to other alters, only in relation to themselves, we do not calculate network density based on emotional closeness between network members. However, network density and other network metrics are captured in a second WHMT diagram, discussed next.

In the current study, we have participants complete a second WHMT diagram, in which they place the physical location of each attachment network figure. In this diagram, the center represents the participant's home, or place of residence, and each of the three concentric circles represents a specific distance from the center: 10 miles, 150 miles, and 500 miles, respectively. The diagram is oriented with north, south, east, and west markings. Participants are instructed to place each network figure into the diagram to show the distance and direction to each figure and the distance and direction between network figures. The result is a two-dimensional map of a person's attachment network with physical distance scores to each network figure and between every pair of network figures. The between network figure scores enables the researcher to calculate the physical density of a person's attachment network, in addition to centrality.

1.3. Current Study

Existing studies on adult attachment networks are limited by a reliance on ordinal measures and consequently provide a limited view of network structure that focuses on network composition and on the primary attachment relationship. The current study greatly expands this approach by using the ratio-scored WHMT to measure five dimensions of adult attachment network structure, including composition and physical distance, as well as three dimensions of network morphology, including hierarchy, centrality, and density. The first aim is to replicate existing findings on attachment network composition. Three hypotheses are proposed:

Hypothesis 1. *Most adults will have, on average, two clear-cut attachment figures, with a minority of adults reporting no clear-cut attachments.*

Hypothesis 2. *Romantic partners will be the primary attachment figure through the adult years.*

Hypothesis 3. *Age, parental status, and/or romantic status will be related to the strength of attachment to friends and parents.*

The second and principal aim of the current study is to extend existing research by exploring new dimensions of adult attachment networks. Four new network dimensions are explored, including physical distance, hierarchy, centrality, and density. Given the lack of previous work in this area, we do not propose specific hypotheses. Instead, we explore these three dimensions as research questions, namely whether hierarchy, centrality, and density are associated with age, parental status, and romantic status.

2. Method

2.1. Sample

Participants included 930 adults (57% female) between 24 and 80 years of age ($M = 42.9$) living in the United States. The majority of participants (77.5%) identified as Caucasian, followed by African American (9.4%), Asian (6.9%), Latino (6%), and the remaining 0.2% identified as other ethnic groups. Based on income and education background, 14.8% of the sample was classified as working class, 48.7% as lower-middle class, 25.8% as middle class, and 10.7% as upper-middle class.

Given our focus on developmental trends in network structure through the adult years, we examined if sample demographics (i.e., gender, romantic status, and parental status) varied significantly by age (see Table 1). Results indicated a similar distribution of gender and romantic status within each age groups. Although the number of people who were married or engaged increased slightly from early adulthood to early middle age, the difference was not statistically significant. Not surprisingly, early adults (22–34 years old) were significantly less likely to be parents compared to older adults, $t(923) = 5.34$, $p < 0.001$.

2.2. Procedure

Participants were recruited through Amazon's Mechanical Turk (MTurk), in conjunction with Cloud Research, a third-party website that interfaces with MTurk through their proprietary toolkit. MTurk is an online crowdsourcing platform where researchers can recruit a diverse and large pool of participants, called MTurk workers, to complete tasks, including surveys and experiments. We used the Cloud Research toolkit to screen MTurk workers on inclusion criteria. Our target population consisted of adults with some residential stability in their lives so that the physical closeness to their social network would vary widely as a function of a recent transition or living in university housing. As such, we stipulated that participants be at least 24 years of age and have lived in the same residence in the USA for the past year. In addition, we used Cloud Research to vet the quality of Mturk participants based on several indicators linked to valid and reliable crowdsourcing data, including HIT acceptance rate (the tasks that require human intelligence and input that are accepted by participants or workers), reliable completion of attention checks, and past completed HITs. A HIT (Human Intelligence Task) refers an Mturk worker who enrolls in the study and completes the study task. Employing these Cloud Research quality control tools has been shown to significantly improve data quality compared to those available on Mturk alone [38]. Once screened and having given consent, participants completed two online measures, including a 10-min WHMT diagrammatic measure, followed by a 10-min Qualtrics survey. Participants who completed both measures and passed attention checks were compensated USD 2.25.

Table 1. Demographic characteristics based on age groups.

		Gender				Romantic Status						Parental Status			
		Male		Female		Single		Dating		Married/ Engaged		No Child		Child	
Age Group	n	n	%	n	%	n	%	n	%	n	%	n	%	n	%
Early Adulthood (ages 22–34)	288	126	43.8	162	56.3	90	31.3	42	14.6	156	54.2	211	73.3	77	26.7
Early Middle Age (ages 35–44)	304	145	47.7	159	52.3	70	23.0	31	10.2	203	66.8	170	55.9	134	44.1
Late Middle Age (ages 45–64)	276	105	38.0	171	62.0	72	26.1	33	12.0	171	62.0	150	54.3	126	45.7
Late Adulthood (ages 65 and older)	62	25	40.3	37	59.7	21	33.9	5	8.1	36	58.1	36	58.1	26	41.9
Total	930	401	43.1	529	56.9	253	27.2	111	11.9	566	60.9	567	61.0	363	39.0

2.3. Measures

Network structure. To measure the attachment network structure, participants completed two versions of the web-based hierarchical mapping technique [18]. The WHMT is a diagrammatic online measure that begins by asking participants to self-select the five most important relationships in their current life from a dropdown menu of 17 possible relationships (e.g., mother, father, sister, aunt, best friend, etc.), including a write-in option. After selecting, participants are taken to a second screen, displaying a target diagram with "you" marked in the center and surrounded by three concentric circles (see Figure 1). The five selected relationships now populate a column outside the diagram, with each relationship represented as a circle icon. Participants are instructed to drag and drop each icon into the diagram so that the distance to the center represents "how close you want to be to that person when you are feeling emotionally insecure, unprotected, or vulnerable." Once submitted, pixel distance between the center and each person is recorded, with scores ranging from 0 (center) to 700 (outside the third circle). Lower scores indicate stronger attachment.

Next, participants completed a second version of the WHMT based on physical distance to and between the same five relationships (see Figure 2). In this second diagram, the three concentric circles represent 10 miles, 250 miles, and 500 miles from the center, marked "home". The diagram is marked with north, south, east and west so that participants can place where each network figure lives geographically in relation to the participant. Participants are instructed to drag and drop each relationship icon into the diagram so that it represents where each person lives relative to the participant and relative to the other network figures. Upon submission of the completed diagram, pixel distances are recorded to each network figure from the center and between each network figure. Pixels distances were transformed into miles to represent physical distances to the participant and between network figures.

Web-Based Hierarchical Mapping Technique (WHMT) Assessment (continued)

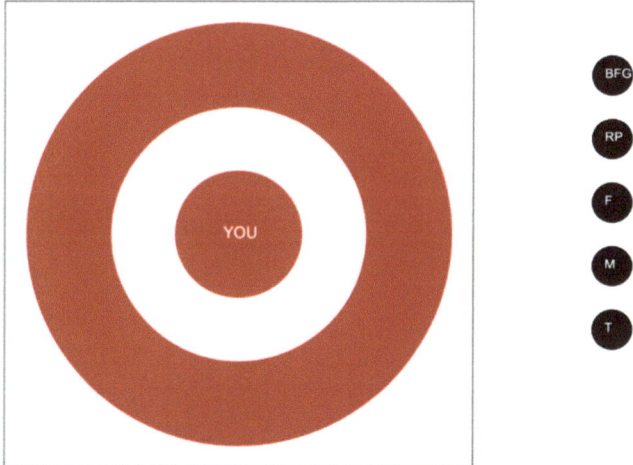

Figure 1. WHMT instructions—emotional distance.

Based on the two WHMT diagrams, we calculated the network composition and three dimensions of the network morphology, including network hierarchy, network centrality, and network density. The measure of each network variable is detailed next.

Network composition. Network composition was measured by identifying who participants selected as their five closest relationships and their attachment strength to each network figure, calculated as the pixel distance to the center of the diagram. Shorter distance corresponds to stronger attachment. In a recent study examining the validity of the WHMT as a measure of attachment strength [18], it was found that participants who placed network figures in the inner circle (60 pixels from the center) consistently met the criteria as clear-cut attachment figures. Using 60 pixels as the cut-off criteria, the number of attachment figures was calculated.

Web-Based Hierarchical Mapping Technique (WHMT) Assessment (continued)

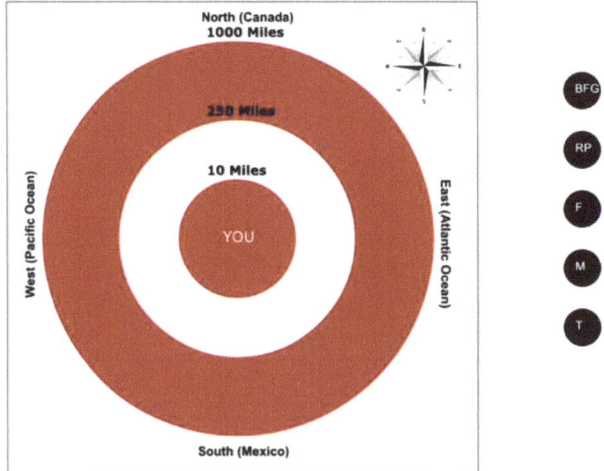

Figure 2. WHMT instructions—physical distance.

Network morphology (shape of the network). Three dimensions of network morphology were determined, including the degree of hierarchy, network centrality, and network density. Network hierarchy describes the extent to which participants perceive a clear order of attachment preference to a primary target for attachment support. We examined this by comparing the difference in attachment strength between the primary and secondary figure and between the primary and tertiary figure, resulting in three ordinal classifications. The first category, monotropic, was marked by the presence of a clear primary attachment figure, who was rated significantly stronger than all the other network figures. A second category, shared primary, was marked by the top two network figures being undifferentiated, but both figures were rated significantly stronger than the remaining network figures. The third category, distributed, was marked by the top three figures, having relatively equal ratings of attachment strength [21]. The network structures were converted and determined based on a cut-off value that indicated a meaningful difference between attachment figures. A clear order of preference between figures was classified based on a clear visual difference in relative position to the center, which was based on the validation study [18]. Each figure icon equaled 18 pixels in radius, and this distance was used as the cut-off score for a visually clear distinction in closeness to center.

The second morphology dimension calculated was network centrality, which corresponds to the average distance of each network figure to the center. Centrality was calculated as the average pixel distance of the five selected close relationships. We chose to include all five figures, given that non-clear-cut attachment figures are often relied on as subsidiary attachment figures under certain conditions.

The third morphology category, network density, refers to the closeness of network figures to each other. This metric was not calculated for attachment strength, given that participants were not asked to place figures in the first WHMT diagram relative to how close network figures were to each other. For this metric, we used the second WHMT diagram that provided information on the physical location of each network figure relative to the participant's home, and relative to the other network figures. Pixel distances were converted to miles, the average distance to the center was computed as the physical centrality of the network, and the average distance between network figures was computed as physical density.

Demographics and normative life events. Following completion of the two WHMT diagrams, participants completed a Qualtrics survey that included the following demographic and life event questions. The descriptions of romantic status included six options: "Not currently romantically involved with someone or dating", "Dating one person but we are not seriously involved", "Dating one person and we are seriously involved, but we are not living together", "Living with my partner, but we are not married", "Engaged to be married", and "Married". For the analysis, options were collapsed into three categories, including single, dating, and married/engaged. For the parental status, participants were asked, "Do you have children, if so, how many children do you have?", and the parental status was eventually coded as a dichotomous variable (0 = no child and 1 = child).

To assess the socioeconomic status (SES), participants were asked about their education background and annual income. We followed Wani's [39] recommendations for weighting these indicators. The total score of income and educational level was calculated, and the average score of the two levels was used and converted into a combined SES.

3. Results

3.1. Descriptive Statistics

Bivariate associations were run between network structure variables and demographic characteristics (see Table 2). Age was significantly and positively associated with parental status, attachment strength to mothers, physical centrality, and physical density, indicating that older participants were more likely to have children, report lower attachment strength to mothers, and to have a social network that, on average, was further from their home (centrality) and more spread apart (i.e., density). Gender was significantly and positively correlated with parental and romantic status, indicating that females were more likely to report having children and being in a romantic relationship. In addition, attachment strength to mothers and romantic partners were both significantly and positively connected with physical centrality and density, as well as attachment strength centrality. Participants with stronger attachments to mothers or romantic partners had a network of figures that tended to live closer, tended to live closer to each other, and tended to provide greater combined attachment support. Interestingly, romantic strength was negatively associated with attachment strength to parents and friends, whereas attachment to fathers, mothers, and friends were all positively related.

3.2. Network Composition

In the first set of inferential analyses, we focused on replicating the existing work on adult network composition. The hypotheses and analytic strategy are primarily based on the work by Doherty and Feeney [16], who examined an adult sample of similar size and similar age range.

Table 2. Correlations between demographics and network structure variables.

Variable	1	2	3	4	5	6	7	8	9	10	11	12
1. Age	-											
2. Gender	0.057	-										
3. Romantic Status	0.003	0.073 *	-									
4. Parental Status	0.123 **	0.069 *	0.489 **	-								
5. Attachment Strength to Romantic Partner	−0.007	−0.035	NA	−0.057	-							
6. Attachment Strength to Mother	0.088 *	0.056	0.101 **	0.036	−0.306 **	-						
7. Attachment Strength to Father	0.041	0.105 *	0.022	−0.034	−0.273 **	0.607 **	-					
8. Attachment Strength to Friend	−0.058	−0.162 *	0.060	0.054	−0.263 **	0.240 **	0.108 *	-				
9. Hierarchy vs. No Hierarchy	0.036	0.005	0.029	0.041	−0.139 **	0.140 **	0.239 **	0.114 **	-			
10. Physical Centrality	0.138 **	0.028	−0.058	−0.104 **	0.212 **	0.284 **	0.230 **	0.146 **	0.058	-		
11. Physical Density	0.114 **	0.021	−0.060	−0.094 **	0.152 **	0.258 **	0.269 **	0.093 *	0.063	0.736 **	-	
12. Attachment Strength Centrality	0.001	−0.058	−0.091 **	−0.080 *	0.563 **	0.675 **	0.645 **	0.586 **	0.171 *	0.290 **	0.288 **	-

Note: n = 657 (participants who rated romantic partners for attachment strength), n = 708 (participants who rated mothers for attachment strength), n = 545 (participants who rated fathers for attachment strength), n = 709 (participants who rated friends for attachment strength). * p < 0.05, ** p < 0.01.

Hypothesis 1: most adults will have, on average, two clear-cut attachment figures, with a minority of adults reporting no clear-cut attachments. Network figures were classified as a "clear-cut attachment" if placed inside the inner circle of the WHMT diagram, a method that was validated based on extensive interviews in a recently published study [18] (see also methods/measures/network composition for more information on how we made this determination).

The results indicated that having two clear-cut attachment figures was average (M = 1.96, SD = 1.2) and the most frequent outcome (33.3%). Nearly a third of participants identified a single clear-cut attachment figure (30.3%), followed by participants reporting three clear-cut figures (18.2%). In sum, 81.8% of participants had one to three clear-cut attachment figures. As predicted, a minority of participants, 8.2% of the sample, had no clear-cut attachment figures, a classification based on placing all five self-selected support figures outside the inner circle. Another 10% of the sample identified either four (5.2%) or five (4.8%) clear-cut attachment figures.

Next, we examined developmental trends associated with attachment network size. The bivariate correlation between age and number of clear-cut attachment figures was close to 0 (r = 0.012). We ran a one-way ANOVA to examine if differences existed between the four age groups (24–34; 35–44; 45–64; ≥65), which also indicated no developmental trends in network size (F(3, 927) = 0.82, p = 0.466).

Hypothesis 2: romantic partners will be the primary attachment figure through the adult years. The primary attachment figure is typically identified as the highest ranked figure. However, this approach applies to studies using traditional Likert-scaled measures, in which independent comparisons between network figures is hampered by ordinal scaling. In the current study, participants indicated their closeness to each figure separately, which allowed for more than one primary figure to be indicated. We classified the first primary figure as the one with the closest pixel score to the center. Given that most individuals have less than three attachment figures, we allowed for up to three primary figures. A second or third primary figure was added if these figures were placed within 15 pixels from the top-rated figure. The 15-pixel cut-off score corresponds to a distance that is visually difficult to differentiate (see Method and the measurement of network hierarchy for more details on this method). Table 3 shows the percentage of each relationship type nominated as a primary attachment figure within each age group. Given that individuals can select more than one primary attachment figure, when all the figures are summed, the total exceeds 100%.

Table 3. Composition of collapsed category results for attachment figures based on age groups.

Age Group	n	Attachment Figure	n	% (Number of Times Selected as the Common Primary Target)
Early Adulthood (ages 22–34)	288	Romantic Partner	158	54.9
		Mother	83	28.8
		Father	36	12.5
		Sibling	33	11.5
		Friend	54	18.8
		Child	4	1.4
		Other	30	10.4
		Total	398	138.2 *
Early Middle Age (ages 35–44)	304	Romantic Partner	180	59.2
		Mother	82	27.0
		Father	42	13.8
		Sibling	33	10.9
		Friend	44	14.5
		Child	17	5.6
		Other	38	12.5
		Total	436	143.4 *
Late Middle Age (ages 45–64)	276	Romantic Partner	144	52.2
		Mother	58	21.0
		Father	20	7.2
		Sibling	38	13.8
		Friend	62	22.5
		Child	29	10.5
		Other	36	13.0
		Total	387	140.2 *
Late Adulthood (ages 65 and older)	62	Romantic Partner	35	56.5
		Mother	7	11.3
		Father	4	6.5
		Sibling	8	12.9
		Friend	14	22.6
		Child	11	17.7
		Other	32	51.6
		Total	111	179.0 *
Total	930			

Note. * Total percent exceeds 100 due to the nomination of multiple primary figures.

The results in Table 3 clearly show the primacy of romantic partners as primary targets for attachment support through the adult years. Romantic partners are nominated twice as often as the next most identified figure, mothers, and three to four times more often compared to the third most rated figures (siblings, friends, and fathers). A series of one-way analysis of variance (ANOVA) procedures were run for each relationship type to examine if the likelihood of being nominated as a primary figure varied between the four age groups. The results were significant for mother ($F(3, 926) = 3.86$, $p = 0.009$), father ($F(3, 926) = 2.82$, $p = 0.038$), and child ($F(3, 926) = 11.25$, $p < 0.001$). Older adults (late middle age and late adulthood) were less likely to nominate mothers and fathers as primary figures compared to early adults or early middle-aged adults. However, the nomination of children as primary figures steadily increased from early adulthood to late adulthood.

Hypothesis 3: age, parental status, and/or romantic status will be related to the strength of attachment to friends and parents. To examine if age, romantic status, and parental status are associated with attachment strength to different relationship types, a series of sequential regression analyses were run. Age, parental status, and romantic status were entered as factors in the first block, and all possible two-way interactions among these variables were added in the second block using centered scores.

The first model of main effects was significant for all relationship types except siblings (see Table 4). Romantic status was statistically and positively predictive of strength to mothers, fathers, and friends, indicated by a stronger attachment to parents and friends among the single participants. Age was statistically and positively predictive of strength to mothers and children. The result suggested that younger adults had stronger attachment strength to their mothers compared to older adults. Surprisingly, the results indicate that the attachment strength to children diminished slightly with age. This finding is counterintuitive and contrasts sharply with Doherty and Feeney's [16] findings. This result may be an artifact of how child strength was included in the networks. "Child" was not a category in the list of available relationships, thus requiring participants to write in this category, which was done so by a minority of participants with children. If we examine who wrote in a child as an attachment figure by age, the significant bivariate correlation (0.225) indicates that older adults were significantly more likely to list a child as a network member. In addition, as presented under hypothesis two, age was positively related to whether the participant viewed their child as a primary attachment figure. Consequently, these findings are consistent with previous work [4,5,15–17]. Lastly, parental status was also a statistically significant predictor of attachment to romantic partners, indicating that the adults with children had stronger attachment to romantic partners compared to their non-parent counterparts.

Table 4. Sequential regression analyses of demographic variables on attachment strength to different attachment figures.

		Attachment Figure										
		Romantic Partner		Mother		Father		Sibling		Friend		Child	
Model	Predictor	R^2ch	β	R^2ch	β	R^2ch	β	R^2ch	β	R^2ch	β	R^2ch	β
1		0.009 *		0.034 **		0.019 *		0.004		0.029 **		0.077 **	
	Age		0.028		0.094 *		0.058		0.021		−0.054		0.195 *
	Parental Status		−0.097 *		−0.027		−0.081		−0.054		0.011		
	Romantic Status				0.167 **		0.135 **		0.053		0.157 **		0.240 **
2		0.001		0.004		0.001		0.005		0.001		0.015	
	Age x Parental Status		−0.044		−0.069		−0.025		−0.064		−0.013		
	Age x Romantic Status				−0.021		0.020		0.033		0.037		−0.196
	Parental Status x Romantic Status				0.016		0.047		0.075		0.041		
R^2		0.010		0.038		0.021		0.008		0.031		0.092	
Adjusted R^2		0.006		0.030		0.010		−0.002		0.023		0.072	
$F_{(df)}$		2.276 (3, 657)		4.583 ** (6, 708)		1.904 (6, 545)		0.838 (6, 594)		3.723 ** (6, 709)		4.519 ** (3, 138)	

Note. Parental status dummy coded as 0 = no child, 1 = child; romantic status dummy coded as 0 = no romantic partner, 1 = romantic partner. * $p < 0.05$. ** $p < 0.01$. R^2ch = R^2 change.

3.3. Moving beyond Network Composition

In this study, we measured and analyzed several new network dimensions to describe more fully the structure of attachment networks through the adult years, including physical proximity to and between network figures, and three dimensions of network morphology, including hierarchy, centrality, and density.

Physical proximity. This network dimension is based on the second WHMT diagram, in which participants placed their five self-selected important relationships in a geographical location in relation to their own home, and thereby, in relation to the other network figures. The average pixel distance of physical proximity to self and to other network figures was transformed and converted to miles (see Table 5). The participants had the closest physical distance to romantic partners, which is not surprising, given that 73% of those in romantic relationships were cohabitating. Of those in relationships but not living with their romantic partner ($n = 172$), 70.3% still lived within 10 miles of their partner.

Table 5. Descriptive statistics for physical proximity to different figures.

Attachment Figure	n	M (miles)	SD	0–10 Miles (%)	11–250 Miles (%)	251–500 Miles (%)	>500 Miles (%)
Romantic Partner	657	6.11	60.45	520 (79.1)	75 (11.4)	37 (5.6)	25 (3.8)
Mother	708	182.71	70.49	296 (41.8)	222 (31.4)	126 (17.8)	64 (9.0)
Father	545	216.58	69.66	163 (29.9)	191 (35.0)	110 (20.2)	81 (14.9)
Sibling	594	197.15	61.65	192 (32.3)	232 (39.1)	108 (18.2)	62 (10.4)
Friend	709	188.29	66.78	255 (36.0)	267 (37.7)	131 (18.5)	56 (7.9)
Child	138	8.19	63.86	102 (73.9)	21 (15.2)	10 (7.3)	5 (3.6)

Research question 1: what is the relationship between age, romantic status, parental status, and physical proximity to each network figure? To investigate whether age, romantic status, and parental status are related to physical proximity to each network figure, we conducted a series of sequential regressions, just as with the attachment strength analysis. The first model of main effects was all significant (see Table 6).

Table 6. Sequential regression analyses of demographic variables on physical proximity to different attachment figures.

		Attachment Figure										
		Romantic Partner		Mother		Father		Sibling		Friend		Child	
Model	Predictor	R^2ch	β	R^2ch	β	R^2ch	β	R^2ch	β	R^2ch	β	R^2ch	β
1		0.026 **		0.069 **		0.035 **		0.034 **		0.028 **		0.248 **	
	Age		0.118 *		0.199 **		0.079		0.069		0.039		0.560 **
	PS		−0.130 **		0.047		−0.077		−0.114		0.039		
	RS				0.248 **		0.169 **		0.182 **		0.209 **		−0.029
2		0.000		0.006		0.005		0.000		0.006		0.005	
	Age x PS		0.006		−0.021		−0.079		−0.011		−0.056		
	Age x RS				0.051		0.069		0.010		0.012		0.114
	PS x RS				−0.118		0.006		−0.003		−0.107		
R^2		0.026		0.075		0.041		0.035		0.033		0.253	
Adjusted R^2		0.021		0.067		0.030		0.025		0.025		0.236	
$F_{(df)}$		5.722 **		9.486 **		3.790 **		3.502 **		4.021 **		15.206	
		(3, 657)		(6, 708)		(6, 545)		(6, 594)		(6, 709)		(3, 138)	

Note. PS = parental status; RS = romantic status; parental status coded as 0 = no child, 1 = child; romantic status coded as 0 = no romantic partner, 1 = romantic partner. * $p < 0.05$. ** $p < 0.01$. R^2ch = R^2 change.

Age was statistically and positively predictive of physical proximity to romantic partners, mothers, and children. The results suggest that older participants, on average, lived further from these figures. Furthermore, parental status statistically and negatively predicted physical proximity to romantic partners, which suggested that having children was related to close physical distance to romantic partners. Finally, romantic status was statistically and positively predictive of physical proximity to mothers, fathers, siblings, and friends. Those who did not have romantic partners had close physical distance to parents, siblings, and friends.

Morphology of attachment network. We examined three dimensions of network morphology, including hierarchical structure, centrality (for both attachment strength and physical distance), and density (for physical distance only). Hierarchical structure was classified into three variations, including the monotropic, shared primary, and distributed attachment categories [21]. Monotropic structure is based on Bowlby's [1–3] assumption of "monotropy", which suggests that humans are predisposed to have a clear primary attachment figure marked by meaningful separation in attachment strength between the highest rated figure and all the other network figures (see the measurement of hierarchy under Method/Measures). Shared primary structure is marked by an undifferentiated rating of the top two figures, which are both rated significantly stronger than the remaining three network figures. This term was used by Schaffer and Emerson [35] to describe the undifferentiated attachment to mothers and fathers that many of their infants showed by 18 months of age. The third classification, distributed attachment, was used by Freeman and Simon [21] to describe a lack of preference between the top three rated figures. The results demonstrated that 69.8% of the sample had the monotropic structure, followed by the shared primary structure (17.2%), and distributed attachment (13%).

Research Question 2: is age, romantic status, or parental status related to the degree of network hierarchy between support figures? To test effects of age, romantic status, and parental status, the same sequential regression analyses as attachment strength and physical proximity were run to predict the degree of network hierarchy between support figures, the emotional or physical centrality of network figures, and the emotional or physical density of network figures (see Table 7). Parental status statistically and negatively predicted the degree of network hierarchy between support figures. Those who have children had non-hierarchical attachment network structures, and they considered that all their support figures were equally significant. Nevertheless, romantic status was statistically and positively predictive of the degree of network hierarchy between attachment figures, which demonstrated that those who have romantic partners had hierarchical network structures. Romantic partners would more likely be identified as the primary figure.

Table 7. Sequential Regression Analyses of Demographic Variables on the Centrality and Density of Attachment Networks.

		Morphology Factors							
		Degree of Network Hierarchy		Emotional Centrality		Physical Centrality		Physical Density	
Model	Predictor	R^2ch	β	R^2ch	β	R^2ch	β	R^2ch	β
1		0.049 **		0.007		0.034 **		0.025 **	
	Age		0.029		0.027		0.164 **		0.092 *
	Parental Status		−0.135 **		−0.125 *		−0.073		−0.089
	Romantic Status		0.163 **		−0.057		0.030		0.016
2		0.007		0.003		0.006		0.002	
	Age × Parental Status		−0.062		0.035		−0.061		−0.049
	Age × Romantic Status		0.026		−0.003		0.072		−0.010
	Parental Status × Romantic Status		0.152 *		0.085		−0.081		−0.038
R^2		0.056		0.010		0.040		0.027	
Adjusted R^2		0.050		0.003		0.034		0.021	
$F_{(df)}$		9.185 ** $_{(6, 930)}$		1.529 $_{(6, 930)}$		6.472 ** $_{(6, 930)}$		4.268 ** $_{(6, 930)}$	

Note. Degree of network hierarchy coded 0 = no hierarchy, 1 = hierarchy; parental status coded 0 = no child, 1 = child; romantic status coded 0 = no romantic partner, 1 = romantic partner.* $p < 0.05$. ** $p < 0.01$. R^2ch = R^2 change.

Emotional and physical centrality and density of network figures. In addition, attachment centrality was calculated as the average attachment strength to all five figures, and physical centrality was calculated as the average physical distance to all five network figures. Physical density was calculated as the average physical distance between every possible pairing of the five network figures. Given that participants were not asked to consider the attachment strength between figures, attachment density was not calculated.

Research Question 3: Is age, romantic status, or parental status related to attachment centrality and physical centrality of network members? To test effects of age, romantic status, and parental status on network centrality (both attachment and physical) two sequential regressions were run. Results are shown in Table 7. Age positively predicted the physical centrality of network member, younger adults, on average, lived closer to their network. Parental status negatively predicted attachment centrality of network figures, indicating that participants with children had stronger attachment networks, and lived closer to their attachment network

Research question 4: is age, romantic status, or parental status related to the emotional or physical density of network figures? An additional sequential regression was run to test the effect of age, romantic status, and parental status on physical density (see Table 7). Only age was statistically and positively related to the physical density variable, indicating that older participants tended to live further away from their attachment network.

4. Discussion

4.1. Network Composition

The network composition findings based on the WHMT diagrammatic measure are highly consistent with previous work using traditional Likert scaled measures, such as the WHO-TO, the IPI, and the ANQ [4,5,15–17]. Attachment network size did not significantly vary by age. Most participants reported one or two clear-cut attachment figures, and about one in five adults indicated three attachment figures. Having more than three or having no attachment figures were both uncommon conditions, each describing approximately 10% of the sample. These results support the view that attachment networks are comprised of a few relationships at any one time from cradle to grave, and that entrance into the inner circle of attachment relationships is highly exclusive, supporting Ainsworth's contention that attachments apply to a limited number of relationships [23]. Within this inner circle of attachment relationships, most adults further differentiated a hierarchy of preference.

The adults in romantic relationships, independent of age, gender, or romantic relationship duration, overwhelmingly identified romantic partners as their primary target for attachment support. Among the single adults less than 44 years of age, mothers were the most common primary target. Mothers remained critical attachment targets into middle adulthood among many single adults between 44 and 64 years of age, being selected as often as friends as the primary figure. The primacy of romantic attachment and the longevity of maternal attachment are consistent with theoretical views on attachment across the life course [11,17,23].

These results strongly support the view that most people continue to rely on mothers as attachment figures through their adult life, and significant disruptions in maternal status are less likely the result of gradual emotional distancing than a function of romantic status, maternal loss through death, or a diminished capacity to fulfill this role. The primacy of romantic partners and mothers suggests that the process of parent-to-peer attachment transfer continues to operate in a bidirectional fashion through most of adulthood, such that a new romantic relationship quickly gives way to prioritizing romantic partners over mothers, after which mothers remain important secondary targets. Given that romantic duration did not mediate the strength of romantic attachment, the process of prioritizing partners over mothers is fairly rapid and not the gradual transfer of attachment provisions observed in adolescence or young adulthood [5,10]. Similarly, in the event of romantic partner loss or dissolution, mothers may immediately resume their original place as the primary figure. Of course, these conclusions are tentative and based on cross-sectional data that preclude a clear understanding of the process and temporal pace of romantic attachment formation.

The shared experience of parenting appears to strengthen reliance on partners for emotional support and possibly promote deeper attachments. Feeney and colleagues [16] reported similar findings in their older adult sample but found the opposite effect for younger parents, in which case having a child strengthened their parental ties, not their romantic relationship. In the current study, the association is weak and may point to the vicissitudes in how parenting influences romantic bonds. In this way, becoming a parent may not be consistently tied to the strengthening or weakening of a specific relationship, but rather signals a redistribution of attachment that is idiosyncratic with respect to individual and contextual factors. This idea is reinforced in the next set of findings on normative life events, including child status, on network centrality.

Being romantically involved and having higher romantic attachment strength predicted less attachment strength to mothers, fathers, friends, and adult children. Beyond middle adulthood, however, other family members, including siblings and adult children, became increasingly common attachment targets. Being a parent was associated with stronger reliance on romantic partners for attachment support, but this life event was not related to attachment strength to other network figures. The adults that did not indicate a preference for romantic partners or mothers identified friends, siblings, or adult children as the most sought primary attachment figures. Fathers, on the other hand, were consistently uncommon primary targets regardless of age, with approximately one out of every twenty participants viewing their fathers in this role.

4.2. Beyond Network Composition

Up until now, research on adult attachment networks has focused on questions of network composition, namely, who the primary attachment figure is and how many social network figures function as "clear-cut" attachment relationships. This work has provided important insights into in size of attachment networks and who function as primary attachment figures through normative adult transitions, but composition alone provides an incomplete understanding of network structure. A major strength of the current study lies in the exploration of novel network structures using the web-based hierarchical mapping technique (WHMT). In addition to composition, The WHMT provides data on whole network dimensions, which we call network morphology, including hierarchical structure, centrality, and density. We explored composition and morphology using both attachment strength and the physical location of network members to provide a fuller understanding of attachment networks through the adult years as a function of parental status and romantic status.

4.3. Physical Proximity to Different Figures

Growing older was associated with greater physical distance to and between attachment network members. This distancing is likely the result of greater mobility in early to midlife transitions, such as leaving school, entering a career, changing vocations, as well as housing transitions and relocations that accompany normative increases in family size (i.e., becoming a parent) [40]. Conversely, relocation in later adulthood may be triggered by life events that reduce household composition, such as romantic relationship dissolution or death, adult children leaving home, and downsizing one's living space after retirement [14,15].

Greater physical centrality and network density were associated with stronger attachments to romantic partners, mothers, fathers, friends, and siblings. These findings underscore the importance of physical availability and access to our closest relationships, even in an age where technology provides instant access to our social network. When coupled with age trends in centrality and density, the developmental trend is toward increasing disconnection from our closest social network, both physically and emotionally. While it is not possible to tease apart the direction of effects, it seems more likely that physical distance due to mobility is the instigating factor for social disconnection.

Romantic status was an important indicator of physical proximity to network members. Single participants lived closer to their parents, siblings, and friends, compared to their coupled counterparts. As discussed, singlehood also corresponded to greater attachment strength to these same figures. Collectively, these findings are consistent with a common perception that spending time together in the same physical space matters more than the same amount of social interaction experienced through distance communication. On the other hand, our data do not provide this fine-grained analysis. An important next step is to document associations between physical centrality and density in relation to interaction context (distance versus in-person). Such a study could lead to a better understanding of how physical closeness directly or indirectly supports emotional closeness.

The romantic and parental status were important, albeit opposite indicators of whether adults indicated a clear preference hierarchy or not. Being in a romantic relationship was associated with a clear monotropic orientation toward one network figure, namely the romantic partner. However, being a parent was associated with a more distributed network. Put another way, romantic relationships tend to pull attachment strength from other network figures, whereas having a child appears to dampen this effect and result in a more equal distribution of attachment preference. This romantic-status-by-parental-status interaction effect was the only interaction effect in all the sequential regressions run with these two life-event factors. At the same time, this effect runs contrary to the child status effect on attachment strength, which suggests that having a child increases romantic partner strength, albeit the association is very small.

According to the attachment and physical centrality of network figures, the findings indicate that individuals tend to have stronger and more consolidated attachments to all network figures when they have children. Parenthood is a shared experience that often brings parents into contact with others who are also going through a similar life event [41]. This shared experience can foster stronger bonds between parents and their peers, as they have a mutual understanding and support system. Moreover, having children often means increased demands on time, energy, and resources. Parents often rely on their social network for practical support, such as help with childcare, advice on parenting issues, and emotional support during challenging times [42]. This reliance may deepen their connections with these individuals.

4.4. Limitations and Future Directions

The limitations of this study are primarily due to a restricted sample (MTurk workers) and the use of cross-sectional data. The respondents in the present study were recruited from a convenience sample of MTurk workers. Although the sample size was fairly large and distributed across the USA, the ethnic diversity was limited and non-representative of the US population, limiting the generalizability to the broader population [43] and especially to non-Western samples. A study in Bangladesh, for instance, found that parents, not romantic partners, remained primary attachment figures for adult women into middle age, an outcome the authors attributed to collectivist cultural values [44]. The reliance on cross-sectional data allows us only to speculate on questions of stability, dynamics, and change in attachment network structures across adulthood.

An important next step is to examine how these same network dimensions, including composition and morphology, operate in diverse cultures, and how these network dimensions predict adult adjustment and physical and mental health. Ideally, such a study could follow participant networks over time to shed light on stability and change in attachment network structures and how these temporal factors are related to well-being and health outcomes.

4.5. Conclusions

These results are the first to examine attachment networks using social network factors including density and centrality. The addition of geographic location of network members also adds to our understanding of how physical distance and emotional connection interrelate within the context of normative adult transitions, including romantic relationship status and parent status. Looking across the three dimensions of morphology, there appears to be a strong dividing line between adults in romantic partnerships and those who are not. Those in romantic relationships are more likely to put their attachment eggs in one basket, live further from their other close relationships, and have a network that is more geographically dispersed. In sum, the more isolated and hierarchical network among romantically involved adults fits the Beatles'[45] refrain, "All You Need is Love". Single adults are more likely to spread their attachment preference equally between two or three closest relationships, often including a friend and a family member. Single adults also tend to live closer to their attachment network. Yet, having a child may lead to some network reorganization by forming new social connections closer to home. In addition to forming romantic partnerships, growing older also contributes to diminished network centrality and density over time. Taken together, these findings reveal a more comprehensive and nuanced look at attachment networks than previous literature has uncovered. Longitudinal research and studies with culturally diverse samples are important avenues for future research.

Author Contributions: Conceptualization, H.F. and J.T.; methodology, H.F. and J.T.; data analysis J.T.; writing—original draft preparation, J.T. and H.F.; review and editing, H.F.; supervision, H.F.; funding acquisition, H.F. All authors have read and agreed to the published version of the manuscript.

Funding: The study was supported by an internal grant to the second author from the School of Education Office of Research at the University of South Dakota.

Institutional Review Board Statement: The study was conducted in accordance with the Declaration of Helsinki, and approved by the University of South Dakota's Institutional Review Board (IRB) (protocol code IRB-20-210).

Informed Consent Statement: Informed consent was obtained from all subjects involved in the study.

Data Availability Statement: The data that support the findings of this study are available from the corresponding author, [HF], upon reasonable request.

Conflicts of Interest: The authors declare no conflicts of interest.

References

1. Bowlby, J. *Attachment and Loss*; Random House: New York, NY, USA, 1969.
2. Bowlby, J. The Making and Breaking of Affectional Bonds: II. Some Principles of Psychotherapy: The Fiftieth Maudsley Lecture (Expanded Version). *Br. J. Psychiatry* **1977**, *130*, 421–431. [CrossRef]
3. Bowlby, J. *Attachment and Loss. Volume I Attachment*; Random House: New York, NY, USA, 1982; Volume I.
4. Feeney, J.; Noller, P. Attachments in Infancy and Beyond. In *Adult Attachment*; Sage Publications: Thousand Oaks, CA, USA, 2012; pp. 1–21. [CrossRef]
5. Fraley, R.C.; Davis, K.E. Attachment Formation and Transfer in Young Adults' Close Friendships and Romantic Relationships. *Pers. Relatsh.* **1997**, *4*, 131–144. [CrossRef]
6. Freeman, H.; Brown, B.B. Primary Attachment to Parents and Peers during Adolescence: Differences by Attachment Style. *J. Youth Adolesc.* **2001**, *30*, 653–674. [CrossRef]
7. Hazan, C.; Shaver, P.R. Attachment as an Organizational Framework for Research on Close Relationships. *Psychol. Inq.* **1994**, *5*, 1–22. [CrossRef]
8. Umemura, T.; Lacinová, L.; Horská, E.; Pivodová, L. Development of multiple attachment relationships from infancy to adulthood: A review of attachment hierarchy. *Ceskosl. Psychol.* **2019**, *63*, 210–225.
9. Hazan, C.; Diamond, L.M. The Place of Attachment in Human Mating. *Rev. Gen. Psychol.* **2000**, *4*, 186–204. [CrossRef]
10. Hazan, C.; Zeifman, D. Pair bonds as attachments. In *Handbook of Attachment: Theory, Research, and Clinical Applications*; Guilford Press: New York, NY, USA, 1999; pp. 336–354.
11. Weiss, R.S. The Attachment Bond in Childhood and Adulthood. In *Attachment across the Life Cycle*; Tavistock Institute: New York, NY, USA, 1991.
12. Pitman, R.; Scharfe, E. Testing the Function of Attachment Hierarchies during Emerging Adulthood. *Pers. Relatsh.* **2010**, *17*, 201–216. [CrossRef]
13. Calvo, V.; Palmieri, A.; Codato, M.; Testoni, I.; Sambin, M. Composition and Function of Women's Attachment Network in Adulthood. *Interdiscip. J. Fam. Stud.* **2012**, *17*, 100–110.

14. Carli, L.L.; Anzelmo, E.; Pozzi, S.; Feeney, J.A.; Gallucci, M.; Santona, A.; Tagini, A. Attachment Networks in Committed Couples. *Front. Psychol.* **2019**, *10*, 1105. [CrossRef]
15. Cicirelli, V.G. Attachment Relationships in Old Age. *J. Soc. Pers. Relat.* **2010**, *27*, 191–199. [CrossRef]
16. Doherty, N.A.; Feeney, J.A. The Composition of Attachment Networks throughout the Adult Years. *Pers. Relatsh.* **2004**, *11*, 469–488. [CrossRef]
17. Fraley, R.C. Attachment in Adulthood: Recent Developments, Emerging Debates, and Future Directions. *Annu. Rev. Psychol.* **2019**, *70*, 401–422. [CrossRef] [PubMed]
18. Freeman, H.; Abdellatif, M.A.; Gnimpieba, E.Z. A Qualitative Validation of Two Diagrammatic Measures of Attachment Network Structure. *Eur. J. Psychol. Assess.* **2021**, *39*, 21–36. [CrossRef]
19. Trinke, S.J.; Bartholomew, K. Hierarchies of Attachment Relationships in Youn Adulthood. *J. Soc. Pers. Relat.* **1997**, *14*, 603–625. [CrossRef]
20. Rosenthal, N.L.; Kobak, R. Assessing Adolescents' Attachment Hierarchies: Differences across Developmental Periods and Associations with Individual Adaptation: Adolescent Attachment Hierachies. *J. Res. Adolesc.* **2010**, *20*, 678–706. [CrossRef] [PubMed]
21. Freeman, H.; Simons, J. Attachment Network Structure as a Predictor of Romantic Attachment Formation and Insecurity. *Soc. Dev.* **2018**, *27*, 201–220. [CrossRef]
22. Hazan, C.; Shaver, P. Romantic Love Conceptualized as an Attachment Process. *J. Pers. Soc. Psychol.* **1987**, *52*, 511–524. [CrossRef]
23. Ainsworth, M.D.S.; Blehar, M.; Waters, E.; Wall, S. *Patterns of Attachment: A Psychological Study of the Strange Situation*; John Wiley & Sons: Nashville, TN, USA, 1978.
24. Freeman, H.; Scholl, J.L.; AnisAbdellatif, M.; Gnimpieba, E.; Forster, G.L.; Jacob, S. I Only Have Eyes for You: Oxytocin Administration Supports Romantic Attachment Formation through Diminished Interest in Close Others and Strangers. *Psychoneuroendocrinology* **2021**, *134*, 105415. [CrossRef]
25. Hazan, C.; Campa, M.; Gur-Yaish, N. Attachment across the lifespan. In *Close Relationships: Functions, Forms and Processes*; Psychology Press: New York, NY, USA, 2006; pp. 189–209.
26. Ainsworth, M.D. Attachments beyond Infancy. *Am. Psychol.* **1989**, *44*, 709–716. [CrossRef]
27. Umemura, T.; Lacinová, L.; Macek, P. Is Emerging Adults' Attachment Preference for the Romantic Partner Transferred from Their Attachment Preferences for Their Mother, Father, and Friends? *Emerg. Adulthood* **2015**, *3*, 179–193. [CrossRef]
28. Umemura, T.; Lacinová, L.; Juhová, D.; Pivodová, L.; Cheung, H.S. Transfer of Early to Late Adolescents' Attachment Figures in a Multicohort Six-Wave Study: Person- and Variable-Oriented Approaches. *J. Early Adolesc.* **2021**, *41*, 1072–1098. [CrossRef]
29. Zhang, H.; Chan, D.K.-S.; Teng, F. Transfer of Attachment Functions and Adjustment among Young Adults in China. *J. Soc. Psychol.* **2011**, *151*, 257–273. [CrossRef] [PubMed]
30. Collins, N.L.; Feeney, B.C. Attachment and Caregiving in Adult Close Relationships: Normative Processes and Individual Differences. *Attach. Hum. Dev.* **2013**, *15*, 241–245. [CrossRef] [PubMed]
31. Feeney, J. *Becoming Parents: Exploring the Bonds between Mothers, Fathers, and Their Infants*; Cambridge University Press: Cambridge, UK, 2001.
32. Carli, L.L.; Alì, P.A.; Anzelmo, E.; Caprin, C.; Crippa, F.; Gallucci, M.; Moioli, L.; Traficante, D.; Feeney, J.A. Attachment Networks in Young Adults. *Front. Psychol.* **2023**, *14*, 1321185. [CrossRef]
33. Rowe, A.C.; Carnelley, K.B. Preliminary Support for the Use of a Hierarchical Mapping Technique to Examine Attachment Networks. *Pers. Relatsh.* **2005**, *12*, 499–519. [CrossRef]
34. Antonucci, T.C. Hierarchical mapping technique. *Generations* **1986**, *10*, 10–12.
35. Schaffer, H.R.; Emerson, P.E. The Development of Social Attachments in Infancy. *Monogr. Soc. Res. Child Dev.* **1964**, *29*, 1–77. [CrossRef]
36. Gillath, O.; Karantzas, G.C.; Lee, J. Attachment and Social Networks. *Curr. Opin. Psychol.* **2019**, *25*, 21–25. [CrossRef]
37. Perry, B.L.; Pescosolido, B.A.; Borgatti, S.P. *Egocentric Network Analysis: Foundations, Methods, and Models*; Cambridge University Press: Cambridge, UK, 2018.
38. Hauser, D.J.; Moss, A.J.; Rosenzweig, C.; Jaffe, S.N.; Robinson, J.; Litman, L. Evaluating CloudResearch's Approved Group as a Solution for Problematic Data Quality on MTurk. *Behav. Res. Methods* **2023**, *55*, 3953–3964. [CrossRef]
39. Wani, R.T. Socioeconomic Status Scales-Modified Kuppuswamy and Udai Pareekh's Scale Updated for 2019. *J. Family Med. Prim. Care* **2019**, *8*, 1846–1849. [CrossRef]
40. Mikulincer, M.; Shaver, P.R. *Attachment in Adulthood: Structure, Dynamics, and Change*; Guilford Publications: New York, NY, USA, 2010.
41. Ainbinder, J.G.; Blanchard, L.W.; Singer, G.H.; Sullivan, M.E.; Powers, L.K.; Marquis, J.G. A Qualitative Study of Parent-to-Parent Support for Parents of Children with Special Needs. *J. Pediatr. Psychol.* **1998**, *23*, 99–109. [CrossRef] [PubMed]
42. Lévesque, S.; Bisson, V.; Charton, L.; Fernet, M. Parenting and Relational Well-Being during the Transition to Parenthood: Challenges for First-Time Parents. *J. Child Fam. Stud.* **2020**, *29*, 1938–1956. [CrossRef]
43. Peer, E.; Vosgerau, J.; Acquisti, A. Reputation as a Sufficient Condition for Data Quality on Amazon Mechanical Turk. *Behav. Res. Methods* **2014**, *46*, 1023–1031. [CrossRef]
44. Flicker, S.M.; Sancier-Barbosa, F.; Afroz, F.; Saif, S.N.; Mohsin, F. Attachment Hierarchies in Bangladeshi Women in Couple-Initiated and Arranged Marriages. *Int. J. Psychol.* **2020**, *55*, 638–646. [CrossRef] [PubMed]

45. The Beatles. *All You Need Is Love*; On Magical Mystery Tour [Album]; Capitol Records: Los Angeles, CA, USA, 1967.

Disclaimer/Publisher's Note: The statements, opinions and data contained in all publications are solely those of the individual author(s) and contributor(s) and not of MDPI and/or the editor(s). MDPI and/or the editor(s) disclaim responsibility for any injury to people or property resulting from any ideas, methods, instructions or products referred to in the content.

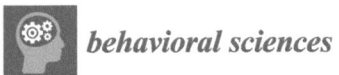

Correction

Correction: Muñoz-Aucapiña et al. (2025). Psychometric Validation of the Dating Violence Questionnaire (DVQ-R) in Ecuadorians. *Behavioral Sciences*, 15(1), 68

Miriam Jacqueline Muñoz-Aucapiña [1], Rosa Elvira Muñoz-Aucapiña [1], Inmaculada García-García [2], María Adelaida Álvarez-Serrano [3,*], Ana María Antolí-Jover [3] and Encarnación Martínez-García [2,4,5]

1. Department of Nursing, Faculty of Health Sciences, University Católica Santiago de Guayaquil, Guayaquil 090615, Ecuador; miriam.munoz@cu.ucsg.edu.ec (M.J.M.-A.); rosa.munoz@cu.ucsg.edu.ec (R.E.M.-A.)
2. Department of Nursing, Faculty of Health Sciences, University of Granada, 18016 Granada, Spain; igarcia@ugr.es (I.G.-G.); emartinez@ugr.es (E.M.-G.)
3. Department of Nursing, Faculty of Health Sciences, University of Granada, 51001 Ceuta, Spain; antolijover@ugr.es
4. Virgen de las Nieves University Hospital, 18014 Granada, Spain
5. Instituto de Investigación Biosanitaria ibs.GRANADA, Granada, Spain
* Correspondence: adealvarez@ugr.es

Updating Affiliation

In the original publication (Muñoz-Aucapiña et al., 2025), the affliation has now been approved for updating as Instituto de Investigación Biosanitaria ibs.GRANADA, Granada, Spain.

Deleting Citation

In the original publication (Muñoz-Aucapiña et al., 2025), Verbeek et al. (2023) was cited. The citation has now been approved for removal in Materials and Methods, *Instrument*, Paragraph Number 1 and the correct text should read as follows:

The questionnaire was divided into two blocks. The first collected information on socio-demographic variables: year of birth; sex (male, female); university (Universidad Católica de Santiago de Guayaquil, Universidad Estatal de Guayaquil); relationship status (No, Yes); relationship duration (1–3 months, 3–6 months, 1–3 years, >3 years). The second block was based on the Dating Violence Questionnaire—Revised (DVQ-R) (Rodríguez Díaz et al., 2017), which was later validated for samples of Ecuadorian women aged 18 to 30 by Cherrez Santos et al. (2022). This study remains the ideal reference for exclusively female samples in this age group and population. This instrument is a simplified version of the Dating Violence Questionnaire (DVQ) (Rodríguez Franco et al., 2010). It is aimed at adolescents involved in dating relationships, or who have been in a relationship in the last six months, with a minimum duration of one month. It includes 20 items and uses a Likert-type scale with five response options (0 = Never to 4 = Always). It can be administered individually or in a group, lasting approximately five to ten minutes. This questionnaire assesses five dimensions of dating violence, which are shown below:

Reference

Muñoz-Aucapiña, M. J., Muñoz-Aucapiña, R. E., García-García, I., Álvarez-Serrano, M. A., Antolí-Jover, A. M., & Martínez-García, E. (2025). Psychometric Validation of the Dating Violence Questionnaire (DVQ-R) in Ecuadorians. *Behavioral Sciences*, *15*(1), 68. [PubMed]

Disclaimer/Publisher's Note: The statements, opinions and data contained in all publications are solely those of the individual author(s) and contributor(s) and not of MDPI and/or the editor(s). MDPI and/or the editor(s) disclaim responsibility for any injury to people or property resulting from any ideas, methods, instructions or products referred to in the content.

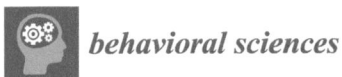

Article

Virtually Connected: Do Shared Novel Activities in Virtual Reality Enhance Self-Expansion and Relationship Quality?

Rhonda N. Balzarini [1,2,*], Anya Sharma [3] and Amy Muise [3]

[1] Department of Psychology, Texas State University, San Marcos, TX 78666, USA
[2] Kinsey Institute, Indiana University, Bloomington, IN 47405, USA
[3] Department of Psychology, York University, Toronto, ON M3J 1P3, Canada; anyashar@yorku.ca (A.S.); muiseamy@yorku.ca (A.M.)
* Correspondence: rbalzarini@txstate.edu

Academic Editors: Bianca P. Acevedo and Adam Bode

Received: 16 October 2024
Revised: 27 December 2024
Accepted: 3 January 2025
Published: 14 January 2025

Citation: Balzarini, R. N., Sharma, A., & Muise, A. (2025). Virtually Connected: Do Shared Novel Activities in Virtual Reality Enhance Self-Expansion and Relationship Quality? *Behavioral Sciences*, 15(1), 67. https://doi.org/10.3390/bs15010067

Copyright: © 2025 by the authors. Licensee MDPI, Basel, Switzerland. This article is an open access article distributed under the terms and conditions of the Creative Commons Attribution (CC BY) license (https://creativecommons.org/licenses/by/4.0/).

Abstract: According to self-expansion theory, sharing novel experiences with a romantic partner can help prevent boredom and maintain relationship quality. However, in today's globalized modern world, partners spend less time together and are more likely to live apart than in previous generations, limiting opportunities for shared novel experiences. In two in-lab experiments, we tested whether shared novel activities in virtual reality (VR) could facilitate self-expansion, reduce boredom, and enhance relationship quality. In Study 1, couples (*N* = 183) engaged in a shared novel and exciting activity in either VR or over video. Participants in the VR condition reported greater presence (i.e., felt like they were in the same space as their partner) and were less bored during the interaction compared to the video condition, though no main effects emerged for reports of self-expansion or relationship quality (relationship satisfaction and closeness). Consistent with predictions, people who reported more presence, in turn, reported greater self-expansion, less boredom, and greater relationship quality. In Study 2, couples (*N* = 141) engaged in a novel and exciting or a mundane experience in VR. Results were mixed such that participants in the novel VR condition reported less boredom and greater closeness post-interaction, though no effects emerged for self-expansion or relationship satisfaction. In exploratory analyses accounting for immersion, couples who engaged in the novel virtual experience reported more self-expansion, less boredom, and greater closeness. The findings suggest that virtual interactions may have less potential than in-person interaction to promote self-expansion but offer interesting future directions given VR's ability to enhance presence beyond video interactions.

Keywords: virtual reality; self-expansion; romantic relationships; relationship satisfaction; intimacy; boredom

1. Introduction

The increasingly globalized modern world means that many people live apart from, or have less time with, those with whom they share the closest relationships (Amato & Hayes, 2013; Flood & Genadek, 2016; Holmes, 2010). In romantic relationships specifically, partners are more likely to live apart for job opportunities and educational pursuits than in previous generations (Hammonds et al., 2020; Holmes, 2010) and even among couples who live together, partners engage in fewer shared activities than they did 40 to 50 years ago (Amato et al., 2007; Dew, 2009; Kaufman-Parks et al., 2023). According to self-expansion theory, shared novel activities with a partner are important for warding off boredom and maintaining relationship quality (Aron & Aron, 1996, 1997; Aron et al., 2022). However, it is not yet clear if couples can engage in these types of experiences virtually. In the current research, we tested the potential of virtual reality (VR) to simulate novel shared experiences between romantic partners. In Study 1, we compared a novel experience in VR to the same experience over video chat to test whether the VR interaction increased presence (i.e., the feeling that they were in the same environment as their partner and experiencing the interaction together) and, in turn, greater self-expansion, lower boredom, and higher relationship quality. In Study 2, mirroring classic self-expansion experiments (Aron et al., 2022), we compared a novel experience in VR to a mundane experience in VR to test whether couples in the novel condition would report higher self-expansion, less boredom, and higher relationship quality. The findings have practical implications for couples seeking novel ways to connect and for researchers seeking ecologically valid ways to manipulate self-expansion.

1.1. Self-Expansion in Relationships

Spending quality time together is important for relationship maintenance (Jaremka et al., 2017), as shared positive leisure time helps couples maintain closeness and satisfaction in their relationships (Aron et al., 2000; Coulter & Malouff, 2013; Ogolsky et al., 2017; Rogge et al., 2013). However, certain activities may have greater potential to enhance relationship quality. Research on self-expansion has consistently shown that when couples engage in novel and exciting activities together (compared to activities that are more familiar or mundane), they experience less boredom and feel closer and more satisfied with their relationship (Aron et al., 2000, 2022).

In the seminal study on self-expansion, Aron and colleagues (Aron et al., 2000) assigned couples to either engage in a novel activity (e.g., an obstacle course) or a mundane activity together and found that couples who participated in novel and arousing activities reported less boredom and in turn, increased closeness and relationship satisfaction. Other experimental studies have shown similar effects; when couples are randomly assigned to engage in novel and exciting activities, they report boosts in their relationship quality compared to a waitlist control (Coulter & Malouff, 2013). In related homework-style studies, couples assigned to engage in novel and exciting (versus mundane but pleasant) activities report greater relationship quality; for a review, see Aron et al. (2022). For example, Reissman et al. (1993) assigned couples to participate in 1.5 h of exciting activities per week or 1.5 h per week of pleasant activities, or couples were assigned to a no-activity control condition for ten weeks. Participants assigned to the novel condition reported greater relationship quality than the other two conditions at the end of the study. Researchers have also used experience sampling designs to track partners' novel shared activities in their daily lives. On days when couples engaged in activities that provided greater self-expansion—such as learning a new skill together (e.g., taking a cooking class), traveling together (e.g., going on a road trip), or engaging in adventurous sports (e.g., rock climbing)—both partners reported feeling more satisfied with their relationship on that day (Muise et al., 2019). In addition, couples who engaged in more self-expanding activities over the three-week study reported greater satisfaction three months later (Muise et al., 2019). Thus, strong support exists for the beneficial role of novel and exciting activities in promoting relationship quality in and outside a controlled laboratory environment.

Although self-expanding activities have been shown to help couples stay connected, maintain relationship satisfaction, and reduce boredom (Aron et al., 2022), previous research examining relational self-expansion has primarily investigated shared novel and exciting activities that involved partners interacting together, in person. Little is known about whether self-expansion can be facilitated virtually. Thus, one aim of the current research was to extend past work to test the potential of VR to facilitate self-expanding experiences for couples.

1.2. The Potential of Virtual Reality for Fostering Self-Expansion

Virtual reality (VR) is increasing in popularity and accessibility. Over 64 million Americans reported using VR in 2022 (Statista, 2024), and VR is projected to have 75.4 million American users by 2025 and 216 million users worldwide by 2025 (Digital in the Round, 2024; Lin, 2024; Sacks, 2024). In the US, the market is expected to keep expanding, especially as more immersive experiences and practical applications emerge (e.g., healthcare and training), helping VR reach a broader audience and drive long-term growth (Lin, 2024). Part of the success of VR has been its ability to immerse users into an experience. That is, VR technology is unique because it places users inside an experience, and users can immerse themselves in realistic simulations with virtual interaction partners. For example, a couple could visit Bali or take a virtual tour of the Taj Mahal together (Tracey, 2024), even from different geographical locations.

Given the immersive quality of VR (Howard et al., 2018; Valtchanov, 2010), researchers have been using VR to induce emotional experiences (Li et al., 2022; Meuleman & Rudrauf, 2018), such as anxiety and relaxation (Riva et al., 2007), fear and disgust (El Bashasse et al., 2023; Inozu et al., 2020; Ji et al., 2016), stress (Himes, 2024), and empathy (Marques et al., 2022; Tay et al., 2003), and simulate the presence of others (Froese et al., 2014; Sanchez-Vives & Slater, 2005; Slater et al., 2009) in a way that other text and video experiences cannot (Baym et al., 2004). Although using VR to facilitate connection in relationships is largely unexplored, in a survey of current VR users, the majority (77%) said they hope their future use of VR would involve more social interaction with other people (Koetsier, 2018). Nevertheless, there is little research on how VR interactions can enhance close relationships. Given the potential of VR to simulate the presence of a partner, there is also potential for relationship researchers to use VR to manipulate relationship-relevant experiences in more realistic ways. As such, understanding how shared experiences can be facilitated in VR has implications for relationship science and the maintenance of relationships more broadly.

1.3. The Current Study

In the current research, we draw on self-expansion theory (Aron & Aron, 1996, 1997) to examine whether VR can facilitate opportunities for couples to engage in novel shared activities. In Study 1, we compared a novel interaction between partners in VR to the same novel interaction over video to test whether VR experiences enhance a partner's presence and, in turn, enhance self-expansion, reduce boredom, and promote higher relationship quality (i.e., closeness and relationship satisfaction). In Study 2, consistent with classic self-expansion experiments (Aron et al., 2000), we compared a novel experience in VR to a mundane experience in VR to test whether couples in the novel condition would report higher self-expansion and, in turn, less boredom and higher relationship quality. Given that shared novel experiences with a partner are a key predictor of closeness and satisfaction (Aron et al., 2022), the findings have practical implications for maintaining relationship quality over time and when partners are geographically distant. The hypotheses for Study 1 and Study 2 were pre-registered on the Open Science Framework (OSF).

2. Study 1

Study 1 aimed to compare people's experience of a novel, shared activity with a romantic partner in VR to the same type of activity over video. Specifically, we tested whether couples who engage in a novel VR experience (compared to video) would report greater presence (H1)—feel like they were actually in the virtual environment with their partner—and higher self-expansion post-interaction (H2) and, in turn, report lower relational boredom and higher closeness and relationship satisfaction (H3). We also explored a series of auxiliary analyses to test whether the findings differed based on participants' age, relationship length, or past VR experience.

2.1. Participants

Participants were recruited through the Undergraduate Research Participant Pool (URPP) at [BLIND FOR REVIEW] University and from the local community. At the time of our pre-registration, no studies had tested differences between shared novel experiences with a partner in VR compared to video interactions. Therefore, we obtained estimates of effect sizes from Campbell et al. (2020), a study of 100 participants that assessed team meetings in VR compared to video conferencing. The most relevant outcomes evaluated by Campbell et al. (2020) for the current study were presence (e.g., how much they felt like they were with the other users) and closeness (e.g., how close they felt to the other users). Presence (assessed on a 9-point scale) was higher in the VR condition (M men = 7.83, M women = 7.80) compared to the video condition (M men = 5.46, M women = 5.84; F = 58.40, d = 1.5284). Closeness (assessed on a 9-point scale) was also higher in the VR condition (M men = 6.61, M women = 6.57) compared to the video condition (M men = 4.66, M women = 4.80; F = 26.93, d = 1.0379). Using G*Power 3.1 (Faul et al., 2009) for a two-tailed test for an effect size of 1.0379 (the most conservation effect) with 99% power and 0.05 alpha, 70 couples (35 per condition) would be needed. However, we oversampled to account for attrition, failed attention checks, or potential technical issues. We initially recruited 111 couples (N = 222). In line with our pre-registration, we removed 18 couples (N = 36) who experienced technical issues during the study, did not follow instructions (i.e., removed headsets, left the virtual area), or failed the attention checks (e.g., a question asking participants to select the type of virtual activity they engaged in).

Our final sample included 186 participants (N = 93 couples), including 92 men, 93 women, and one non-binary participant. The final sample was racially diverse, though most participants identified as white (37.1%) or black (16.7%). The majority of participants identified as straight/heterosexual (74.7%) and reported "seriously dating" their partners (88.2%). Participants were in established relationships with their partners for approximately two years (M = 2.22 years, SD = 2.50) and were in their early 20s (M = 20.2, SD = 3.81) on average. See Table 1 for sample demographics.

Table 1. Demographic information for Study 1 and Study 2.

	Study 1	Study 2
	Mean (SD) or N (%)	Mean (SD) or N (%)
Age	20.20 (3.81)	20.30 (3.64)
Relationship Length	2.22 (2.50)	1.83 (1.77)
Gender		
Man	92 (49.46%)	128 (44.60%)
Woman	93 (50.00%)	156 (54.36%)
Non-Binary	-	3 (1.05%)
No response	1 (0.50%)	-
Race/Ethnicity		
White	69 (37.10%)	70 (24.39%)
South Asian	29 (15.59%)	74 (25.78%)
East Asian	-	30 (10.45%)
Black	31 (16.7%)	30 (10.45%)
Latin American	16 (8.60%)	23 (8.01%)
Native American/First Nation	1 (0.54%)	-

Table 1. *Cont.*

	Study 1	Study 2
	Mean (SD) or N (%)	Mean (SD) or N (%)
Bi- or multi-racial	19 (10.22%)	30 (10.45%)
Self-identified	21 (11.29%)	43 (14.98%)
Sexual Orientation		
Heterosexual	139 (74.73%)	216 (75.26%)
Lesbian/Gay	4 (2.15%)	5 (1.74%)
Bisexual	32 (17.20%)	48 (16.72%)
Pansexual	6 (3.23%)	4 (1.39%)
Queer	1 (0.54%)	1 (0.35%)
Questioning	2 (1.08%)	8 (2.79%)
Asexual	-	1 (0.35%)
No response	2 (1.08%)	2 (0.70%)
Relationship Status		
Casually dating	4 (2.15%)	34 (11.85%)
Seriously dating	164 (88.17%)	227 (79.09%)
Engaged	4 (2.15%)	-
Common-law	5 (2.69%)	6 (2.09%)
Married	8 (4.30%)	17 (5.92%)
No response	1 (0.54)	3 (1.05%)
Past VR Experience		
None	36 (19.4%)	105 (36.6%)
Used it once	51 (27.4%)	79 (27.5%)
Used it a few times	73 (39.2%)	86 (30.0%)
I own a VR/use it regularly	15 (8.1%)	16 (5.6%)
Missing	11 (5.9%)	1 (0.3%)

2.2. Procedures

Before enrollment in the study, informed consent was obtained from all participants. Once both partners agreed to participate, they were asked to complete a 20 min online survey before attending the in-lab session, which included demographic and general relationship questions, and questions about previous experiences with VR. For the in-lab session, couples were randomly assigned to one of two conditions: (1) the novel VR experience condition ($N = 82$; 41 couples) in which participants took a virtual hot air balloon ride over a Kenyan safari, or (2) the novel video experience condition ($N = 104$; 52 couples), in which participants watched a video of a hot air balloon ride over a Kenyan safari (via a video chat with their partner). In both conditions, partners were taken to separate rooms and interacted virtually using VR or video chat. The interactions lasted approximately six minutes in both conditions. Following the interaction, participants completed a post-manipulation survey asking about their feelings during the interaction. Partners were then reunited and debriefed.

2.3. Measures

After exposure to the experimental condition, participants were asked to respond to a series of post-manipulation questions outlined below. Table 2 shows correlations between variables within each condition, and Figure 1 reports means across conditions.

Table 2. Correlations among focal variables in Study 1.

	1	2	3	4	5	6
Novel Video Condition						
1. Presence	-					
2. Self-Expansion	0.45 ***	-				
3. Boredom	−0.35 **	−0.28 **	-			
4. Closeness	0.52 ***	0.34 ***	−0.42 ***	-		
5. Relationship Sat.	0.40 ***	0.38 ***	−0.32 ***	0.46 ***	-	
6. Relationship Length	−0.05	−0.12	0.15	−0.09	−0.08	-
Novel VR Condition						
1. Presence	-					
2. Self-Expansion	0.48 ***	-				
3. Boredom	−0.41 **	−0.36 **	-			
4. Closeness	0.60 ***	0.51 ***	0.45 ***	-		
5. Relationship Sat.	0.43 ***	0.44 ***	−0.30 ***	0.57 ***	-	
6. Relationship Length	−0.02	−0.15	0.22 *	−0.11	−0.14	-

Note: *** $p < 0.001$, ** $p < 0.01$, * $p < 0.05$. Rel Sat = relationship satisfaction.

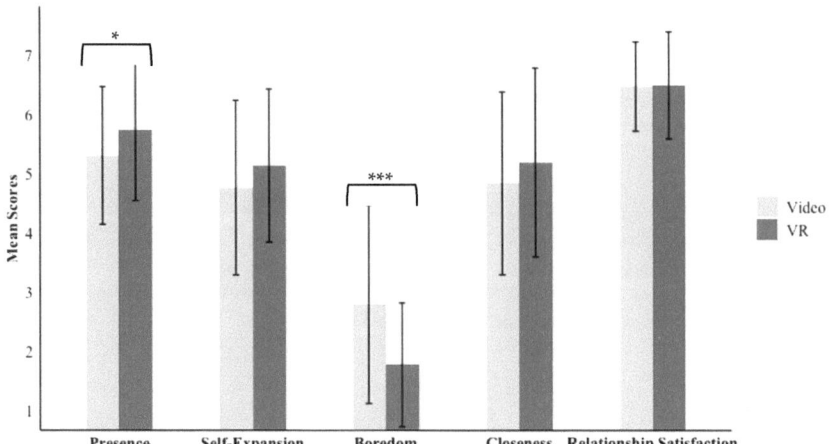

Figure 1. Descriptive statistics between conditions for Study 1 focal variables. Note: The error bars represent standard deviations, and significance is denoted with *** $p < 0.001$ and * $p < 0.05$.

2.3.1. Presence

Participants reported their sense of their partner's presence during the interaction, e.g., "How much did you have the sense that you were in the environment with your partner?"; "How much did you feel like you and your partner were having a shared experience (i.e., experiencing the same thing at the same time)?", and "During the interaction, did you feel you were with your partner (like your partner was present)?", adapted from the Networked Minds Social Presence Inventory (NMSPI) (Biocca & Harms, 2024). Possible responses were on a 7-point scale (Q1, 1 = *not at all*, 7 = *completely*; Q2–3, 1 = *never*, 7 = *all the time*), and the items were mean aggregated, with higher scores indicating higher perceived presence.

2.3.2. Self-Expansion

Participants were asked to rate their perceptions of self-expansion with their partner during the interaction. Participants were provided the following instructions: "Thinking about the experience you and your partner just had together, answer each question according to the way you personally feel, using the following scale". Participants were then asked to rate six items that were adapted from the Self-Expansion Scale (Lewandowski & Aron,

2002) (e.g., "How much did your interaction with your partner result in your having new experiences?"; "How much has the experience with your partner today resulted in your learning new things?"). Responses were provided on a 7-point scale (1 = *not very much*, 7 = *very much*), and the items were mean aggregated, with higher scores indicating higher self-expansion post-interaction (α VR = 0.90; α video = 0.90).

2.3.3. Boredom

Post-interaction, participants were asked to indicate how bored they felt during the interaction (e.g., "To what extent did you feel bored during the interaction?"). Responses were provided on a 7-point scale (1 = *not very much*, 7 = *a great deal*) with higher scores indicating higher boredom.

2.3.4. Closeness

The Inclusion of Other in the Self Scale (IOS) (Aron et al., 1992) was used to assess perceptions of closeness and intimacy with their partner during the interaction. Participants were asked to indicate how close they were with their partner (e.g., "How interconnected were you and your partner during your interaction?") using a widely used single-item pictorial scale that provides partially overlapping circles to indicate closeness with the circles increasing in closeness as they become more inclusive of the other in their self. Participant's selections were assigned a value that ranged from 1 (indicating the "*most distant*" via the overlapping circles) to 7 (indicating the "*most close*" via the overlapping circles). This scale has shown test–retest reliability as well as convergent, divergent, and criterion validity (Aron et al., 1992).

2.3.5. Relationship Satisfaction

Post-interaction, participants were asked to indicate their satisfaction with their romantic partner. One item assessed relationship satisfaction (e.g., "How satisfied were you with your relationship?"). Possible responses were on a 7-point scale (1 = *not at all*, 7 = *extremely*), with higher scores indicating more satisfaction.

2.3.6. Experience with VR

Participants were asked to indicate their previous VR experience on a 4-point scale (e.g., "Besides today, how much experience have you had with virtual reality?"; 0 = *none*, 1 = *used it once*, 2 = *used it a few times*, 3 = *I own a VR/use VR frequently*) post-interaction, with higher scores indicating more experience using VR. Most participants had some experience with VR, with only 19.4% of participants indicating no prior experience, 27.4% indicated using it once before, 39.2% indicating that they had used it a few times, and 8.1% indicated that they either owned a VR headset or used VR frequently (with 5.9% not answering the question).

2.4. Analytic Approach

To examine whether people in the novel VR condition (compared to those in the novel video condition) reported greater presence (H1) and self-expansion (H2), and to exploratorily examine the effects on boredom, closeness, and relationship satisfaction (E1–3), we conducted a series of multilevel models in which partners were nested within couples.[1] We used multilevel modeling (mlm) to test the effect of the condition on the outcomes of interest to account for the fact that our data include both partners in a relationship having a shared interaction. In these analyses, we tested whether the experimental condition (0 = *video*, 1 = *VR*, a dyadic variable given that partners are assigned to the same condition) predicted our outcomes of interest (examining each outcome individually). Then, we tested whether couples in the novel VR condition reported greater self-expansion, less boredom, and greater relationship quality post-interaction through presence (H3). To do so, we conducted a series of multilevel mediation models using the Monte Carlo Method for Assessing Mediation (MCMAM) (Selig & Preacher, 2024). Indirect effects were deemed significant if the 95% CI did not contain zero. In auxiliary analyses, we examined whether the effect of the condition on our key outcomes was moderated by relationship length, age, or previous experience with VR. This involved adding an interaction between the condition and each moderator (examined individually). If the interaction was significant, we interpreted the effects at high and low levels of the moderator. The data and syntax for all analyses reported for this paper can be found on the OSF.

2.5. Results

2.5.1. Shared Novel Experiences in VR Versus Video

Consistent with our pre-registered predictions, people who engaged in a brief novel interaction with their partner in VR ($M = 5.74$, $SD = 1.19$) reported a greater sense of presence than people in the video condition ($M = 5.31$, $SD = 1.16$; $b = 0.41$, $t(84.42) = 2.01$, $p = 0.048$, 95% CI [0.004, 0.81]). However, inconsistent with our predictions, although people in the VR condition reported higher self-expansion ($M = 5.14$, $SD = 1.30$) compared to those in the video condition ($M = 4.77$, $SD = 1.47$), the difference between the conditions was not significant ($b = 0.37$, $t(88.68) = 1.60$, $p = 0.113$, 95% CI [−0.09, 0.83]).

Next, in exploratory analyses, we examined the effect of the condition on boredom, closeness, and relationship satisfaction post-interaction. We found significant differences in condition for people's reports of relational boredom ($b = -1.03$, $t(91.14) = -4.72$, $p < 0.001$, 95% CI [−1.46, −0.60]), such that people in the VR condition reported lower boredom ($M = 1.78$, $SD = 1.04$) than people in the video condition ($M = 2.80$, $SD = 1.68$) post-interaction, but no significant differences emerged between the conditions and people's reports of closeness ($p = 0.213$) or relationship satisfaction ($p = 0.909$) post-interaction.

2.5.2. Mediation Through Presence

Next, consistent with our pre-registration, we tested whether people benefit from novel virtual experiences with their partner (compared to novel experiences over video chat) because their partner was perceived to be more present in VR (i.e., they felt more like they were with a partner). We examined whether the greater presence reported by participants in the novel VR condition would, in turn, be associated with higher self-expansion, less boredom, higher relationship satisfaction, and greater closeness. Consistent with predictions, people in the VR condition reported more presence than those in the video condition, which was, in turn, lower boredom (95% CI [−0.40, −0.004]). Although there were no direct effects on self-expansion, relationship satisfaction, and closeness, there were indirect effects via greater presence on higher self-expansion (95% CI [0.01, 0.64]), greater closeness (95% CI [0.01, 0.52]), and higher relationship satisfaction (95% CI [0.004, 0.24]) post-interaction. (See Figure 2A–D).

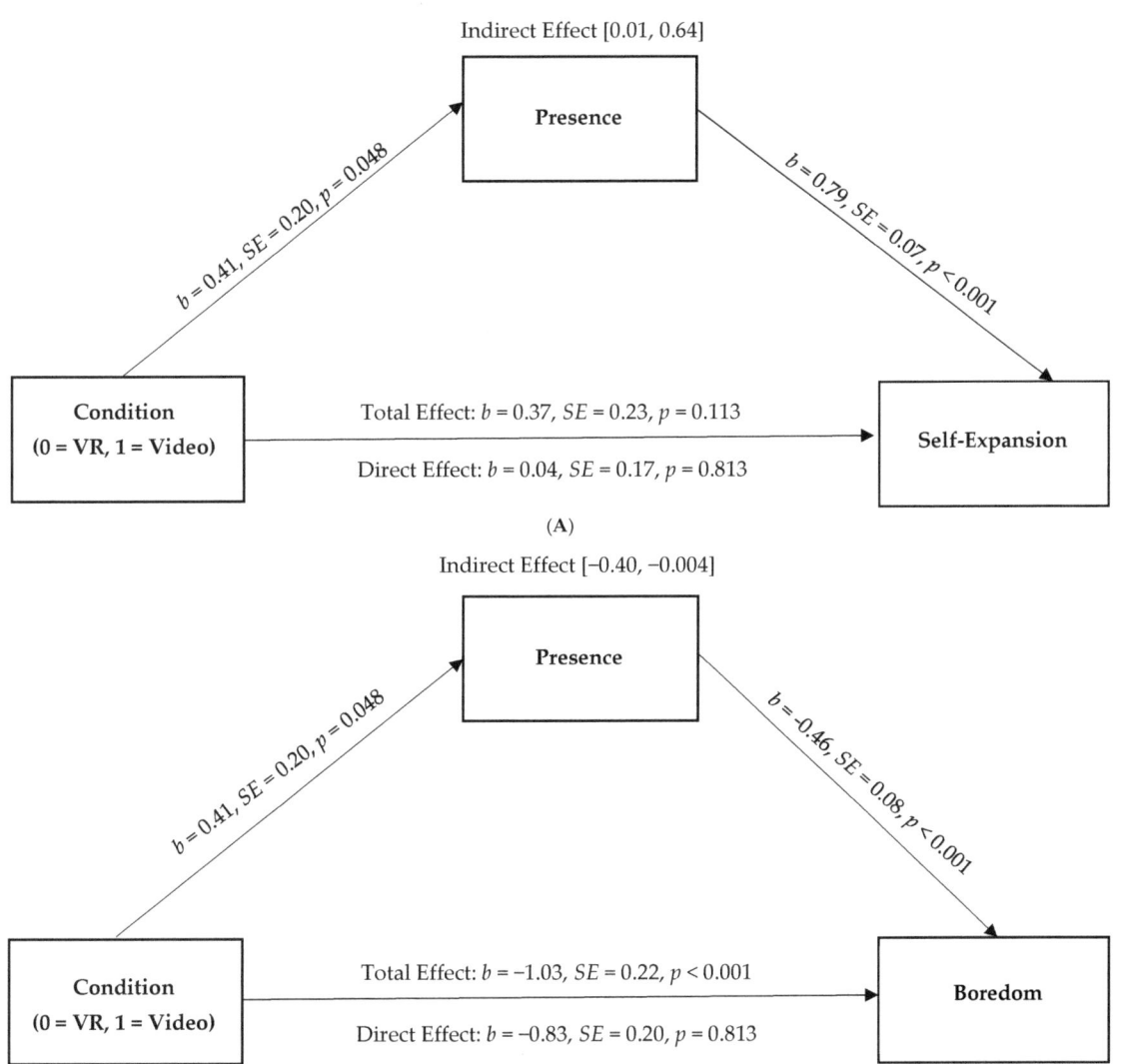

Figure 2. *Cont.*

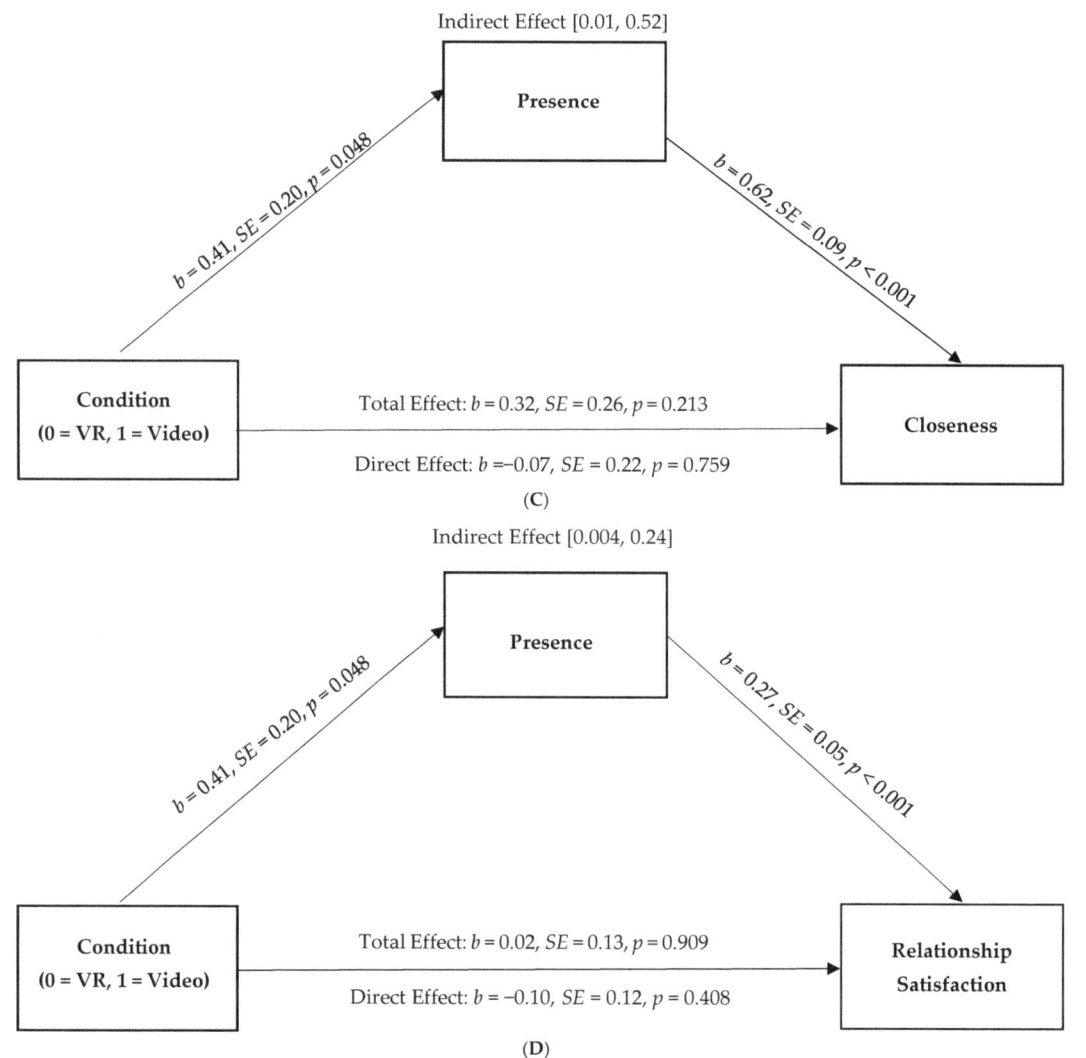

Figure 2. Perceived partner presence as a mediator of the association between condition (0 = VR, 1 = video) on reports of (**A**) self-expansion, (**B**) boredom, (**C**) closeness, and (**D**) relationship satisfaction in Study 1.

2.5.3. Considering the Role of Relationship Length, Age, and Experience with VR

In auxiliary analyses, we explored the role of relationship length, age, and experience with VR in the effect of the condition on our key outcomes. We examined each as a separate moderator. No significant differences by relationship length emerged (all $p > 0.05$). However, we found that the association between condition and closeness was moderated by age ($b = 0.23$, $t(114.92) = 3.06$, $p = 0.003$, 95% CI [0.08, 0.38]), such that older participants (+1 SD) reported greater closeness in the VR condition compared to the video condition ($b = 1.05$, $t(97.09) = 2.63$, $p = 0.010$, 95% CI [0.26, 1.84]), whereas there was no effect of the condition for younger participants (−1 SD; $b = -0.71$, $t(100.75) = -1.81$, $p = 0.073$, 95% CI [−1.50, 0.07]). Participants' age did not moderate the association between the condition and other focal variables. The effect of the condition on self-expansion was moderated by having prior experience with VR ($b = -0.53$, $t(170.11) = -2.25$, $p = 0.026$, 95% CI [-0.99, -0.06]), such that people with less experience with VR (-1 SD) reported greater self-expansion in the VR condition compared to the video condition ($b = 0.74$, $t(122.69) = 2.31$, $p = 0.022$, 95% CI [0.11, 1.37]), whereas there was no effect of the condition on reports of self-expansion among people who had more experience with VR (+1 SD; $b = -0.22$, $t(124.13) = -0.68$, $p = 0.499$, 95% CI [-0.85, 0.42]). We also found that the effect of the condition and closeness was moderated by past VR experience ($b = -0.57$, $t(168.91) = -2.18$, $p = 0.031$, 95% CI [-1.09, -0.05]), such that people with less experience with VR (-1SD) reported greater closeness in the VR condition compared to the video condition ($b = 0.73$, $t(121.05) = 2.06$, $p = 0.031$, 95% CI [0.03, 1.43]), but, there was no effect of the condition on people who had more (+ 1SD) experience with VR ($b = -0.31$, $t(122.51) = -0.87$, $p = 0.388$, 95% CI [-1.01, 0.40]).

2.6. Study 1 Discussion

The results from Study 1 suggest that people who engaged in a brief novel interaction with their partner in VR experienced a greater sense of presence than people who had a novel interaction over video. However, inconsistent with our predictions, people in the VR condition did not report greater self-expansion post-interaction. It is possible that participants' experiences in the novel VR and video condition did not result in differences in self-expansion because both experiences were "novel". However, participants reported less boredom during the VR experience compared to the video interaction with their partner. Greater presence in the VR (versus video) condition accounted for the lower boredom reported in the VR condition. There were significant indirect effects via presence on self-expansion, relationship satisfaction, and closeness, but these emerged without significant direct effects. Importantly, however, in exploratory analyses testing the role of relationship length, age, and VR experience, people in the VR condition did report greater self-expansion and closeness with their partner, but only when they had less experience with VR; there were no effects for those with more experience. Also, participants who were older reported greater closeness following the interaction in the VR versus video condition, but there was no effect for younger participants. Therefore, the VR condition may have been more novel for people with limited previous experience with VR or for those who were older, leading to stronger effects on self-expansion and closeness.

3. Study 2

Study 1 demonstrated that a VR interaction could enhance the presence of a partner (feeling like you are having a shared experience with a partner) compared to a video interaction and that perceiving a partner to be more present, in turn, was associated with higher self-expansion, less boredom, and higher relationship quality post-interaction. However, when we examined the main effects in the overall sample, people in the novel virtual condition did not differ in their reports of self-expansion from participants in the video condition. It is possible we did not find the expected main effect of the condition on self-expansion overall because both conditions involved a novel experience with a partner, or differences may exist between conditions but not captured with our current sample size (we based the sample size on a study examining VR versus video interactions among work colleagues and the effects on closeness and related outcomes might be smaller for romantic partners). As such, in our next study, we aimed to manipulate the novelty of a shared interaction rather than the communication technology and to recruit a larger sample. In Study 2, all participants interacted using VR, and we manipulated the type of interaction (novel versus mundane) to mirror previous in-lab studies of self-expansion (Aron et al., 2000). We aimed to test whether engaging in a novel and exciting activity compared to a mundane but pleasant activity with a romantic partner (both of which occurred in VR) would enhance self-expansion and, in turn, reduce boredom and enhance relationship quality. More specifically, we predicted that couples in the novel condition would report greater self-expansion (H1), less boredom, greater closeness, and greater relationship satisfaction (H2) than people in the mundane VR condition. We also predicted that higher self-expansion in the novelty versus the mundane VR condition would mediate (account for) the effect of the condition on lower boredom, greater closeness, and greater relationship satisfaction.

Results from Study 1 suggest that VR enhances feelings of presence; however, in Study 2, both conditions were in VR, and thus, we expected presence to be high and not differ across conditions. As such, in this study, we were interested in whether differences emerged among those who had a novel versus mundane experience with their romantic partner in VR. We pre-registered our predictions before data collection (see the OSF); however, we also tested a series of exploratory analyses that deviated from the pre-registered hypotheses. To start, we assessed immersion, the extent to which people feel engaged in the virtual environment and can block out the physical world, which is important for people's experiences in VR (Berkman & Akan, 2019; Cummings & Bailenson, 2016; Maymon et al., 2023). In these auxiliary analyses, we sought to account for immersion (Berkman & Akan, 2019) and examine whether the effects of interest emerged when the participant's engagement with the task was held constant. Lastly, as in Study 1, we also explored a series of auxiliary analyses to test whether the findings differed based on participants' age, relationship length, or past VR experience.

3.1. Participants

Participants were recruited through the Undergraduate Research Participant Pool (URPP) at York University. At the time of our pre-registration, no studies had tested differences between self-expansion in relationships in VR. However, a previous in-lab study compared couples' reports of relationship satisfaction after engaging in a novel and exciting versus a mundane activity in person. This study reported large effect sizes ($d = 0.93$) on relationship satisfaction (Aron et al., 2000). When we estimated an effect of $d = 0.93$ with 80% power and an alpha of 0.05 using G*Power 3.1 (Faul et al., 2009), it was estimated that we would need 40 couples (20 per condition). However, because this effect size is derived from a study in the lab (and not in VR), we wanted to estimate a more conservative, medium effect size. With a medium effect (0.5) with 80% power and 0.05 alpha, 128 couples (64 per condition) would be needed. We oversampled by approximately 10% to account for attrition, failed attention checks, or potential technical issues.

We initially recruited 159 couples ($N = 318$); however, we removed 14 couples ($N = 28$) who experienced technical issues during the study or did not follow instructions (i.e., removed headset, left virtual area). In line with our pre-registration, we removed three participants for failing the attention check to ask them to select the type of virtual activity they engaged in and one participant whose post-manipulation data were not saved. In these four cases, their partner's data was retained. Our final sample included 287 participants ($N = 142$ couples, three individuals), 128 men, 156 women, and three non-binary people. The final sample was racially diverse, though most participants identified as South Asian (25.78%) or white (24.39%). Most of the participants identified as straight/heterosexual (75.26%) and reported "seriously dating" their partners (79.09%). Participants were in established relationships with their partners of nearly two years ($M = 1.83$ years; $SD = 1.77$ years) and in their early 20s (ranging from 17 to 41, $M = 20.3$, $SD = 3.64$) on average. See Table 1 for demographic information.

3.2. Procedure

Once both partners agreed to participate in the study, they were asked to complete a 20 min online survey before attending the in-lab session. The online survey included demographic and general relationship questions, and questions about previous experiences with VR. Couples were then asked to attend an in-lab session. Once in the lab, partners were taken to separate rooms and were randomly assigned to have one of two types of interactions using VR: (1) a shared novel experience (a gondola ride in the Swiss Alps) ($N = 148$; 73 couples, two individuals) or (2) a shared mundane experience (a virtual porch which overlooked a scenic environment) ($N = 138$; 68 couples, two individuals). The interactions lasted approximately 6 min in both conditions and following the interaction, participants completed a post-manipulation survey asking about their feelings during the interaction. Partners were then reunited and debriefed.

3.3. Measures

After exposure to the experimental condition, participants were asked to respond to a series of post-manipulation questions outlined below. Table 3 shows correlations between variables within each condition, and Figure 3 reports the means across conditions.

Table 3. Correlations among focal variables in Study 2.

	1	2	3	4	5	6
Mundane VR Condition						
1. Immersion	-					
2. Self-Expansion	0.52 ***	-				
3. Boredom	−0.51 ***	−0.34 ***	-			
4. Closeness	0.23 **	0.27 ***	−0.24 **	-		
5. Relationship Sat.	0.40 ***	0.34 ***	−0.43 ***	0.38 ***	-	
6. Relationship Length	−0.20 *	−0.16	0.26 **	0.02	−0.12	-
Novel VR Condition						
1. Immersion	-					
2. Self-Expansion	0.69 ***	-				
3. Boredom	−0.51 ***	−0.50 ***	-			
4. Closeness	0.19 *	0.18 *	−0.22 **	-		
5. Relationship Sat.	0.18 *	0.26 **	−0.26 **	0.32 ***	-	
6. Relationship Length	0.03	0.05	−0.05	0.02	0.07	-

Note: *** $p < 0.001$, ** $p < 0.01$, * $p < 0.05$. Rel Sat = relationship satisfaction.

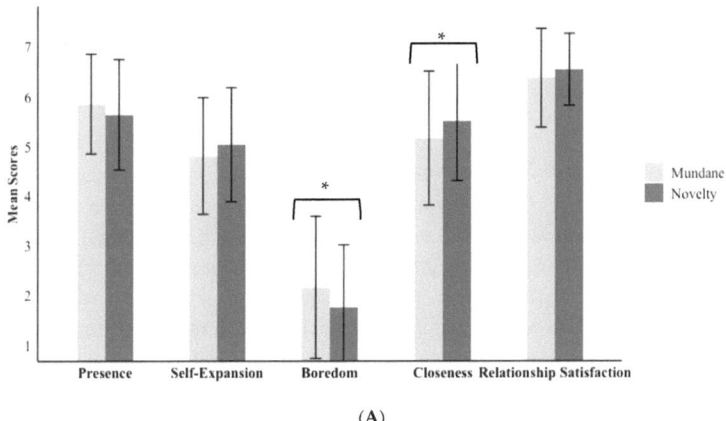

(A)

Figure 3. Cont.

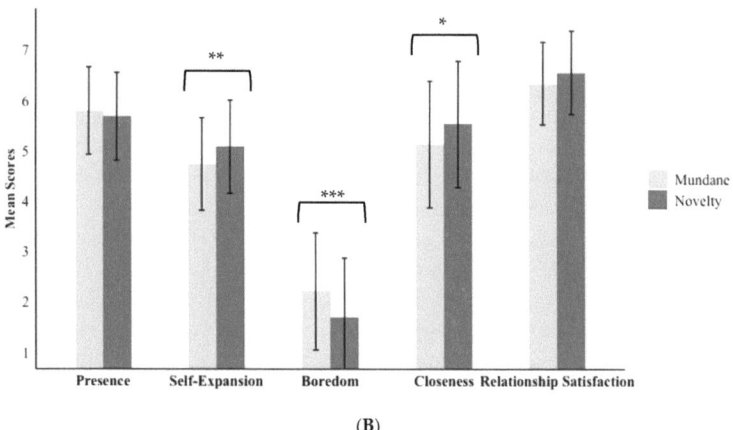

(B)

Figure 3. Descriptive statistics between conditions for Study 2 focal variables with (**A**) raw means and (**B**) adjusted means (controlling for reports of immersion). Note. The error bars represent standard deviations, and significance is denoted with *** $p < 0.001$, ** $p < 0.01$, and * $p < 0.05$.

3.3.1. Manipulation Check

Participants were asked two questions immediately after the interaction, which served as manipulation checks. The first questions read as follows: "You were asked to use virtual reality with your partner, what did you and your partner do?" with options including "Sat on a porch outside", "Went on a virtual tour of the Swiss Alps", or "Swam with sharks". The second item asked participants to indicate, "How well do the following statements characterize the virtual experience you just had with your partner"?, "dull", "exciting", "fun", and "interesting", with response options ranging from 1 (*not at all*) to 7 (*extremely*). For the first item, participants who were in the mundane condition should have selected the first option, that they "sat on a porch outside", and participants who were in the novelty condition should have selected the second option, indicating that they "went on a virtual tour of the Swiss Alps". In line with our pre-registration, participants who incorrectly identified their condition were removed from data analyses. The second set of items (ratings of the experience as "dull", "exciting", "fun", and "interesting") served as additional manipulation checks (each item examined separately). We expected participants in the novelty condition to indicate that the experience was less dull and more fun, exciting, and interesting than participants in the mundane condition.

3.3.2. Presence

Participants were asked to indicate presence using the same measure as in Study 1 (α novel = 0.78; α mundane = 0.77).

3.3.3. Immersion

Post-interaction, participants were asked to answer two questions to assess their immersion during the interaction (e.g., "During our interaction, I was immersed in the environment"; "Our interaction was realistic"). Possible responses were on a 7-point scale (1 = *not at all*, 7 = *completely*), and the items were mean aggregated, with higher scores indicating greater perceived immersion (mundane $r = 0.39$, $p < 0.001$, novel $r = 0.54$, $p < 0.001$).

3.3.4. Self-Expansion

Post-interaction, participants were asked to rate their perceptions of self-expansion with their partner during the interaction. Participants were provided the following instructions, "Thinking about the experience you and your partner just had together, answer each question according to the way you personally feel, using the following scale". Participants were then asked to rate six items that were adapted from a measure of self-expansion (Lewandowski & Aron, 2002; e.g., "To what extent did this interaction feel like a new experience?"; "Did you learn new things during your experience?"; "How much did this experience expand your sense of the kind of person you are?"). Responses were provided on a 7-point scale (1 = *not very much*, 7 = *very much*), and the items were mean aggregated, with higher scores indicating higher self-expansion (α novel = 0.85; α mundane = 0.82).

3.3.5. Boredom

Participants were asked to indicate how bored they were post-interaction using the scale employed in Study 1.

3.3.6. Closeness

Participants were asked to indicate how close they felt to their partner after the interaction using the same item (i.e., the IOS) from Study 1 (Aron et al., 1992).

3.3.7. Relationship Satisfaction

After the interaction, participants were asked to indicate their satisfaction with their partner using the same item as in Study 1.

3.3.8. Experience with VR

Participants were asked to indicate their previous VR experience on a 4-point scale, as in Study 1. Many participants had some experience with VR, though, in Study 2, 36.6% of participants indicated no prior experience, 27.5% indicated using it once before, 30% indicated that they had used it a few times, and 5.6% indicated that they either owned a VR headset or used VR frequently (with one person, 0.3%, not answering the question).

3.4. Analytic Approach

As in Study 1, to examine whether people in the novel condition (compared to those in the mundane condition) reported greater self-expansion (H1), lower boredom, greater closeness, and relationship satisfaction (H2), we conducted a series of multilevel models with partners nested within couples. We tested whether the experimental condition (0 = mundane, 1 = novel) predicted our variables of interest. We then examined whether individuals in the novel VR condition reported less boredom and greater relationship quality post-interaction through self-expansion (H3). As in Study 1, to test our mediation models, we conducted a series of multilevel mediation models using the Monte Carlo Method for Assessing Mediation (MCMAM) (Selig & Preacher, 2024). We tested whether there were significant indirect effects, with indirect effects being deemed significant if the 95% CI did not contain zero in the analyses controlling for immersion. To account for individual differences in immersion, we controlled for the participant's reports of immersion in the analyses. Importantly, reports of immersion did not differ by condition. That is, in an exploratory analysis, we found that reports of immersion did not differ in the novel ($M = 5.22$, $SD = 1.24$) and mundane ($M = 5.42$, $SD = 1.10$) conditions ($p = 0.188$). We conducted additional auxiliary exploratory analyses as in Study 1 to examine whether age, relationship length, or experience with VR moderated the effects of interest. The data and syntax needed to reproduce the results can be found on the OSF.

3.5. Results

3.5.1. Manipulation Check

As expected, participants in the novelty condition reported a less dull (novel $M = 1.70$, $SD = 1.26$, mundane $M = 2.04$, $SD = 1.45$; $b = -0.35$, $SE = 0.17$, $t(143.29) = -2.08$, $p = 0.039$, CI $[-0.68, -0.02]$) and marginally more exciting experience than those in the mundane condition (novel $M = 5.62$, $SD = 1.26$, mundane $M = 5.28$, $SD = 1.47$; $b = 0.35$, $SE = 0.18$, $t(142.93) = 1.90$, $p = 0.059$, CI $[-0.01, 0.70]$). However, participants in the novel and mundane conditions did not differ in their reports of how fun ($b = 0.05$, $SE = 0.16$, $t(143.03) = 0.32$, $p = 0.747$, CI $[-0.27, 0.37]$) or interesting the experience was ($b = -0.06$, $SE = 0.13$, $t(143.36) = -0.49$, $p = 0.626$, CI $[-0.32, 0.19]$). Overall, participants found both conditions exciting, fun, interesting, and not dull, and when differences did emerge, they were small or marginal.

3.5.2. The Effect of Novel Versus Mundane Virtual Experiences

As expected, participants in the novel ($M = 5.64$, $SD = 1.11$) and mundane conditions ($M = 5.86$, $SD = 1.00$) did not differ in their reports of perceived presence with their partner ($b = -0.22$, $SE = 0.14$, $t(143.31) = -1.61$, $p = 0.109$, 95% CI $[-0.49, 0.05]$, given that both interactions were in VR. We then tested whether people in the novel condition reported more self-expansion than people in the mundane condition. Although participants in the novel condition did report higher self-expansion ($M = 5.03$, $SD = 1.15$) than those in the mundane condition ($M = 4.81$, $SD = 1.17$), differences between the conditions were not significant ($b = 0.23$, $SE = 0.15$, $t(143.24) = 1.48$, $p = 0.140$). However, consistent with our pre-registered predictions, people in the novel condition ($M = 1.76$, $SD = 2.16$) reported less boredom compared to those in the mundane condition ($M = 2.16$, $SD = 1.43$; $b = -0.40$, $SE = 0.18$, $t(143.27) = -2.25$, $p = 0.026$). Also, in line with our predictions, people in the novel condition ($M = 5.51$, $SD = 1.21$) reported greater closeness with their partner post-interaction compared to those in the mundane condition ($M = 5.16$, $SD = 1.35$; $b = 0.35$, $SE = 0.17$, $t(144.01) = 2.03$, $p = 0.044$). However, contrary to our predictions, there were no significant differences between groups on relationship satisfaction ($b = 0.17$, $SE = 0.12$, $t(142.4) = 1.37$, $p = 0.17$). Given that the condition did not significantly predict differences in self-expansion, we did not test indirect effects.

3.5.3. Considering the Role of Immersion

In a series of exploratory analyses, we assessed the predicted associations controlling for participants' reports of immersion during their virtual experience. Controlling for immersion, participants in the novel ($M = 5.69$ $SE = 0.07$) and mundane conditions ($M = 5.80$, $SE = 0.07$) did not differ in their reports of perceived presence with their partner ($b = -0.12$, $SE = 0.11$, $t(143.69) = -1.06$, $p = 0.290$, 95% CI $[-0.33, 0.10]$), as expected. However, effects did emerge for self-expansion, with participants in the novel virtual condition ($M = 5.09$, $SE = 0.08$) reporting more self-expansion after the interaction than people in the mundane condition ($M = 4.74$, $SE = 0.08$; $b = 0.35$, $SE = 0.12$, $t(143.58) = 2.94$, $p = 0.004$, 95% CI $[0.11, 0.58]$). In addition, controlling for immersion, people in the novel condition ($M = 1.71$, $SE = 0.10$) reported less boredom than people in the mundane condition ($M = 2.22$, $SE = 0.10$; $b = -0.51$, $SE = 0.14$, $t(141.78) = -3.55$, $p < 0.001$, 95% CI $[-0.80, -0.23]$). Participants in the novel condition ($M = 5.54$, $SE = 0.10$) also reported more closeness than those in the mundane condition ($M = 5.14$, $SE = 0.11$; $b = 0.39$, $SE = 0.17$, $t(143.67) = 2.33$, $p = 0.021$, 95% CI $[0.06, 0.73]$). Finally, although participants in the novel condition reported greater relationship satisfaction ($M = 6.56$, $SE = 0.07$) compared to those in the mundane condition ($M = 6.35$, $SE = 0.07$), the effect was not significant ($b = 0.21$, $SE = 0.12$, $t(143.12) = 1.80$,

$p = 0.075$, 95% CI [−0.02, 0.44]), with both groups reporting high levels of relationship satisfaction (see Figure 3).

Lastly, we examined the mediation effects controlling for participant's reports of immersion in the analyses. Results suggest that there were significant indirect effects of the condition on boredom (95% CI [−0.16, −0.02]), closeness (95% CI [0.001, 0.13]), and relationship satisfaction (95% CI [0.01, 0.11]) post-interaction through self-expansion (see Figure 4A–C). Although the effects are small, and the association between the condition and relationship satisfaction was not significant, this pattern of results suggests that novel (vs. mundane) experiences in VR can influence reports of self-expansion and have downstream effects on people's reports of boredom, closeness, and satisfaction with their partners when accounting for immersion.

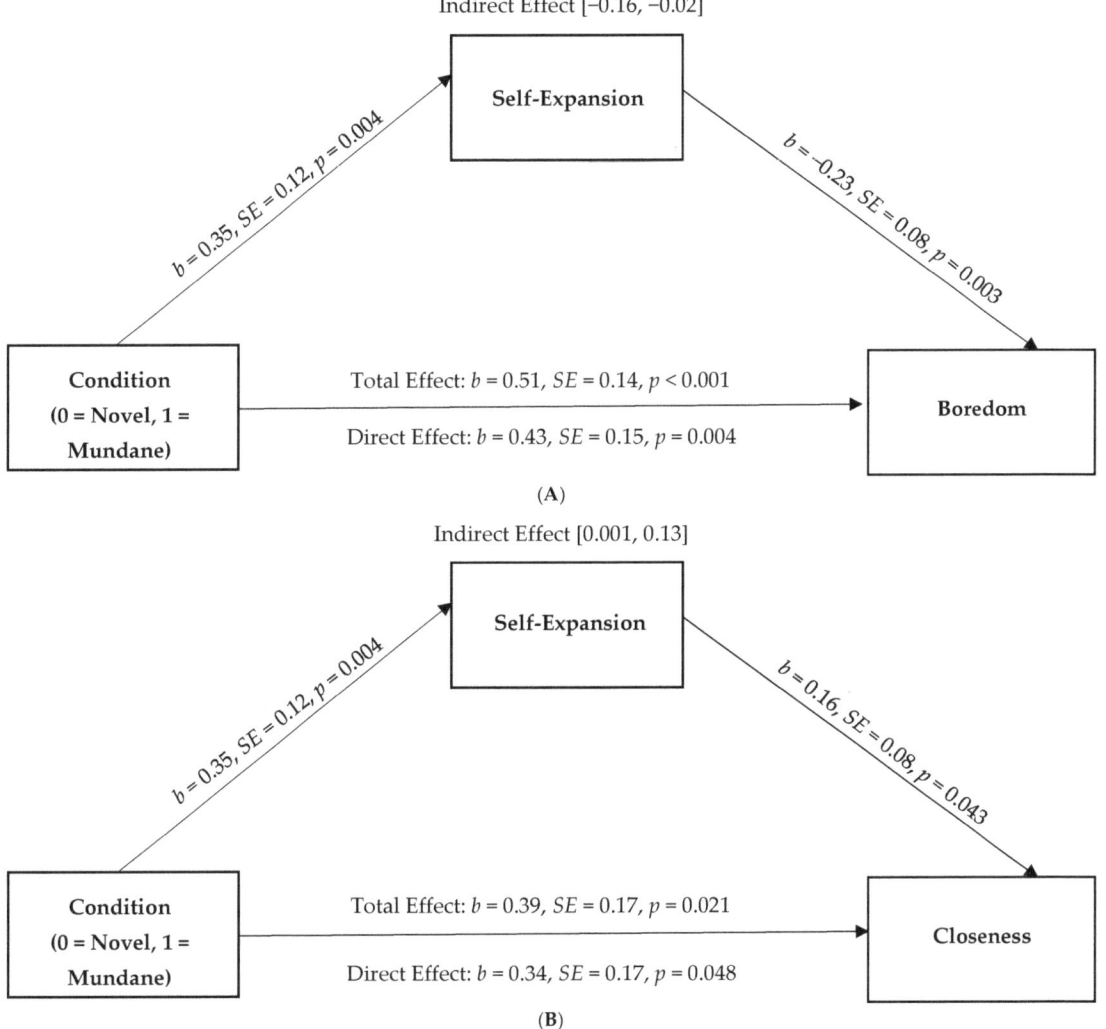

Figure 4. Cont.

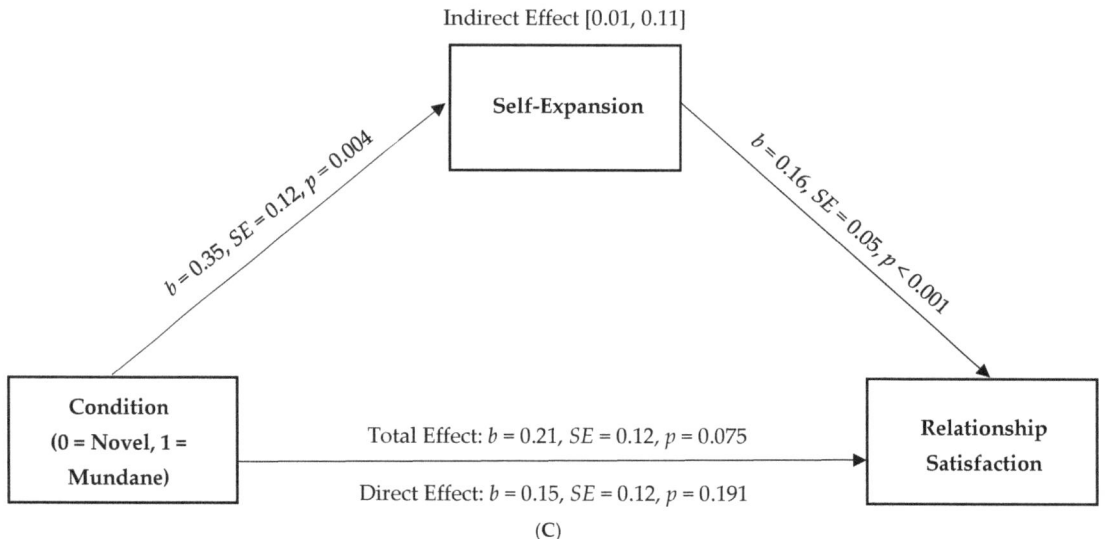

Figure 4. Self-expansion as a mediator of the association between the condition (0 = novel, 1 = mundane) on reports of (**A**) boredom, (**B**) closeness, and (**C**) relationship satisfaction controlling for immersion.

3.5.4. Considering the Role of Relationship Length, Age, and Experience with VR

We conducted auxiliary analyses to test whether people in the novel (compared to the mundane) virtual experience differed on key demographics (e.g., age, relationship length) or experience with VR. We found no significant differences between conditions (in all cases, $p > 0.05$). Despite this, and consistent with Study 1, we explored if any of the effects differed based on participants' age, length of the relationship, or past VR experience via moderation analyses. No significant interactions for relationship length, age, or experience with VR emerged (all $p > 0.05$).

3.6. Study 2 Discussion

Contrary to our hypotheses, differences did not emerge across conditions for self-expansion or relationship satisfaction. However, people in the novel VR condition reported lower boredom and greater closeness post-interaction compared to those in mundane VR condition. In exploratory analyses accounting for immersion (i.e., the extent to which they were engaged in the virtual environment), people in the novel condition reported greater self-expansion than those in the mundane condition and, in turn, lower boredom and greater relationship quality post-interaction. There were no significant differences based on relationship length, age, or previous experience with VR. The findings suggest challenges of manipulating virtual self-expanding experiences, as VR experiences (even more mundane ones) may be novel for most people, and hint that future research designing manipulations using VR should consider the role of immersion.

4. General Discussion

Self-expansion, which can be facilitated through shared novel activities in romantic relationships, is associated with lower boredom and greater relationship quality among romantic partners (Aron & Aron, 1996, 1997; Aron et al., 2022). However, in the globalized, modern world, many couples will experience periods in which they are apart (e.g., pursuing educational and vocational opportunities), and shared novel activities might be limited, thus hindering opportunities for couples to stay connected. Two dyadic experimental studies examined whether VR could simulate shared virtual couple activities. In Study 1, participants who engaged in a brief, novel virtual interaction with their partner (compared to participants who engaged in a brief, novel video interaction) experienced greater presence (i.e., felt they had a shared experience with their partner) and reported less boredom. Participants in the novel VR condition did not differ in their reports of self-expansion, relationship satisfaction, or closeness from those in the video condition. However, these effects worked indirectly through a greater sense of presence with a partner in the VR (versus) condition. In Study 2, couples engaged in either a novel and exciting or mundane experience in VR. Results were mixed. Contrary to our predictions, there were no differences between the condition on self-expansion or relationship satisfaction. However, participants in the novel VR condition reported less boredom and greater closeness post-interaction than those in the virtual mundane condition. In auxiliary analyses, we tested the role of immersion—the extent to which people feel engaged in the virtual environment and can block out the physical world. Past research demonstrates that there are individual differences in the extent to which people can block out the physical world and engage with a virtual world and this can be important for people's experiences in VR (Berkman & Akan, 2019; Cummings & Bailenson, 2016; Maymon et al., 2023). Accounting for immersion in the virtual world, people in the novel VR condition reported greater self-expansion, less boredom, and greater closeness than those in the mundane VR condition. Additionally, holding immersion constant, results suggest that people who had a novel virtual interaction with their partner reported greater self-expansion and greater self-expansion was, in turn, associated with less boredom, greater closeness, and higher relationship satisfaction (although there were no main effects on relationship satisfaction). In Study 1, results suggested that people who were older and had less experience using VR benefitted more from novel interactions in VR than those who were younger or had more VR experience. There were no differences in Study 2 based on age or VR experience and no differences across studies for relationship duration.

Examining Whether VR Can Enhance Relational Self-Expansion

Extending previous research examining self-expansion in relationships, the results from the current research demonstrate that shared novel and exciting activities in VR can provide opportunities for reducing boredom in romantic relationships. These findings are consistent with research showing that couples who engage in novel and exciting experiences together report less boredom (Aron et al., 2022). Contrary to our predictions and past research on self-expansion theory, the effects of novel virtual experiences on reports of self-expansion and relationship quality compared to novel video experiences (Study 1) or mundane virtual experiences (Study 2) were not significant in most instances (e.g., direct effects did not emerge, with the exception to Study 2, when immersion was controlled for). Thus, despite designing studies premised on self-expansion theory, the findings suggest that novel virtual experiences may help reduce boredom, although results for self-expansion and relationship quality are less promising.

The current research extends past research on self-expansion in relationships by examining novel experiences in VR. Most of the past research has focused on shared, in-person, novel and exciting activities among couples. Here, we tested whether self-expansion can be experienced virtually and have downstream consequences for relationship quality. The findings were mixed. The findings from Study 1 suggests VR has the potential (compared to video interactions) to simulate presence between partners, but there were no differences in self-expansion. Therefore, VR might provide new opportunities for partners to connect (i.e., feel like they are together) when in different geographical locations or when separated for extended periods of time. Also, given the range of activities available in VR (the full range was not tested in the current study), the findings from Study 2 suggest that some shared virtual activities (i.e., novel experiences such as a virtual gondola ride over the Swiss Alps) can foster closeness and reduce boredom compared to other virtual interaction (i.e., familiar scenery such as sitting on a virtual porch). However, more work is needed to understand how these experiences can promote self-expansion and further boost relationship quality.

The current research also has implications for researchers looking for novel ways to manipulate shared couples' experiences in the lab. Past research on shared self-expansion in relationships has often focused on assessing naturalistic self-expanding experiences in couples' daily lives (Coulter & Malouff, 2013; Harasymchuk et al., 2021; Muise et al., 2019) or manipulating novel (versus mundane) activities in the lab (Aron et al., 2000), the motivation to self-expand (Dys-Steenbergen et al., 2016), or need for self-expansion (Tsapelas et al., 2020). However, although more work is needed, VR presents an opportunity to develop experimental manipulations of shared activities that can occur in the lab but feel more realistic. Indeed, this research provides some initial evidence that VR technology can simulate the presence of a partner, unlike video chat, which leads to several possibilities for simulating or manipulating shared interactions or emotional experiences.

While the findings from these studies provide initial support for the promise of virtual reality for simulating a romantic partner's presence (based on Study 1) and reducing boredom (based on Studies 1–2), more work is needed. More specifically, many of the effects across studies were small, and in some instances, indirect effects emerged in the absence of main effects. For instance, in Study 1, the main effect of the condition was only significant for reports of presence and boredom, not for reports of self-expansion, closeness, or relationship satisfaction post-interaction. Furthermore, there was no main effect on relationship satisfaction across both studies, despite past research showing a strong association between self-expansion and relationship satisfaction (Aron et al., 2022). The most consistent, strongest effect across studies was that the novel VR condition was associated with less boredom than the novel video condition (Study 1) and the mundane VR condition (Study 2). Although the effects of the condition on relationship quality did not emerge, it is possible that it was difficult to enhance relationship satisfaction because, in the current studies, couples were already highly satisfied; they did not have much room to grow. Future research might target more diverse samples and aim to refine the manipulations of shared experiences in VR.

Overall, these initial studies taught us some helpful lessons about using VR to manipulate self-expansion or other relationship constructs. From the results of Study 1, VR is able to simulate presence more than video interactions with a partner, which is important and suggests the ability to simulate shared couple activities or interactions in VR. Past research has shown that people report more presence (like they are really in the environment) in VR compared to other commonly used technologies (Baym et al., 2004; Froese et al., 2014; Meuleman & Rudrauf, 2018), but to our knowledge, the current research is the first to demonstrate participants' perceptions of the presence of a romantic partner in VR.

It is also noteworthy that past research (Berkman & Akan, 2019; Howard et al., 2018; Maymon et al., 2023) has consistently demonstrated individual differences in people's immersion in VR experiences, which could be important to account for in future research. More specifically, in Study 2, we found that many of the results of interest were nonsignificant when examined independently, though when we controlled for immersion, differences emerged across the groups, as discussed above. VR is widely considered to be more immersive than other technologies, allowing users to feel deeply "present" within a virtual environment, which in turn can lead to a stronger ability to induce emotions, both positive and negative, compared to traditional screens or other mediums (Li et al.,

2022; Meuleman & Rudrauf, 2018; Riva et al., 2007). However, people differ in how much they engage with virtual environments and suspend their attention to the physical world (Berkman & Akan, 2019). Therefore, unique to VR studies, interactions should be designed with presence and immersion in mind, and these constructs should be assessed in VR research examining relational processes in VR.

5. Limitations and Future Direction

Across two experimental lab studies examining novel and exciting virtual interactions among romantic couples, it seems possible to enhance people's perceptions of their partner's presence by having them engage in novel virtual experiences (as seen in Study 1). Additionally, the finding from Study 2 suggests that people who engaged in a novel virtual experience with their partner did not report greater self-expansion unless immersion was controlled. However, when immersion was controlled for, people reported greater self-expansion and, in turn, reported lower boredom and higher levels of closeness and satisfaction compared to people who had a mundane virtual experience with their partner (Study 2). Importantly, in both studies, reports of boredom and relationship quality were assessed after one brief interaction in the lab, and we did not compare virtual experiences to in-person novel experiences. Future work could consider how couples might use VR outside of a lab environment and compare experiences in VR to in-person experiences. As such, using more ecologically valid methods (i.e., having geographically distant couples communicate with VR versus other technologies) could provide more insight into the potential uses of VR for connection with close others.

It is also important to note that the current studies included relatively homogenous samples of mostly mixed-sex, college-aged couples. Although the sample was racially diverse, participants were relatively young, and many were in the early stages of their relationship (e.g., on average, less than three years together). Past research shows that although opportunities for self-expansion are heightened in the early stages of relationships (Aron et al., 2022), the association between self-expansion and relationship quality can be stronger for couples in longer relationships (Muise et al., 2019). In the current studies, exploratory analyses indicate that the effects for reports of closeness differed based on age (e.g., an association between condition and closeness emerged among older but not younger participants in Study 1 only). Differences did not arise based on relationship length, although there was insufficient diversity in relationship length (as well as a restricted age range). We also could not adequately test whether the association between virtual self-expansion and reports of boredom and relationship quality were widely generalizable (e.g., across diverse sexual and relationship orientations). Thus, these findings should only be generalized to a heterosexual, college-aged sample of couples in relatively short-term relationships. Future research would benefit from examining the effects among a more diverse and representative sample and across a wider age and relationship length range, as some of the auxiliary analyses suggested that differences may emerge among those who are older or who have been with their partner for more time.

Finally, a practical consideration of this work is finding appropriate stimuli to manipulate shared novel activities. We used an existing application (i.e., Alcove) and piloted different experiences (mostly related to travel) from the options. At the time that this research was being conducted (2022–2023), Alcove was one of the main options for multiplayer VR applications that would allow people to have a shared experience with an interaction partner while restricting access to others. In future work, researchers could program their own stimuli to control the interaction's specific features. For example, in a recent study of individuals, the researchers designed a manipulation to induce fear in which participants walked along a plank in the lab while in a VR headset. In the fear group, participants were 80 stories high. In contrast, in the control group, they were at ground level (El Basbasse et al., 2023). This is an excellent example of how VR can be used to conduct ecologically valid experiments and successfully induce emotions. Moving forward, there are many exciting directions to pursue, but related to the current study and thinking about dyadic research in VR, the early research examining the misattribution of arousal (e.g., when people mistakenly attribute their physiological arousal to an interaction partner on a scary bridge versus a safe bridge) could be replicated using virtual reality with a similar design to the fear manipulation.

6. Concluding Remarks

In the globalized, modern world, where couples spend less time with each other and are more likely to live apart than in past generations, finding ways for couples to stay connected is more important than ever. Based on the findings from Study 1, engaging in novel, virtual interactions with a romantic partner (compared to video interaction) simulated greater partner presence, which, in turn, was associated with higher reports of self-expansion, less boredom, and higher relationship quality (e.g., relationship satisfaction and closeness) post-interaction. Furthermore, across the two experimental studies, we found that engaging in a novel virtual interaction was consistently associated with lower reports of boredom, and was, at times, associated with greater closeness (e.g., Study 2). However, contrary to our predictions, engaging in novel virtual experiences with a partner was not associated with reports of self-expansion or relationship satisfaction in either study. For example, in Study 2, in which we compared mundane to novel virtual interactions, we found no association between condition and self-expansion, though when we controlled for reports of immersion, this effect became significant, and self-expansion was, in turn, associated with lower boredom and greater relationship quality. According to this research, while virtual novel experiences with a romantic partner may help partners feel like they are in each other's presence and protect against boredom, the condition has limited effects on self-expansion and relationship quality. This suggests that research examining the effects of VR on relationships should carefully consider the role of presence and immersion in the study design and the effects. Overall, this research supports the idea that VR might offer people new opportunities to engage in shared activities with close others and raises some promising directions for future research using VR to manipulate shared experiences. That said, more work is needed to understand when and under what conditions virtual experiences can promote self-expansion and bolster the relationship quality among romantic partners.

Author Contributions: R.N.B. and A.M. conceptualized the studies and methodology. R.N.B. conducted the analyses, A.M. verified the results, and A.S. assisted with data visualization. R.N.B. and A.M. acquired funding for the study, and all authors trained research assistants to collect data and follow the study's procedures. R.N.B. drafted the initial manuscript and created the necessary files to ensure data access via the OSF, with A.M. providing feedback along the way. All authors have read and agreed to the published version of the manuscript.

Funding: This research was supported by the Insight Development Grant (awarded to Amy Muise and Rhonda Balzarini), a Mitacs Elevate Grant (awarded to Rhonda Balzarini and Amy Muise), a Canadian Foundation for Innovation Grant, and a York Research Chair award granted to Amy Muise.

Institutional Review Board Statement: The study was conducted in accordance with the Declaration of Helsinki, and approved by the Institutional Review Board of York University (#2020-078, approved on 5 March 2021) and Texas State University (#7972, approved on 31 December 2023).

Informed Consent Statement: Informed consent was obtained from all subjects involved in this study.

Data Availability Statement: Study 1 and Study 2 were pre-registered on the Open Science Framework (OSF). We have also provided our anonymized data and syntax on the OSF. As this paper is under review, the data component is currently private, though we are happy to grant access to it upon request. We are committed to making all these components public with the final published paper to increase transparency and reliability and facilitate the replicability of the current findings.

Acknowledgments: We want to thank Heesoo Choi, Joshua Coignet, Oscar Fumero Gonzalez, Madison Green, Danielle Fitzpatrick, Jordan Frank, McKenna Hildebrandt, Olivia Honest, Chantelle Ivanski, Shahmir Khan, Evan Nares, Megan Nguyen, Nathan Smith, Olivia Smith, and Faith Swanson for their assistance in conducting the research.

Conflicts of Interest: The authors declare no conflicts of interest.

Note

[1] In the pre-registration for Studies 1–2, we indicated that regression analyses would be used for the analyses. However, as the data comprise romantic couples, we modified the approach to use mlms instead, as this analytic strategy accounts for the interdependence among partners. Results for regression analyses overlap substantially with the mlm analyses.

References

Amato, P. R., Booth, A., Johnson, D. R., & Rogers, S. J. (2007). *Alone together: How marriage in America is changing*. Harvard University Press.

Amato, P. R., & Hayes, L. N. (2013). 'Alone together' marriages and 'living apart together' relationships. In *Contemporary issues in family studies* (pp. 31–45). John Wiley & Sons.

Aron, A., & Aron, E. N. (1996). Self and self-expansion in relationships. In *Knowledge structures in close relationships: A social psychological approach* (1st ed., pp. 325–344). Psychology Press.

Aron, A., & Aron, E. N. (1997). Self-expansion motivation and including other in the self. In S. Duck (Ed.), *Handbook of personal relationships: Theory, research and interventions* (2nd ed., pp. 251–270). John Wiley & Sons.

Aron, A., Aron, E. N., & Smollan, D. (1992). Inclusion of the other in the self scale and the structure of interpersonal closeness. *Journal of Personality and Social Psychology*, 63(4), 596–612. [CrossRef]

Aron, A., Lewandowski, G., Branand, B., Mashek, D., & Aron, E. (2022). Self-expansion motivation and inclusion of others in self: An updated review. *Journal of Social and Personal Relationships*, 39(12), 3821–3852. [CrossRef]

Aron, A., Norman, C. C., Aron, E. N., McKenna, C., & Heyman, R. E. (2000). Couples' shared participation in novel and arousing activities and experienced relationship quality. *Journal of Personality and Social Psychology*, 78(2), 273–284. [CrossRef] [PubMed]

Baym, N. K., Zhang, Y. B., & Lin, M. C. (2004). Social interactions across media: Interpersonal communication on the internet, telephone and face-to-face. *New Media and Society*, 6(3), 299–318.

Berkman, M. I., & Akan, E. (2019). Presence and immersion in virtual reality. In *Encyclopedia of computer graphics and games* (pp. 1461–1470). Springer International Publishing.

Biocca, F., & Harms, C. (2024). *Networked minds social presence inventory* (Version 1.2). Michigan State University. Available online: http://cogprints.org/6742/ (accessed on 24 December 2024).

Campbell, A. G., Holz, T., Cosgrove, J., Harlick, M., & O'Sullivan, T. (2020). Uses of virtual reality for communication in financial services: A case study on comparing different telepresence interfaces: Virtual reality compared to video conferencing. In K. Arai, & R. Bhatia (Eds.), *Advances in information and communication. FICC 2019. Lecture notes in networks and systems* (Vol. 69). Springer.

Coulter, K., & Malouff, J. M. (2013). Effects of an intervention designed to enhance romantic relationship excitement: A randomized-control trial. *Couple and Family Psychology: Research and Practice*, 2(1), 33–34. [CrossRef]

Cummings, J. J., & Bailenson, J. N. (2016). How immersive is enough? A meta-analysis of the effect of immersive technology on user presence. *Media Psychology*, 19(2), 272–309. [CrossRef]

Dew, J. (2009). Has the marital time cost of parenting changed over time? *Social Forces*, 88(2), 519–542. [CrossRef]

Digital in the Round. (2024). *Virtual reality statistics*. Available online: https://digitalintheround.com/virtual-reality-statistics/ (accessed on 24 December 2024).

Dys-Steenbergen, O., Wright, S. C., & Aron, A. (2016). Self-expansion motivation improves cross-group interactions and enhances self-growth. *Group Processes and Intergroup Relations*, 19(1), 60–71. [CrossRef]

El Basbasse, Y., Packheiser, J., Peterburs, J., Maymon, C., Güntürkün, O., Grimshaw, G., & Ocklenburg, S. (2023). Walk the plank! Using mobile electroencephalography to investigate emotional lateralization of immersive fear in virtual reality. *Royal Society Open Science*, 10(5), 221239. [CrossRef] [PubMed]

Faul, F., Erdfelder, E., Buchner, A., & Lang, A.-G. (2009). Statistical power analyses using G*Power 3.1: Tests for correlation and regression analyses. *Behavior Research Methods, 41*, 1149–1160. [CrossRef] [PubMed]

Flood, S. M., & Genadek, K. R. (2016). Time for each other: Work and family constraints among couples. *Journal of Marriage and Family, 78*(1), 142–164. [CrossRef] [PubMed]

Froese, T., Iizuka, H., & Ikegami, T. (2014). Embodied social interaction constitutes social cognition in pairs of humans: A minimalist virtual reality experiment. *Scientific Reports, 4*(1), 3672. [CrossRef]

Hammonds, J. R., Ribarsky, E., & Soares, G. (2020). Attached and apart: Attachment styles and self-disclosure in long-distance romantic relationships. *Journal of Relationships Research, 11*, e10. [CrossRef]

Harasymchuk, C., Walker, D. L., Muise, A., & Impett, E. A. (2021). Planning date nights that promote closeness: The roles of relationship goals and self-expansion. *Journal of Social and Personal Relationships, 38*(5), 1692–1709. [CrossRef] [PubMed]

Himes, T. (2024). *Virtual reality and the co-regulation of stress in romantic relationships* [Master's thesis, Texas State University].

Holmes, M. (2010). Intimacy, distance relationships and emotional care. *Sociological and Anthropological Research, 41*(41-1), 105–123. [CrossRef]

Howard, S., Serpanchy, K., & Lewin, K. (2018). Virtual reality content for higher education curriculum. In *VALA2018 proceedings: 19th biennial conference and exhibition* (pp. 1–15). VALA-Libraries, Technology and the Future Inc.

Inozu, M., Celikcan, U., Akin, B., & Cicek, N. M. (2020). The use of virtual reality (VR) exposure for reducing contamination fear and disgust: Can VR be an effective alternative exposure technique to in vivo? *Journal of Obsessive-Compulsive and Related Disorders, 25*, 100518. [CrossRef]

Jaremka, L. M., Sunami, N., & Nadzan, M. A. (2017). Eating moderates the link between body mass index and perceived social connection. *Appetite, 112*, 124–132. [CrossRef] [PubMed]

Ji, J. L., Heyes, S. B., MacLeod, C., & Holmes, E. A. (2016). Emotional mental imagery as simulation of reality: Fear and beyond—A tribute to Peter Lang. *Behavior Therapy, 47*(5), 702–719. [CrossRef] [PubMed]

Kaufman-Parks, A. M., Longmore, M. A., Manning, W. D., & Giordano, P. C. (2023). The influence of peers, romantic partners, and families on emerging adults' sexual behavior. *Archives of Sexual Behavior, 52*(4), 1561–1573. [CrossRef] [PubMed]

Koetsier, J. (2018). *VR needs more social: 77% of virtual reality users want more social engagement*. Forbes. Available online: https://www.forbes.com/sites/johnkoetsier/2018/04/30/virtual-reality-77-of-vr-users-want-more-social-engagement-67-use-weekly-28-use-daily/ (accessed on 24 December 2024).

Lewandowski, G. W., & Aron, A. (2002, February 20–25). *The self-expansion scale: Construction and validation*. Third Annual Meeting of the Society of Personality and Social Psychology (Vol. 1,), Savannah, GA, USA.

Li, M., Pan, J., Gao, Y., Shen, Y., Luo, F., Dai, J., & Qin, H. (2022). Neurophysiological and subjective analysis of VR emotion induction paradigm. *IEEE Transactions on Visualization and Computer Graphics, 28*(11), 3832–3842. [CrossRef] [PubMed]

Lin, Y. (2024). *10 virtual reality statistics every marketer should know in 2023*. Oberlo. Available online: https://www.oberlo.com/blog/virtual-reality-statistics (accessed on 24 December 2024).

Marques, A. J., Gomes Veloso, P., Araújo, M., de Almeida, R. S., Correia, A., Pereira, J., & Silva, C. F. (2022). Impact of a virtual reality-based simulation on empathy and attitudes toward schizophrenia. *Frontiers in Psychology, 13*, 814984. [CrossRef]

Maymon, C., Wu, Y. C., & Grimshaw, G. (2023). The promises and pitfalls of virtual reality. *Current Topics in Behavioral Neurosciences, 65*(3), 3–23. [PubMed]

Meuleman, B., & Rudrauf, D. (2018). Induction and profiling of strong multi-componential emotions in virtual reality. *IEEE Transactions on Visualization and Computer Graphics, 12*(1), 189–202. [CrossRef]

Muise, A., Harasymchuk, C., Day, L. C., Bacev-Giles, C., Gere, J., & Impett, E. A. (2019). Broadening your horizons: Self-expanding activities promote desire and satisfaction in established romantic relationships. *Journal of Personality and Social Psychology, 116*(2), 237–258. [CrossRef] [PubMed]

Ogolsky, B. G., Monk, J. K., Rice, T. M., Theisen, J. C., & Maniotes, C. R. (2017). Relationship maintenance: A review of research on romantic relationships. *Journal of Family Theory and Review, 9*(3), 275–306. [CrossRef]

Reissman, C., Aron, A., & Bergen, M. R. (1993). Shared activities and marital satisfaction: Causal direction and self-expansion versus boredom. *Journal of Social and Personal Relationships, 10*(2), 243–254. [CrossRef]

Riva, G., Mantovani, F., Capideville, C. S., Preziosa, A., Morganti, F., Villani, D., & Alcañiz, M. (2007). Affective interactions using virtual reality: The link between presence and emotions. *Cyberpsychology and Behavior, 10*(1), 45–56. [CrossRef]

Rogge, R. D., Cobb, R. J., Lawrence, E., Johnson, M. D., & Bradbury, T. N. (2013). Is skills training necessary for the primary prevention of marital distress and dissolution? A 3-year experimental study of three interventions. *Journal of Consulting and Clinical Psychology, 81*(6), 949–961. [CrossRef] [PubMed]

Sacks, G. (2024). *6 VR & AR statistics: Shaping the future of augmented reality with data*. NewsGenApps. Available online: https://www.newgenapps.com/blog/6-vr-and-ar-statistics-shaping-the-future-of-augmented-reality-with-data (accessed on 24 December 2024).

Sanchez-Vives, M. V., & Slater, M. (2005). From presence to consciousness through virtual reality. *Nature Reviews Neuroscience*, *6*(4), 332–339. [CrossRef] [PubMed]

Selig, J. P., & Preacher, K. J. (2024). *Monte Carlo method for assessing mediation: An interactive tool for creating confidence intervals for indirect effects* [Computer software]. Available online: http://quantpsy.org/ (accessed on 24 December 2024).

Slater, M., Lotto, B., Arnold, M. M., & Sanchez-Vives, M. V. (2009). How we experience immersive virtual environments: The concept of presence and its measurement. *Anuario de Psicologia*, *40*(2), 193–210.

Statista. (2024). *VR statistics*. Available online: https://www.statista.com (accessed on 24 December 2024).

Tay, J. L., Xie, H., & Sim, K. (2003). Effectiveness of augmented and virtual reality-based interventions in improving knowledge, attitudes, empathy and stigma regarding people with mental illnesses—A scoping review. *Journal of Personalized Medicine*, *13*(1), 112. [CrossRef] [PubMed]

Tracey, R. (2024). *20 real-world examples of virtual reality. E-learning provocateur*. Available online: https://ryan2point0.wordpress.com/2016/03/22/20-real-world-examples-of-virtual-reality/ (accessed on 24 December 2024).

Tsapelas, I., Beckes, L., & Aron, A. (2020). Manipulation of self-expansion alters responses to attractive alternative partners. *Frontiers in Psychology*, *11*, 938. [CrossRef] [PubMed]

Valtchanov, D. (2010). *Physiological and affective responses to immersion in virtual reality: Effects of nature and urban settings* [Master's thesis, University of Waterloo].

Disclaimer/Publisher's Note: The statements, opinions and data contained in all publications are solely those of the individual author(s) and contributor(s) and not of MDPI and/or the editor(s). MDPI and/or the editor(s) disclaim responsibility for any injury to people or property resulting from any ideas, methods, instructions or products referred to in the content.

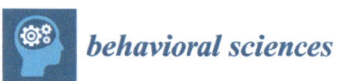 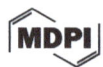

Article

Coupling Up: A Dynamic Investigation of Romantic Partners' Neurobiological States During Nonverbal Connection

Cailee M. Nelson [1,2,3,*], Christian O'Reilly [2,3,4,5], Mengya Xia [6] and Caitlin M. Hudac [1,2,3,*]

1. Department of Psychology, University of South Carolina, 1512 Pendleton Street, Columbia, SC 29208, USA
2. Carolina Autism and Neurodevelopment Research Center, University of South Carolina, 1800 Gervais Street, Columbia, SC 29201, USA; christian.oreilly@sc.edu
3. Institute for Mind and Brain, University of South Carolina, 1800 Gervais Street, Columbia, SC 29201, USA
4. Artificial Intelligence Institute, University of South Carolina, 1112 Greene Street, Columbia, SC 29208, USA
5. Department of Computer Science and Engineering, University of South Carolina, 1244 Blossom Street, Columbia, SC 29208, USA
6. T. Denny Sanford School of Social and Family Dynamics, Arizona State University, Wilson Hall, Floor 3, Tempe, AZ 85287, USA; mengya.xia@asu.edu
* Correspondence: caileen@mailbox.sc.edu (C.M.N.); chudac@mailbox.sc.edu (C.M.H.)

Abstract: Nonverbal connection is an important aspect of everyday communication. For romantic partners, nonverbal connection is essential for establishing and maintaining feelings of closeness. EEG hyperscanning offers a unique opportunity to examine the link between nonverbal connection and neural synchrony among romantic partners. This current study used an EEG hyperscanning paradigm to collect frontal alpha asymmetry (FAA) signatures from 30 participants (15 romantic dyads) engaged in five different types of nonverbal connection that varied based on physical touch and visual contact. The results suggest that there was a lack of FAA while romantic partners were embracing and positive FAA (i.e., indicating approach) while they were holding hands, looking at each other, or doing both. Additionally, partners' FAA synchrony was greatest at a four second lag while they were holding hands and looking at each other. Finally, there was a significant association between partners' weekly negative feelings and FAA such that as they felt more negative their FAA became more positive. Taken together, this study further supports the idea that fleeting moments of interpersonal touch and gaze are important for the biological mechanisms that may underlie affiliative pair bonding in romantic relationships.

Keywords: romantic love; electroencephalography (EEG); hyperscanning neuroscience; frontal alpha asymmetry; nonverbal connection

Citation: Nelson, C.M.; O'Reilly, C.; Xia, M.; Hudac, C.M. Coupling Up: A Dynamic Investigation of Romantic Partners' Neurobiological States During Nonverbal Connection. *Behav. Sci.* **2024**, *14*, 1133. https://doi.org/10.3390/bs14121133

Academic Editors: Bianca P. Acevedo and Adam Bode

Received: 27 September 2024
Revised: 15 November 2024
Accepted: 22 November 2024
Published: 26 November 2024

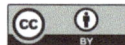

Copyright: © 2024 by the authors. Licensee MDPI, Basel, Switzerland. This article is an open access article distributed under the terms and conditions of the Creative Commons Attribution (CC BY) license (https://creativecommons.org/licenses/by/4.0/).

1. Introduction

Every day, romantic partners use communication to initiate or maintain closeness. Nonverbal connections can be initiated through actions, such as interpersonal touch, postural changes, and shared gaze, and these actions serve as an important aspect of communication that aids in bonding between romantic partners. In fact, more nonverbal connection between romantic partners is associated with greater intimacy [1,2], sexual interest and arousal [3,4], and relationship satisfaction [5,6]. Even though these moments occur rapidly and may be fleeting, nonverbal connections and cues (or a relative lack of connection) can provide evidence of a partner's romantic feelings and have lasting effects [7,8]. For instance, memories of simple nonverbal cues, such as eye gaze, facial expression, and touch, can serve as important "turning points" in relationships [9].

Despite the short-term and long-term socioemotional and relational implications of nonverbal communication on romantic relationships [6,10], it is unclear how nonverbal connections (even brief moments) may relate to current experiences and biological mechanisms of positive feeling or love. Longstanding evidence from animals and humans suggests that loving attachments are subserved by instantaneous, biobehavioral synchrony wherein biological signals co-relate [11]. To that extent, synchronized physiology may subserve increased feelings of closeness between romantic partners engaged in nonverbal connection. Indeed, romantic partners sharing interpersonal touch demonstrate increased synchronization of electrodermal [12], heart rate [13], and brain activity [14,15]. However, interpersonal touch is only one type of nonverbal connection important to romantic relationships. Shared gaze and close proximity are other examples of nonverbal connection that occur more often in romantic relationships compared to other social partnerships (e.g., friendships) [16]. Yet it is currently unclear whether there are differences in physiological synchrony among romantic partners across varied nonverbal connections. Examining these relationships is important for understanding how brief moments of nonverbal connection aid in developing and maintaining romantic feelings, building successful romantic relationships, and bolstering an individual's wellbeing. In fact, synchrony is thought to be greatest among romantic partners compared to other relationships [17–20] and could be responsible for influencing feelings of intimacy and social connection occurring in moments of nonverbal connection that aid in romantic relationship success [1,2,6]. Therefore, this current study sets out to investigate how gaze, interpersonal touch, and the combination of both between romantic partners may differ in the way they influence neurobiological and psychological states (e.g., approach motivation) relevant to building loving connections.

"Hyperscanning" describes the dual collection of biological processes during dyadic interaction and is often used to measure neural synchrony during dynamic and real-time social interactions [21]. Electroencephalography (EEG) hyperscanning research using phase coupling or power correlational approaches is particularly relevant for evaluating neural synchrony between romantic partners engaged in nonverbal connection. For instance, Kinreich and colleagues [22] found that gamma frequencies (30–90 Hz) occurring in temporoparietal regions of the brain (i.e., regions implicated in social skills) are significantly more correlated in romantic couples compared to strangers. Importantly, they also found that this synchrony was greatest during moments of shared gaze. This suggests that nonverbal connection influences neural synchrony between partners; however, this finding was specific to romantic partners engaged in conversation. Indeed, most hyperscanning research on romantic partners examining neural synchrony uses verbal or non-interactive tasks (i.e., joint video watching). This body of literature indicates that neural synchrony is influenced by creativity [18], honesty [20], interpersonal conflict [19], and relationship quality [17], but there still remains a need to understand how nonverbal connection alone influences neural synchrony between romantic partners.

1.1. Frontal Alpha Asymmetry as a Proxy of Approach Motivation in Romantic Partners

Social approach and its counterpart (social avoidance) describes the neurobiological and psychological instinct to engage (or disengage) with selected people [23]. Considering the nature of affiliative pair bonding [24], neural mechanisms that modulate social approach/avoidance [25] are likely synchronized between romantic partners [11]. One important EEG measurement of social approach is known as frontal alpha asymmetry (FAA), which reflects approach or avoidant motivational states in the brain [26,27]. FAA is calculated by the ratio of natural logarithm of alpha power occurring at the right relative to left frontal scalp electrodes (i.e., FAA = ln(right) − ln(left)) [28]. As brain activity measured via the blood-oxygen-level-dependent (BOLD) signal is negatively correlated with alpha power in many social brain regions (e.g., orbitofrontal cortex, superior frontal gyrus), it is thought that decreases in alpha power indicate increases in hemodynamic activity of the brain [29]. Therefore, approach motivation (i.e., the desire to go toward something) [30,31] is generally linked to more positive FAA scores (i.e., left hemodynamic activity) while avoidance motivation (i.e., the desire to move away from something) is linked to more negative FAA scores (i.e., right hemodynamic activity) [32,33]. It is hypothesized that romantic love would elicit more positive FAA due to romantic partners' motivation to approach one another [34], yet very little empirical work has examined this explicitly. Evidence of alpha asymmetry is present during passive viewing of affiliative movies [35], across occipital regions during a love induction task [36], and while romantic partners are embracing and kissing [37]. However, there is limited work examining approach/avoidance states and the synchronization of these neurobiological states over time during dyadic nonverbal connection. Furthermore, while FAA may become more positive during certain types of interpersonal touch (e.g., massage therapy, embracing) [37,38], it remains unclear if FAA is present in varied nonverbal connections among romantic partners and whether FAA dynamically shifts or synchronizes between romantic partners during nonverbal connection.

1.2. Current Study Objectives

This current study examines the biological mechanisms and psychological states underlying nonverbal connections between romantic partners through multiple objectives. First, we aimed to better understand the neural correlates supporting nonverbal connections in dynamic, real-time social interactions between romantic partners. Given that previous research has established that varied types of interpersonal touch and shared gaze are important types of nonverbal connection for romantic relationships [9] and may in-fluence FAA [37], we evaluated FAA across five types of nonverbal connection, varying on elements of interpersonal touch (e.g., holding hands, embracing) and visual contact (e.g., mutual gaze) using a hyperscanning approach. Considering that more positive FAA (i.e., increased left hemodynamic activity) is associated with approach processes [32,33], we hypothesized that participants would demonstrate more positive FAA during in-stances of connection (e.g., mutual gaze and touch) relative to no connection (e.g., no gaze or touch).

Second, to better characterize synchrony among romantic partners while engaged in nonverbal connection, we analyzed correlations of partners' FAA across time. As research suggests that neural synchrony is greatest among romantic partners compared to other social relationships [17–20], we believed FAA synchrony would be present across all levels of nonverbal connection. However, as FAA is largest for romantic partners who are embracing and kissing [37] and neural synchrony among romantic partners might be related to arousal [19] that is likely present during an embrace, we hypothesized that FAA would become most concordant while embracing. More specifically, we predicted that while participants were embracing, they would exhibit more positive patterns of FAA (i.e., more approach) that would match their partner's FAA patterns more closely than the other conditions.

Finally, there is limited research targeting why dyadic nonverbal connections may vary across people, particularly given the variability in how a person perceives their relationship and ongoing, lived experiences. Yet a better understanding of these underlying biological mechanisms may aid in strengthening the connections and bonds within a couple. For instance, nonverbal behavior may strengthen intimate relationships [7], but it is still unclear how the biological mechanisms that underlie moments of nonverbal connection in romantic relationships are linked to other predictors of relationship outcomes (e.g., relationship duration, feelings of intimacy). To initiate this work, we explored associations between multiple individual factors (age, relationship duration, time spent together, romantic/loving feelings, wellbeing) and subject-level biological correlates (FAA, synchrony with their partner). This aim was largely exploratory; therefore, we did not have specific predictions but expected general correlations between biological mechanisms and individual factors. For instance, it would be reasonable to predict people would exhibit more positive FAA following more positive romantic feelings, and that couples that spend more time together may be more attuned to each other's nonverbal communication. Given the preliminary nature of this work, we conducted this post hoc analysis on the conditions and moments when FAA and synchrony were the greatest, following the first two analyses.

2. Materials and Methods

2.1. Participants

Fifteen dyads (N = 30; 15 females; see Table 1 for characterization) aged 18–40 years that were in a self-affirmed romantic relationship completed several experiments related to a larger study being conducted at a university in the Southeastern United States. Relationship status was best described as dating exclusively or cohabitating (n = 20) and married (n = 10); no dyad identified as casual dating (i.e., dating multiple people). On an open-ended question about sexuality, a majority (n = 25, 83%) of the participants identified as heterosexual or straight, and five others identified as queer, bisexual, omnisexual, or straight/trans. Most participants identified as White (n = 22, 76%) and eight others identified as Asian, Lebanese/Arab, or Black. Two participants were left-handed. The local ethical review board approved this project, and all participants gave written informed consent.

Table 1. Demographic Information for Romantic Partners. Baseline and weekly averaged descriptive statistics for individual factors are reported for the entire sample. Items used to generate individual factor scores for each construct can be found in Table S1.

Baseline (Visit 1)	Mean (SD)	Range
Age (Years)	28.03 (5.05)	21–40
Relationship duration (Years)	7.41 (5.99)	1–20
Weekday time (Hours)	40.8 (19.18)	10–90
Weekend time (Hours)	75.9 (19.07)	10–97
Perceived love	9.03 (1.03)	7–10
Wellbeing	6.65 (1.36)	3.59–9.39
Weekly Mean Across 7 Days	**Mean (SD)**	**Range**
Perceived love	8.31 (1.33)	5.7–10
Loving feelings	7.07 (1.47)	4.07–9.93
Negative feelings	1.9 (0.67)	1–3.5
Positive feelings	6.86 (1.68)	3.14–10
Wellbeing	6.07 (0.88)	4.61–7.85
Shared time together (Hours/day)	5.83 (2.29)	1.5–10
Communication time (Hours/day)	5.46 (3.63)	1.52–17.57

2.2. General Procedures

Participants attended two in-person visits. During the first visit, they completed a battery of surveys to capture basic demographic information and questions about their partner. During the second visit, participants completed brief surveys to report on their current loving feelings towards their partner and then completed a set of EEG hyperscanning experiments, including the Nonverbal Connections Paradigm (described below). During the week between visits, participants completed a set of surveys that addressed constructs of perception of love, loving feelings, negative feelings toward their romantic partner, positive feelings toward their romantic partner, and general wellbeing (full survey items available in Table S1). We characterize the individual difference factors used in this study in Table 1. Except for time questions that were reported in hours, all items were recoded so that values of 1 equaled "strongly disagree" and values of 10 equaled "strongly agree". We generated subject-level scores by averaging across items based upon the construct.

2.3. Nonverbal Connections Paradigm

Participants were asked to interact nonverbally with their partner in five specific ways while EEG was recorded. Conditions varied based upon physical touch (no touch, holding hands, standing embrace) and visual contact (no gaze with eyes closed, shared gaze; Figure 1). The researcher instructed the pair about which condition was next and left the room to start EEG recording for 2 min. The order of condition was consistent across dyads—(1) No Connection, (2) Gaze Only, (3) Hands Only, (4) Gaze and Hands, and (5) Embrace. The first two pairs scheduled (Pair 1, 4) completed 1.5 min of each condition before the duration of each condition was extended to 2 min. One pair (Pair 1) did not complete the Embrace condition due to scheduling constraints. All participants complied with the nonverbal instruction. Post-task feedback indicated that most participants felt focused ($M = 7.54$, $SD = 1.93$, range 2–10), on a scale of 1–10, where 10 indicated full focus. Most participants ($n = 27$) identified at least one positive feeling (e.g., love, happiness, contentment, safety, warmth) during the task, but three participants described only negative feelings (e.g., boredom, awkwardness, pressure; Supplemental Information 1.1). Nine participants specifically described thinking about being or feeling "connected", and five participants described thinking about their mutual physical connection (e.g., smell, breathing rate; Supplemental Information 1.2).

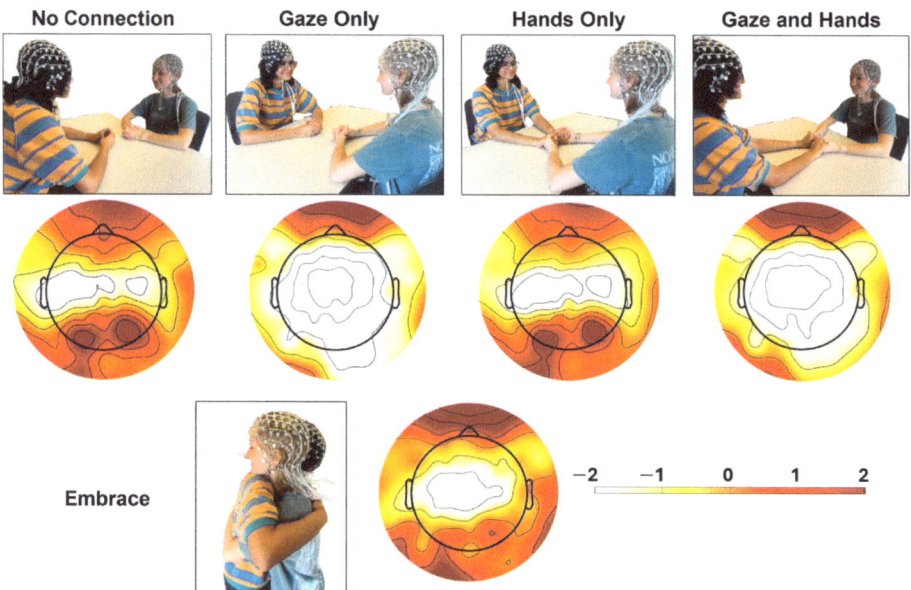

Figure 1. Nonverbal Connection Conditions and Topographic Maps for Corresponding Conditions. Topographic maps represent the power spectral density of alpha (8–12 Hz) across all channels for each condition, where darker colors indicate greater power and lighter colors indicate lesser power.

2.4. EEG Acquisition, Processing, and FAA Computation

Continuous EEG was recorded from high-density 128-channel geodesic sensor nets using Net Station 5.3 software integrated with two identical EEG high-impedance 400-series amplifiers (Magstim-EGI, Eugene, OR, USA). During acquisition, EEG signals were referenced to the vertex electrode, analog filtered (0.1 Hz high-pass, 100 Hz elliptical low-pass), amplified, and digitized with a sampling rate of 250 Hz. Standard post-processing procedures included bandpass filtering between 0.1–40 Hz and automated artifact rejection using the clean_rawdata plugin in EEGLAB [39]. In line with Delorme's [40] examination of preprocessing standards, channels were rejected using a rejection threshold of 0.9. Large artifacts were then removed via spectrum thresholding using the pop_rejcont function of EEGLAB (frequency range: 20–40 Hz, threshold: 10 dB). All removed channels were interpolated, and data were re-referenced to average.

EEG for the entire duration of the nonverbal connection conditions was epoched with 500 ms windows and decomposed by frequency using the default EEGLAB settings for time-frequency analyses. Relative and absolute alpha (8–12 Hz) power was then averaged across channels into two frontal clusters (left channels = E23, E24, E26, E27, E33 right channels = E2, E3, E122, E123, E124) for each trial. FAA was calculated by subtracting the natural log-transformed alpha of the left cluster from the right [i.e., ln(right) − ln(left)]. Preliminary models indicated that both relative and absolute alpha exhibited significant condition differences between left and right hemispheres ($p < 0.0001$ for both). To be consistent with the literature [28], relative alpha was utilized throughout the remainder of the study (see Figure 1).

2.5. Analytic Plan

All statistical analyses were performed using R (version 4.3.1). Linear mixed-effects models were computed using restricted maximum likelihood with Nelder–Mead optimization via the "lme4" package [41]. Estimated marginal means (EMMs) and 95% confidence intervals (CIs) are reported for post hoc testing with false discovery rate correction [42] applied for multiple comparisons. A pictorial representation of the analytic plan and model equations are available in Figure 2.

1. Group-level FAA across condition and time

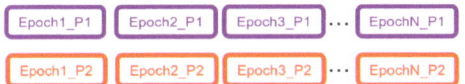

Linear mixed-effects model

$FAA_{tci} = \beta_0 + \beta_1(Condition_c) + \beta_2(Time_t) + \beta_3(Time_t^2) + \beta_4(Condition_c)(Time_t) + \beta_5(Condition_c)(Time_t^2) + U_{0i} + e_{tci}$

2. Concordance of FAA to partner's FAA across condition and lag

Concurrent (2a) and lagged (2b) coupling

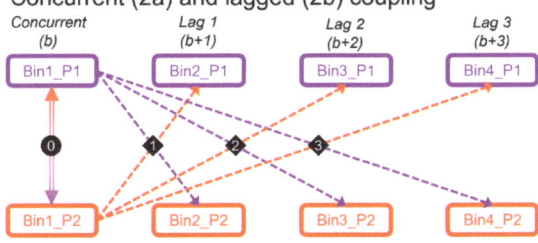

Concordance correlation coefficient (CCC)

$CCC(P1, P2) = \dfrac{2\, Corr(P1, P2)\sigma_{P1}\sigma_{P2}}{\sigma^2_{P1} + \sigma^2_{P2} + (\mu_{P1} - \mu_{P2})^2}$

Linear mixed-effects model

$CCC_{tci} = \beta_0 + \beta_1(Condition_c) + \beta_2(Lag_t) + \beta_3(Condition_c)(Lag_t) + U_{0p} + e_{tci}$

Figure 2. Analytic Plan. Graphical representation and model equations for analytic plan to assess (1) group-level frontal alpha asymmetry (FAA) effects across condition and time, and (2) within-dyad FAA effects across condition and temporal lag (1-lag, 2-lag, and 3-lag). Epochs are extracted every 500 ms from continuous EEG. Bins are computed as the average across 4 contiguous epochs (e.g., 2 s). P1 and P2 represent partner one and two, respectively, within a pair.

First, mixed-linear-effects models tested group-level (i.e., across all individuals) FAA differences related to condition and dynamic shifts over the two-minute experience by including effects of time to assess a linear slope and quadratic slope across epoch. A random intercept for each person was included to account for repeated measures. Missing data (e.g., due to artifacts) was ignored at the epoch level. Each participant contributed at least 38 valid epochs per condition, with most participants contributing over 200 valid epochs per condition (M = 218.7, SE = 3.1 500 ms epochs). Dynamic shift characterization was confirmed by extracting model-estimated time features (linear slope, quadratic slope) every 60 epochs (30 s increments) and verifying non-zero values (e.g., confidence intervals do not cross zero) for each condition using lstrends() from the "emmeans" package in R [43].

Second, we examined within-dyad effects of FAA across condition and temporal lag by converting FAA scores into within-dyad concordance values. To do this, within each person, we averaged FAA values across four contiguous epochs that generated 60 non-overlapping bins (2 s each bin). Epochs included only data surviving artifact detection and correction; thus, any bin-level missing data were due to missing data (e.g., due to artifacts) across the full 2 s bin. Note that there were 45 bins for the two pairs that only completed 1.5 min per condition. These bins were then used to examine concurrent and lagged coupling (i.e., neural synchrony) of FAA within dyads. Then, we examined concurrent and lagged similarities between the two people within the dyad using concordance correlation coefficients (CCCs; scale limits = −1 to 1) [44,45] at each bin. Positive CCC values indicate strong concordance of FAA (e.g., both FAA reflective of approach), and negative CCC values indicate strong discordance of FAA (e.g., FAA reflects approach in one partner and avoidance in the other partner). Close-to-zero CCC values reflect no linear relationship between partners' FAA. Although the CCC is more commonly used to validate against a gold-standard measure, it has proved useful in prior dyadic EEG and biological measurement studies [46,47]. In addition to concurrent coupling across bins, we examined whether each person's FAA was predicted by their partner's previous FAA values at a 1-bin, 2-bin, and 3-bin lag (see Figure 2). CCC was estimated separately for each condition, only including bins where FAA was available for both partners. Average CCC values were extracted for the entire sample first to describe overall trends, such that computation was tested on data from each participant relative to their partner for each lag and condition, across all available epochs. Then, CCC values were extracted to generate each person's unique CCC value for each lag and condition to be used for statistical models. In this way, concurrent lag was identical for a participant and their partner (i.e., FAA similarity at the same time point); subsequent lags were not identical because one partner may respond to their partner's nonverbal cues differently or at different rates. These individually derived CCC values were input into linear mixed effects models to predict CCC differences by included fixed effects of condition, lag, and a random intercept for each person to account for repeated measures. A priori pairwise comparisons were planned to examine condition differences at each lag level.

Finally, as a post hoc exploratory analysis we used Pearson correlations with FDR-corrections to estimate how subject-level FAA and within-dyad CCCs related to baseline individual differences in age, relationship duration, estimate of weekday and weekend hours spent with their romantic partner, perception of love, and wellbeing. Given that participants responded to individual difference measures for a week, we also evaluated relationships between FAA, CCCs, and weekly mean and variability from evening daily diary reports of perception of love, loving feelings, positive feelings, negative feelings, wellbeing, and amount of time shared together. For exploratory analyses, we opted to retain all data points as a first step to learn about the variability and potential relationships within data [48]; however, model results where outliers were winsorized can be found in supplemental information (Figures S4–S7).

3. Results

3.1. General FAA Differences Related to Condition and Time

Results for the linear mixed-effects model are reported in Table 2 and illustrated in Figure 3.

Table 2. Linear Mixed-Effects Model Results Predicting Frontal Alpha Asymmetry (FAA). Model predicting FAA included single-epoch FAA values for each person ($N = 30$), condition (No Connection, Gaze only, Hands only, Gaze and Hands, and Embrace), and epoch (up to 240 epochs).

Effect	F	(df1, df2)	p-Value
Random intercept	2.99	(1, 32319)	0.0835
Condition	8.27	(4, 32319)	**<0.0001**
Time (slope)	1.62	(1, 32319)	0.2031
Time (quadratic)	1.94	(1, 32319)	0.1639
Condition × Time (slope)	4.09	(4, 32319)	**0.0026**
Condition × Time (quadratic)	6.13	(4, 32319)	**0.0001**

Note: Bolded p-values indicate significant effects.

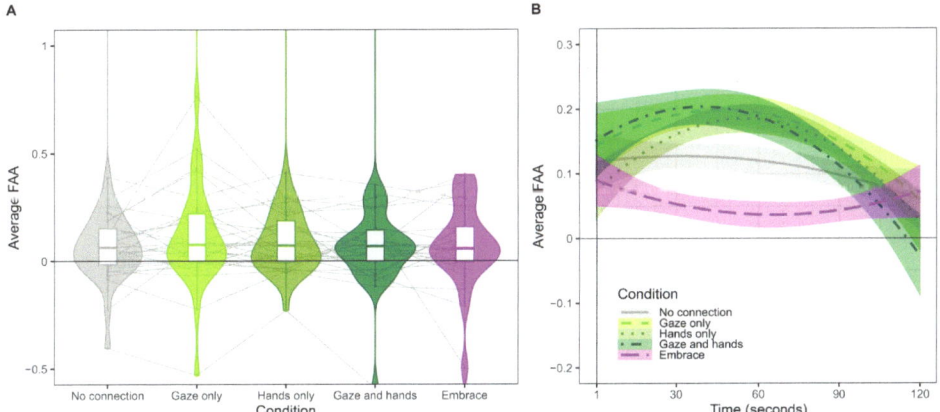

Figure 3. Average Frontal Alpha Asymmetry (FAA). Positive FAA values reflect approach processes, zero-like FAA values reflect neutral processes, and negative FAA values reflect avoidance processes. Panel (**A**) illustrates group-level FAA as violin plots to describe variability and boxplots to describe quartile ranges per condition. Gray lines reflect within-person individual differences across condition. Panel (**B**) illustrates group-level average FAA across epoch.

3.1.1. Lack of FAA for No Connection and Embrace Conditions

Post hoc testing following a main effect of the condition indicated positive but non-significant FAA values (i.e., neutral neurobiological state) for both the No Connection condition (EMM = 0.120, CI = −0.06–0.3) and the Embrace condition (EMM = 0.116, CI = −0.06–0.3). Both conditions were less positive than the other conditions, $p < 0.0001$, that indicated positive FAA: Gaze Only (EMM = 0.184, CI = 0.002–0.37), Hands Only (EMM = 0.184, CI = 0.002–0.37), and Gaze and Hands (EMM = 0.182, CI = 0.0008–0.36).

3.1.2. Dynamic Shifts Across Epoch Varied by Condition

The results for the omnibus model are reported in Table 2, and patterns are illustrated in Figure 3B. As described above, statistical verification of dynamic shifts was computed via testing linear trends from estimated marginal means in 60-epoch (30 s) increments. With minor exceptions, FAA was stable for two conditions: No Connection and Embrace conditions (negative slope slowing down due to negative quadratic term at epoch 180 and epoch 60, respectively). The other conditions (Gaze Only, Hands Only, Gaze and Hands) exhibited an initial increase in FAA (positive slope) that decreased by epoch 120 (negative quadratic term).

3.2. Interplay of FAA Responses Within Romantic Partner Dyads

Descriptively (group-level; see Figure 4), conditional CCC values ranged from −0.68 to 0.42, negatively skewed for the Gaze Only condition, and kurtosis values greater than 2 indicated a more peaked distribution (i.e., relative to normal) for all conditions except Hands Only. As illustrated in Figure 4, CCCs were weakly negative (i.e., −0.05 to −0.2) at concurrent, Lag 1, and Lag 3. At Lag 2, group-level CCCs were positive for all conditions, indicating that FAA values were concordant with partner's FAA values at a 4 s lag.

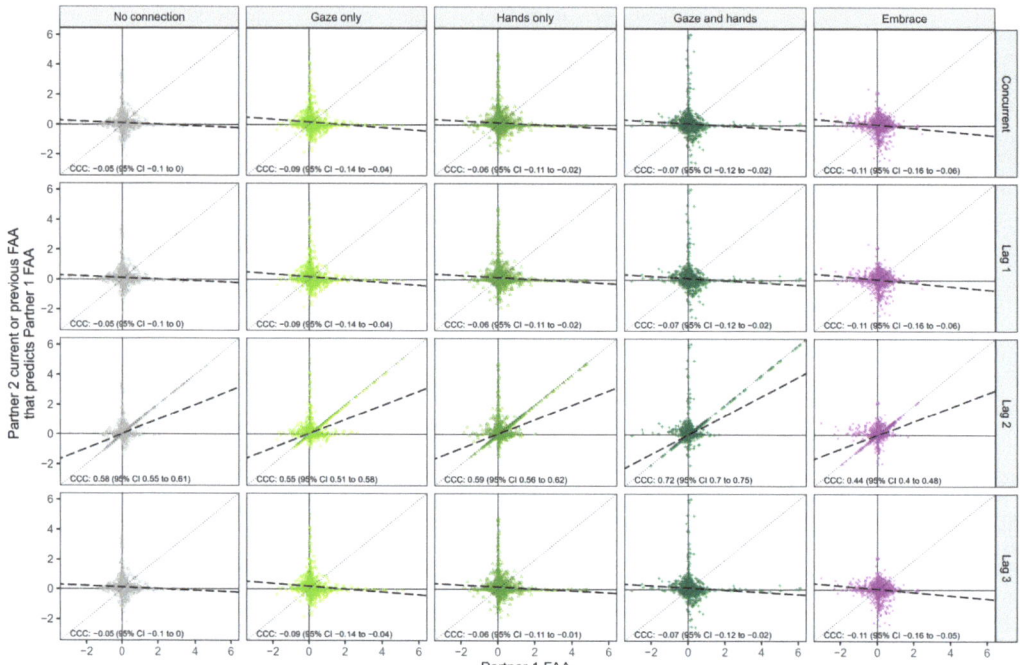

Figure 4. Evidence of Within-Dyad Concordance Across Condition and Epoch Lag. Concordance correlation coefficients (CCCs) and 95% confidence intervals are computed and reported. Perfect concordance occurs at CCC = 1 (all points perfectly aligned on the dotted line at 45 degree) and perfect discordance occurs at CCC = −1. Within a dyad, Partner 1 and Partner 2 designations were randomly assigned, as CCCs are symmetric with respect to these attributions (i.e., CCC(P1, P2) = CCC(P2, P1)). Dots illustrate the dyad- and bin-level, such that each dot indicates the concordance between each partner at each bin with valid data. The thick dashed line represents the slope concordance between Partner 1 and 2. Panel rows reflect bin-lag; for example, in row two for Lag 1, Partner 1's FAA is predicted by Partner 2's previous bin FAA.

For subject-level descriptives (i.e., each person in reference to their partner), see Table 3 (lag-level descriptives available in Table S2). Results for the linear mixed-effects model indicated a main effect of condition, $F(4, 543) = 4.10$, $p = 0.003$, and highlighted several patterns—(1) more negative CCCs for No Connection and Embrace, relative to Gaze and Hands, $p < 0.043$; (2) more negative CCCs for Gaze Only relative to No Connection and Hands Only, $p < 0.02$. Effects of lag, $F(3, 543) = 2.37$, $p = 0.07$, and the condition by lag interaction, $F(12,543) = 1.44$, $p = 0.14$, were not significant; however, planned comparisons of condition across lag indicated the condition differences described were present only for Lag 2, $p < 0.005$, but no other lag, $p > 0.13$.

Table 3. Descriptive Statistics of Concordance Correlation Coefficients (CCCs) for Each Condition at the Subject Level. CCC values were computed for each subject in reference to their partner and are described as collapsed across persons and lag.

	Mean	SD	Min	Max	Skew	Kurtosis
No Connection	0.01	0.102	−0.254	0.389	0.749	2.855
Gaze Only	−0.024	0.109	−0.682	0.228	−1.994	9.742
Hands only	0.011	0.088	−0.213	0.33	0.308	1.415
Gaze and Hands	0.014	0.082	−0.238	0.404	0.792	4.266
Embrace	−0.016	0.102	−0.417	0.293	−0.245	2.642

3.3. Influence of Individual Differences

As FAA was approach-like and CCCs at Lag 2 were most concordant during the Gaze and Hands condition, we only report results specific to this condition. Pearson correlations with FDR corrections revealed no significant relationships between FAA and baseline individual differences (see Figure S1). However, there was a positive correlation between FAA and weekly mean negative feelings, $r(28) = 0.49$, $p = 0.042$ (Figure 5). No Pearson correlations were significant with FDR correction for any of the variables and CCCs. Statistical results for weekly and baseline values are reported in Figures S2 and S3.

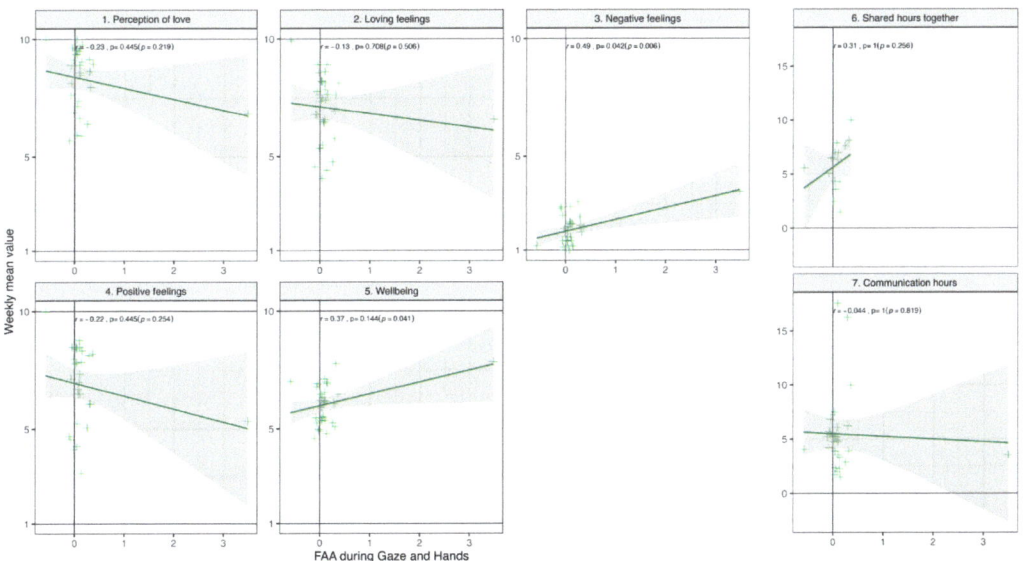

Figure 5. Relationship Between FAA and Average Weekly Means. FAA values are extracted as each person's average FAA value during Gaze and Hand condition, as the condition by which FAA was positive, reflecting more approach-like neurobiological states. Individual difference factors are computed as the weekly means from daily surveys, and specific questions are available in Table S1. For panels 1–5, items are scored from strongly disagree (1) to strongly agree (10).

4. Discussion

In this study, we used an EEG hyperscanning task to evaluate how nonverbal connections influence individual and concordant neurobiological states between romantic partners. Specifically, we investigated how neurobiological states of approach/avoidance as reflected by FAA shifted and synchronized between partners across different levels of nonverbal connection (e.g., hand holding, embracing, mutual gaze). While some of the literature has examined either neural synchrony or FAA between romantic partners, to our knowledge, this is the first study to examine FAA synchrony in the context of nonverbal connection. Our results suggest that FAA varies based on the type of nonverbal connection and how long partners are engaged in nonverbal connection. Additionally, we found that FAA becomes synchronized between romantic partners at a four second lag, particularly when holding hands and looking at each other.

4.1. Approach-like Neural Correlates Vary over Different Types of Nonverbal Connection and Time

In general, group-level FAA was positive for all conditions, suggesting that there was some level of approach for romantic partners across all types of nonverbal connection. While it was initially surprising that there was positive FAA (i.e., indicating approach-like signatures) for the No Connection condition, further examination of participants' thoughts and feelings during the experiment might best explain these results (see Supplemental Information 1.1 and 1.2). For example, after completing this experiment, one participant indicated that during this condition they were trying to listen to their partner's breath and make their own breathing patterns apparent to their partner. As such, positive FAA in the No Connection condition might have been caused by participants being in close proximity with their partners in a loving context.

Results indicated significantly less positive group-level FAA (i.e., less approach) in the No Connection and Embrace conditions compared to the other three conditions (i.e., Gaze Only, Hands Only, Gaze and Hands). Additionally, while our analyses did not reveal a significant main effect of time on FAA, there was a significant interaction term between time and condition. This may suggest that FAA changes dynamically over time based on the type of nonverbal connection romantic partners are engaged in. While FAA was quickly extinguished for the No Connection and Embrace conditions, FAA remained steady until about halfway through the experiment for the other conditions, as confirmed with testing the linear trends in 30 s increments. This may suggest that FAA became increasingly more approach-like as participants engaged in shared gaze, interpersonal touch via hand holding, or both. However, time alone was not a significant predictor, and these results should be interpreted with caution.

The lack of positive FAA and early decrease to FAA below statistically significant levels in the Embrace condition was not in line with our hypothesis nor previous research that suggests alpha asymmetry for romantic partners is largest while embracing or kissing [37]. Even though hyperscanning allows for more naturalistic measurement of dynamic social situations, there are still methodological constraints that might explain the lack of approach signatures during the Embrace condition. For example, unlike previous research (e.g., [37]), partners were asked to embrace longer (i.e., two minutes), which may have felt a little unnatural. Likewise, Packheiser and colleagues [37] conducted their study in partners' homes, which may have allowed for more comfort between partners. While most of our participants ($n = 27$) indicated positive feelings post-experiment, some ($n = 3$) indicated that they felt awkward, bored, and frustrated. Finally, previous research examining alpha asymmetry during embrace has yet to compare this condition to other types of nonverbal connection (e.g., shared gaze, hand holding), which proved in this current study to elicit stronger approach-like signatures. In fact, Packheiser and colleagues [37] had participants look at each other while embracing, which may suggest that gaze could have been influencing the alpha asymmetry in their study. As our findings support previous research that has demonstrated approach signatures during interpersonal touch [15] and shared gaze [22] separately, there is a need for future research to further distinguish the biological mechanisms underlying differing nonverbal connections in ecologically valid ways.

4.2. Partners' Brains Couple-Up at a Lagged Offset During Nonverbal Connection

Condition effects of FAA concordance between partners revealed larger concordance (i.e., coupling or synchrony) during the Gaze and Hands condition specifically compared to the No Connection and Embrace conditions. While it was surprising that embracing did not elicit the greatest synchronization of FAA between partners, this may have been due to the weak approach-like neurobiological states (i.e., positive FAA) in general during this condition. Stronger concordance during moments of mutual gaze and interpersonal touch, however, is supported by previous research. For example, greater neural synchronization between romantic partners during interpersonal touch compared to vocal communication has been reported in an fNIRS study [15]. Additionally, it has been reported that synchrony between romantic partners having a conversation was greatest during moments of shared gaze [22].

The current results also suggest that concordance effects were greatest at a four second lag. In other words, one participant's current FAA was most in-sync with their partner's FAA from four seconds ago. While this was not necessarily expected, given that nonverbal connection occurs rapidly, varied lagged inter-brain concordance ranging anywhere from 1.55 [49] to 12.5 s [50] is reported in hyperscanning studies investigating social interactions [51] and can develop as a result of experimental settings or external environmental changes regardless of social interaction [52]. Additionally, memories of eye gaze, facial expression, and touch are particularly salient in romantic relationships [9]. Therefore, the lagged synchrony might be a result of deeper encoding of the nonverbal connection occurring between romantic partners. For instance, if participant A, in a state of approach, tried to make their partner (i.e., participant B) laugh or smile while engaged in nonverbal connection, participant B's brain might have been delayed in reaching a state of approach due to encoding and information processing of participant A's behavior. Additionally, one participant reported initially feeling awkward during the different nonverbal connection conditions but "slowly [...] felt more admiration and compassion for my partner thereafter", as they remained engaged in the nonverbal connection (see Supplemental Information 1.2). This may indicate that because partners initially felt uncomfortable during each nonverbal connection, the synchrony of their neurobiological states might have been delayed and dependent on each other, feeling more comfortable as time went on.

4.3. Negative Feelings May Influence Partners' Approach-like Neural Correlates

As a preliminary analysis, we explored associations between individual differences and romantic partners' FAA and CCC values, which revealed only one significant positive correlation between weekly mean negative feelings and FAA. This suggests that as partners' negative feelings increased, neurobiological states became more approach-like. Considering this measure described negative feelings like anger and tension, these results are in line with evidence that suggests certain negative emotions (e.g., anger), elicit approach-like states [53–55]. A visual examination of this relationship demonstrates one outlier that had much more positive FAA and more negative feelings than the sample, however. Thus, we caution against overinterpretation of this relationship and encourage deeper future examinations. Additionally, while no other significant relationships survived corrections for multiple comparisons, there was an uncorrected trend between average weekly negative feelings and CCCs, in line with the FAA association. Here, partners that reported more negative feelings had more concordant neurobiological states. These exploratory findings may be in line with previous research suggesting that romantic partners that are distressed or in moments of conflict are more neurally synced [17,19] but also deserve further exploration in the future.

4.4. Limitations and Future Directions

The order of nonverbal connection conditions was fixed across participants, such that No Connection was always presented first, and Embrace was always presented last. This fixed order may have contributed to the lack of positive FAA in the Embrace condition, as participants may have been fatigued by the time they met this condition. Additionally, EEG data are particularly sensitive to body and head movements that occur naturally when people embrace. While we attempted to mitigate this noise during the experiment (i.e., asking participants to hold the same embrace the entire time, reminding participants to move as little as possible) and in preprocessing of the data (e.g., artifact detection/rejection described in Section 2.5), it is possible that noisy data may have influenced our results. Given that other studies have found positive FAA while romantic partners are embracing, future research should aim to investigate randomized or different orders of nonverbal connections to better understand the relationship between FAA and embracing among romantic partners.

The sample size in this current study is representative of other within-subject studies investigating FAA [37,56,57]; however, a larger sample size may produce larger variability of FAA and CCCs between nonverbal connection conditions and will be better suited to improve our understanding of the relationship between individual differences, FAA, and CCCs associated with nonverbal connection. Similarly, individual differences at the neural level (e.g., skull thickness, baseline alpha power) and demographic level (e.g., race, relationship type) may influence FAA scores [58]. As such, investigating these constructs in a more diverse sample of romantic partners (e.g., non-white, Hispanic/Latine) and romantic partnership types (e.g., non-monogamous, casually dating) while correcting for overall alpha power within an individual could strengthen the generalizability of these conclusions.

While we chose to focus on concordance of partners' neurobiological states via FAA to clarify how partners were aligned in terms of approach and avoidance during nonverbal connection, continued work utilizing more sophisticated signal-processing techniques is needed. For example, Granger Causality or Partial Directed Coherence may be particularly helpful in understanding the directionality by which information is sent between people [21]. These techniques would offer more sophisticated insight into the biological process, which could aid in a deeper understanding of individual differences that may influence neural synchrony and co-occurring psychological states. One study examining neural synchrony underlying cooperation between romantic partners using Granger Causality analyses found that there was stronger directional synchronization from females to males during a cooperative task [59]. Future research may also consider incorporating other physiological measures to better understand the relationship between biological synchrony and relationship outcomes. For instance, research has demonstrated that synchronous electrodermal activity predicts mutual romantic and sexual interest [60], and sexual satisfaction moderates heart rate synchrony [61]. While understanding causal interactions and how neurobiological synchrony aligns with the synchronization of other physiological rhythms among romantic partners engaged in nonverbal connection was outside the scope of this current study, the presence of lagged synchrony in our results demonstrates a need to better understand this in future research.

5. Conclusions

This study was one of the first to dynamically examine the impact of various nonverbal connections on romantic partners' neurobiological states. Our results suggest that all types of nonverbal connection elicit approach-like neurobiological states among romantic partners. Importantly, these neurobiological states appear to synchronize between romantic partners specifically when holding hands and looking at each other. Additionally, this synchrony may be delayed as one partner encodes and processes their partner's behavior and nonverbal cues. Finally, approach-like neurobiological states seem to be positively related to negative feelings between partners. These findings are particularly relevant to understanding the underlying relationships between nonverbal connections and romantic relationship success. More specifically, this current study may inform future studies interested in investigating how neurobiological states of nonverbal connection influence short- and long-term romantic outcomes.

Supplementary Materials: The following supporting information can be downloaded at https://www.mdpi.com/article/10.3390/bs14121133/s1, Supplemental Information 1.1: Post-experiment responses to "What were you thinking about during this task?"; Supplemental Information 1.2: Post-experiment responses to "What were you feeling during this task?"; Figure S1: Relationship between FAA and baseline characteristics; Figure S2: Relationship between concordance and baseline characteristics; Figure S3: Relationship between concordance and average weekly characteristics; Figure S4: Relationship between FAA and baseline characteristics with winsorized outliers; Figure S5: Relationship between FAA and average weekly experiences with winsorized outliers; Figure S6: Relationship between concordance and baseline characteristics with winsorized outliers; Figure S7: Relationship between concordance and average weekly experiences with winsorized outliers; Table S1: Daily items from evening survey; Table S2: Descriptive statistics of concordance correlation coefficients (CCCs) for each condition at the subject-level.

Author Contributions: Conceptualization, C.M.H. and M.X.; methodology, C.M.H. and M.X.; software, C.M.H.; validation, C.M.H. and C.M.N.; formal analysis, C.M.H. and C.O.; investigation, C.M.H. and M.X.; resources, C.M.H. and M.X.; data curation, C.M.H., M.X. and C.M.N.; writing—original draft preparation, C.M.N. and C.M.H.; writing—review and editing, C.M.N., C.M.H., M.X. and C.O.; visualization, C.M.H. and C.M.N.; supervision, C.M.H. and M.X.; project administration, C.M.H. and M.X. All authors have read and agreed to the published version of the manuscript.

Funding: This research received no external funding.

Institutional Review Board Statement: This study was conducted in accordance with the Declaration of Helsinki and approved by the Institutional Review Board (or Ethics Committee) of the University of Alabama (protocol #22-02-5365, approved 26 April 2022).

Informed Consent Statement: Written informed consent has been obtained from the patient(s) to publish this paper.

Data Availability Statement: The raw data supporting the conclusions of this article will be made available by the authors on request.

Acknowledgments: We would like to thank each of our participants. We are grateful to our colleagues who helped with recruitment, coordination of the session, and EEG net application, including Victoria Ward, Nicole Friedman, Pratibha Gautam, Ja'Lynn Harris, and Skyler Hughes.

Conflicts of Interest: The authors declare no conflicts of interest.

References

1. Burgoon, J.K.; Le Poire, B.A. Nonverbal cues and interpersonal judgements: Participant and observer perceptions of intimacy, dominance, composure, and formality. *Commun. Monogr.* **1999**, *66*, 105–124. [CrossRef]
2. Jones, S.E.; Yarbrough, A.E. A naturalistic study of the meanings of touch. *Commun. Monogr.* **1985**, *52*, 19–56. [CrossRef]
3. Jarick, M.; Laidlaw, K.E.; Nasiopoulos, E.; Kingstone, A. Eye contact affects attention more than arousal as revealed by prospective time estimation. *Atten. Percept. Psychophys.* **2016**, *78*, 1302–1307. [CrossRef] [PubMed]
4. Vannier, S.A.; O'sullivan, L.F. Communicating interest in sex: Verbal and nonverbal initiation of sexual activity in young adults' romantic dating relationships. *Arch. Sex. Behav.* **2011**, *40*, 961–969. [CrossRef]
5. Noller, P. *Nonverbal Communication and Marital Interaction*; Pergamon Press: Oxford, UK, 1984.
6. Schrage, K.M.; Maxwell, J.A.; Impett, E.A.; Keltner, D.; MacDonald, G. Effects of verbal and nonverbal communication of affection on avoidantly attached partners' emotions and message receptiveness. *Personal. Soc. Psychol. Bull.* **2020**, *46*, 1567–1580. [CrossRef]
7. Andersen, P.A.; Guerrero, L.K.; Jones, S.M. Nonverbal behavior in intimate interactions and intimate relationships. In *The Sage Handbook of Nonverbal Communication*; Manusov, V., Patterson, M.L., Eds.; Sage Publications, Inc.: Thousand Oaks, CA, USA, 2006; pp. 259–277. [CrossRef]
8. Horgan, T.G. The verbal and nonverbal communication of romantic interest. In *Nonverbal Communication of Our Gendered and Sexual Selves*; Palgrave Macmillan: Cham, Switzerland, 2024; pp. 203–235. [CrossRef]
9. Docan-Morgan, T.; Manusov, V.; Harvey, J. When a small thing means so much: Nonverbal cues as turning points in relationships. *Interpersona Int. J. Pers. Relatsh.* **2013**, *7*, 110–124. [CrossRef]
10. Frank, M.G.; Solbu, A.; Glowacki, Z.R.; Toh, Z.; Neurohr, M. The look of love: Evolution and nonverbal signs and signals of attraction. In *Nonverbal Communication in Close Relationships: What Words Don't Tell Us*; Sternberg, R.J., Kostić, A., Eds.; Springer International Publishing: Cham, Switzerland, 2022; pp. 75–104.
11. Feldman, R. The neurobiology of human attachments. *Trends Cogn. Sci.* **2017**, *21*, 80–99. [CrossRef]
12. Chatel-Goldman, J.; Congedo, M.; Jutten, C.; Schwartz, J. Touch increases autonomic coupling between romantic partners. *Front. Behav. Neurosci.* **2014**, *8*, 95. [CrossRef]
13. Goldstein, P.; Weissman-Fogel, I.; Shamay-Tsoory, S.G. The role of touch in regulating inter-partner physiological coupling during empathy for pain. *Sci. Rep.* **2017**, *7*, 3252. [CrossRef]
14. Goldstein, P.; Weissman-Foge, I.; Dumas, G.; Shamay-Tsoory, S.G. Brain-to-brain coupling during handholding is associated with pain reduction. *Proc. Natl. Acad. Sci. USA* **2018**, *115*, E2528–E2537. [CrossRef]

15. Long, Y.; Zheng, L.; Zhao, H.; Zhou, S.; Zhai, Y.; Lu, C. Interpersonal neural synchronization during interpersonal touch underlies affiliative pair bonding between romantic couples. *Cereb. Cortex* **2021**, *31*, 1647–1659. [CrossRef] [PubMed]
16. Guerrero, L.K. Nonverbal involvement across interactions with same-sex friends, opposite-sex friends and romantic partners: Consistency or change? *J. Soc. Pers. Relatsh.* **1997**, *14*, 31–58. [CrossRef]
17. Chen, Y.; Liu, S.; Hao, Y.; Zhao, Q.; Ren, J.; Piao, Y.; Wang, L.; Yan, Y.; Jin, C.; Wang, H.; et al. Higher emotional synchronization is modulated by relationship quality in romantic relationships and not in close friendships. *NeuroImage* **2024**, *297*, 120733. [CrossRef] [PubMed]
18. Duan, H.; Yang, T.; Wang, X.; Kan, Y.; Zhao, H.; Li, Y.; Hu, W. Is the creativity of lovers better? A behavioral and functional near-infrared spectroscopy hyperscanning study. *Curr. Psychol.* **2022**, *41*, 41–54. [CrossRef]
19. Long, Y.; Chen, C.; Wu, K.; Zhou, S.; Zhou, F.; Zheng, L.; Zhao, H.; Zhai, Y.; Lu, C. Interpersonal conflict increases interpersonal neural synchronization in romantic couples. *Cereb. Cortex* **2022**, *32*, 3254–3268. [CrossRef]
20. Shao, C.; Zhang, X.; Wu, Y.; Zhang, W.; Sun, B. Increased interpersonal brain synchronization in romantic couples is associated with higher honesty: An fNIRS hyperscanning study. *Brain Sci.* **2023**, *13*, 833. [CrossRef]
21. Czeszumski, A.; Eustergerling, S.; Lang, A.; Menrath, D.; Gerstenberger, M.; Schuberth, S.; Schreiber, F.; Rendon, Z.Z.; König, P. Hyperscanning: A valid method to study neural inter-brain underpinnings of social interaction. *Front. Hum. Neurosci.* **2020**, *14*, 39. [CrossRef]
22. Kinreich, S.; Djalovski, A.; Kraus, L.; Louzoun, Y.; Feldman, R. Brain-to-brain synchrony during naturalistic social interactions. *Sci. Rep.* **2017**, *7*, 17060. [CrossRef]
23. Nikitin, J.; Schoch, S. Social approach and avoidance motivations. In *Handbook of Solitude: Psychological Perspectives on Social Isolation, Social Withdrawal, and Being Alone*, 2nd ed.; Coplan, R.J., Bowker, J.C., Eds.; Wiley Blackwell: New York, NY, USA, 2021; pp. 191–208.
24. Johnson, Z.V.; Young, L.J. Neurobiological mechanisms of social attachment and pair bonding. *Curr. Opin. Behav. Sci.* **2015**, *3*, 38–44. [CrossRef]
25. Porges, S.W. The polyvagal theory: Phylogenetic substrates of a social nervous system. *Int. J. Psychophysiol.* **2001**, *42*, 123–146. [CrossRef]
26. Kelley, N.J.; Hortensius, R.; Schutter, D.J.L.G.; Harmon-Jones, E. The relationship of approach/avoidance motivation and asymmetric frontal cortical activity: A review of studies manipulating frontal asymmetry. *Int. J. Psychophysiol.* **2017**, *119*, 19–30. [CrossRef] [PubMed]
27. Reznik, S.J.; Allen, J.J. Frontal asymmetry as a mediator and moderator of emotion: An updated review. *Psychophysiology* **2018**, *55*, e12965. [CrossRef] [PubMed]
28. Vincent, K.M.; Xie, W.; Nelson, C.A. Using different methods for calculating frontal alpha asymmetry to study its development form infancy to 3 years of age in a large longitudinal sample. *Dev. Psychobiol.* **2021**, *63*, e22163. [CrossRef] [PubMed]
29. Gonçalves, S.I.; de Munck, J.C.; Pouwels, P.J.W.; Schoonhoven, R.; Kuijer, J.P.A.; Maurits, N.M.; Hoogduin, J.M.; Van Someren, E.J.W.; Heethaar, R.M.; Lopes da Silva, F.H. Correlating the alpha rhythm to BOLD using simultaneous EEG/fMRI: Inter-subject variability. *NeuroImage* **2006**, *30*, 203–213. [CrossRef]
30. Harmon-Jones, E.; Gable, P.A. On the role of asymmetric frontal cortical activity in approach and withdrawal motivation: An updated review of the evidence. *Psychophysiology* **2018**, *55*, e12879. [CrossRef]
31. Schöne, B.; Schomberg, J.; Gruber, T.; Quirin, M. Event-related frontal alpha asymmetries: Electrophysiological correlates of approach motivation. *Exp. Brain Res.* **2016**, *234*, 559–567. [CrossRef]
32. Deng, X.; Zhang, S.; Chen, X.; Coplan, R.J.; Xiao, B.; Ding, X. Links between social avoidance and frontal alpha asymmetry during processing emotional facial stimuli: An exploratory study. *Biol. Psychol.* **2023**, *178*, 108516. [CrossRef]
33. Sobotka, S.S.; Davidson, R.J.; Senulis, J.A. Anterior brain electriacl asymmetries in response to reward and punishment. *Electroencephalography Clin. Neurophysiol.* **1992**, *83*, 236–247. [CrossRef]
34. Langeslag, S.J.E. Electrophysiological correlates of romantic love: A review of EEG and ERP studies with beloved-related stimuli. *Brain Sci.* **2022**, *12*, 551. [CrossRef]
35. Quirin, M.; Gruber, T.; Kuhl, J.; Düsing, R. Is love right? Prefrontal resting brain asymmetry is related to the affiliation motive. *Front. Hum. Neurosci.* **2013**, *7*, 902. [CrossRef]
36. Aghedu, F.C.; Sarlo, M.; Zappasodi, F.; Acevado, B.P.; Bisiacchi, P.S. Romantic love affects emotional processing of love-unrelated stimuli: An EEG/ERP study using a love induction task. *Brain Cogn.* **2021**, *151*, 105733. [CrossRef] [PubMed]
37. Packheiser, J.; Berretz, G.; Rook, N.; Bahr, C.; Schockenhoff, L.; Güntürkün, O.; Ocklenburg, S. Investigating real-life emotions in romantic couples: A mobile EEG study. *Sci. Rep.* **2021**, *11*, 1142. [CrossRef] [PubMed]
38. Jones, N.A.; Field, T. Massage and music therapies attenuate frontal EEG asymmetry in depressed adolescents. *Adolescence* **1999**, *34*, 529–534. [PubMed]
39. Delorme, A.; Makeig, S. EEGLAB: An open source toolbox for analysis of single-trial EEG dynamics including independent component analysis. *J. Neurosci. Methods* **2004**, *134*, 9–21. [CrossRef]
40. Delorme, A. EEG is better left alone. *Sci. Rep.* **2023**, *13*, 2372. [CrossRef]
41. Bates, D.M. *lme4: Mixed-Effects Modeling with R*; Springer: Berlin/Heidelberg, Germany, 2010.
42. Benjamini, Y.; Hochberg, Y. Controlling the false discovery rate: A practical and powerful approach to multiple testing. *J. R. Stat. Soc. Ser. B* **1995**, *57*, 289–300. [CrossRef]

43. Lenth, R.V. emmeans: Estimated Marginal Means, aka Least-Squares Means. R Package Version 1.7.2. 2021. Available online: https://CRAN.R-project.org/package=emmeans (accessed on 22 November 2024).
44. Lin, L. A concordance correlation coefficient to evaluate reproducibility. *Biometrics* **1989**, *45*, 255–268. [CrossRef]
45. Lin, L. A note on the concordance correlation coefficient. *Biometrics* **2000**, *56*, 324–325.
46. Fatima, S.N.; Erzin, E. Use of affect context in dyadic interactions for continuous emotion recognition. *Speech Commun.* **2021**, *132*, 70–82. [CrossRef]
47. Quinn, C.; Haber, M.J.; Pan, Y. Use of the concordance correlation coefficient when examining agreement in dyadic research. *Nurs. Res.* **2009**, *58*, 368–373. [CrossRef]
48. Tabachnick, B.G.; Fidell, L.S. *Using Multivariate Statistics*, 6th ed.; Pearson: Boston, MA, USA, 2013.
49. Goelman, G.; Dan, R.; Stößel, G.; Tost, H.; Meyer-Lindenberg, A.; Bilek, E. Bidirectional signal exchanges and their mechanisms during joint attention interaction—A hyperscanning fMRI study. *Neuroimage* **2019**, *198*, 242–254. [CrossRef] [PubMed]
50. Kuhlen, A.K.; Allefeld, C.; Haynes, J.D. Content-specific coordination of listeners' to speakers' EEG during communication. *Front. Hum. Neurosci.* **2012**, *6*, 266. [CrossRef] [PubMed]
51. Misaki, M.; Kerr, K.L.; Ratliff, E.L.; Cosgrove, K.T.; Simmons, W.K.; Morris, A.S.; Bodurka, J. Beyond synchrony: The capacity of fMRI hyperscanning for the study of human social interaction. *Soc. Cogn. Affect. Neurosci.* **2021**, *16*, 84–92. [CrossRef]
52. Stolk, A.; Noordzij, M.L.; Verhagen, L.; Volman, I.; Schoffelen, J.-M.; Oostenveld, R.; Hagoort, P.; Toni, I. Cerebral coherence between communicators marks the emergence of meaning. *Proc. Natl. Acad. Sci. USA* **2014**, *111*, 18183–18188. [CrossRef]
53. Carver, C.S.; Harmon-Jones, E. Anger is an approach-related affect: Evidence and implications. *Psychol. Bull.* **2009**, *135*, 183–204. [CrossRef]
54. Harmon-Jones, E. Anger and the behavioral approach system. *Personal. Individ. Differ.* **2003**, *35*, 995–1005. [CrossRef]
55. Harmon-Jones, E.; Allen, J.J.B. Anger and frontal brain activity: EEG asymmetry consistent with approach motivation despite negative affective valence. *J. Personal. Soc. Psychol.* **1998**, *74*, 1310–1316. [CrossRef]
56. Flo, E.; Steine, I.; Blågstad, T.; Grønli, J.; Pallesen, S.; Portas, C.M. Transient changes in frontal alpha asymmetry as a measure of emotional and physical distress during sleep. *Brain Res.* **2011**, *1367*, 234–249. [CrossRef]
57. Mikutta, C.; Altorfer, A.; Strik, W.; Koenig, T. Emotions, arousal, and frontal alpha rhythm asymmetry during Beethoven's 5th symphony. *Brain Topogr.* **2012**, *25*, 423–430. [CrossRef]
58. Smith, E.E.; Reznik, S.J.; Stewart, J.L.; Allen, J.J.B. Assessing and conceptualizing frontal EEG asymmetry: An updated primer on recording, processing, analyzing, and interpreting frontal alpha asymmetry. *Int. J. Psychophysiol.* **2017**, *111*, 98–114. [CrossRef]
59. Pan, Y.; Cheng, X.; Zhang, Z.; Li, X.; Hu, Y. Cooperation in lovers: An fNIRS-based hyperscanning study. *Hum. Brain Mapp.* **2017**, *38*, 831–841. [CrossRef] [PubMed]
60. Zeevi, L.; Selle, N.K.; Kellmann, E.L.; Boiman, G.; Hart, Y.; Atzil, S. Bio-behavioral synchrony is a potential mechanism for mate selection in humans. *Sci. Rep.* **2022**, *12*, 4786. [CrossRef] [PubMed]
61. Freihart, B.K.; Meston, C.M. Preliminary evidence for a relationship between physiological synchrony and sexual satisfaction in opposite-sex couples. *J. Sex. Med.* **2019**, *16*, 2000–2010. [CrossRef] [PubMed]

Disclaimer/Publisher's Note: The statements, opinions and data contained in all publications are solely those of the individual author(s) and contributor(s) and not of MDPI and/or the editor(s). MDPI and/or the editor(s) disclaim responsibility for any injury to people or property resulting from any ideas, methods, instructions or products referred to in the content.

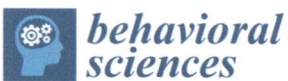 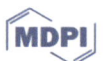

Article

Romantic Love and Behavioral Activation System Sensitivity to a Loved One

Adam Bode [1,*] and Phillip S. Kavanagh [2,3]

[1] School of Archaeology and Anthropology, ANU College of Arts and Social Sciences, The Australian National University, Canberra, ACT 2601, Australia
[2] Discipline of Psychology, Faculty of Health, University of Canberra, Bruce, ACT 2617, Australia; phil.kavanagh@canberra.edu.au
[3] Justice and Society, University of South Australia, Magill, SA 5072, Australia
* Correspondence: adam.bode@anu.edu.au

Abstract: Research investigating the mechanisms that contribute to romantic love is in its infancy. The behavioral activation system is one biopsychological system that has been demonstrated to play a role in several motivational outcomes. This study was the first to investigate romantic love and the behavioral activation system. In study 1, the Behavioral Activation System—Sensitivity to a Loved One (BAS-SLO) Scale was validated in a sample of 1556 partnered young adults experiencing romantic love. In study 2, hierarchical linear regression was used to identify BAS-SLO Scale associations with the intensity of romantic love in a subsample of 812 partnered young adults experiencing romantic love for two years or less. The BAS-SLO Scale explained 8.89% of the variance in the intensity of romantic love. Subject to further validation and testing, the BAS-SLO Scale may be useful in future neuroimaging and psychological studies. The findings are considered in terms of the mechanisms and evolutionary history of romantic love.

Keywords: BAS-SLO Scale; behavioral activation system; CFA; evolution; romantic love; Romantic Love Survey 2022

Citation: Bode, A.; Kavanagh, P.S. Romantic Love and Behavioral Activation System Sensitivity to a Loved One. *Behav. Sci.* **2023**, *13*, 921. https://doi.org/10.3390/bs13110921

Academic Editor: Heidi Kloos

Received: 6 September 2023
Revised: 31 October 2023
Accepted: 7 November 2023
Published: 10 November 2023

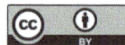

Copyright: © 2023 by the authors. Licensee MDPI, Basel, Switzerland. This article is an open access article distributed under the terms and conditions of the Creative Commons Attribution (CC BY) license (https://creativecommons.org/licenses/by/4.0/).

1. Introduction

Research investigating the mechanisms that contribute to romantic love is in its infancy. The behavioral activation system (BAS) is one biopsychological system that has been demonstrated to play a role in several motivational outcomes. To our knowledge, no studies have investigated the role the BAS may play in romantic love. Using a biological conceptualization of romantic love, we develop a means of assessing BAS sensitivity to a loved one and assess its association with the intensity of romantic love. The result is the formulation of a new means of assessing one biopsychological system that may contribute to the expression of romantic love.

1.1. Romantic Love

The topic of love in romantic relationships is riddled with definitional inconsistency and ambiguity. Sociological [1,2], anthropological [3], psychological [4,5], and biological [6] conceptions of love in romantic relationships all have their own terminology and formulations. While in many such disciplines, it is common to refer to all types of love within romantic relationships as "romantic love," the biopsychological focus of this article leads us to choose a different approach. In the discipline of biology, "romantic love" tends to refer to the period of intense feelings that often accompanies the early stages of romantic relationships [6,7]. As such, we use the term "romantic love" to refer to a motivational state associated with a range of reproductive functions, including mate choice, courtship, sex, and pair bonding [6] (p. 21). It is the basis of long-term romantic relationships and family formation throughout much of the world. It is associated with a range of cognitive, emotional, and behavioral activities in both sexes. It is sometimes referred to as "passionate love" in certain areas of psychology [8]. The expression of romantic love is partly socially or culturally influenced, and differences in its presentation are found across cultures (e.g., [1–3,9–12]).

Cognitive activity of romantic love includes intrusive thinking or preoccupation with the partner, idealization of the other in the relationship, and desire to know the other and to be known. Emotional activity includes attraction to the other, especially sexual attraction, negative feelings when things go awry, longing for reciprocity, desire for complete union, and physiological arousal. Behavioral activity includes actions toward determining the other's feelings, studying the other person, service to the other, and maintaining physical closeness.

Romantic love often happens at the early stages of a romantic relationship (referred to as early-stage romantic love) and usually lasts months or years (see [13,14]) but can sometimes last many years or decades (referred to as long-term romantic love) [15–17]. The psychological characteristics of both types of romantic love are similar, except that long-term romantic love is not characterized by intrusive thinking or preoccupation with the partner [15,16]. The neural mechanisms that cause each type of romantic love are similar but are not identical.

Romantic love is most strongly associated with neural activity in systems associated with reward and motivation (e.g., ventral tegmental area, nucleus accumbens, amygdala, and medial prefrontal cortex), emotions (e.g., amygdala, anterior cingulate cortex, and the insula), sexual desire and arousal (e.g., caudate, insula, putamen, and anterior cingulate cortex), and social cognition (e.g., amygdala, insula, and medial prefrontal cortex), as well as higher-order cortical brain areas that are involved in attention, memory, mental associations, and self-representation [6,18]. Functional connectivity is increased in people experiencing early-stage romantic love within the reward, motivation, and emotion regulation network (dorsal anterior cingulate cortex, insula, caudate, amygdala, and nucleus accumbens) as well as the social cognition network (temporo-parietal junction, posterior cingulate cortex, medial prefrontal cortex, inferior parietal, precuneus, and temporal lobe [19]. Early-stage romantic love is also associated with lower network segregation and altered connectivity degree [20] and with the endocrine activity of sex hormones, serotonin, dopamine, cortisol, oxytocin, and nerve growth factor [6]. To our knowledge, no research has investigated the endocrinological correlates of long-term romantic love.

1.2. The Behavioral Activation System (BAS)

One biological mechanism that is thought to play a role in the promotion of behavior is the BAS. This system is believed to be associated with dopaminergic reward and motivation circuitry [21–24]. The BAS works as a system that involves both inputs and outputs. Inputs are stimuli that serve as cues for goal-directed behavior. They include life events involving goal salience or goal attainment. Behavioral activation system outputs include motor activity, energy, confidence, interest, pleasure in rewards, and, potentially, sociability and exploration. The general outputs of the BAS have been compared with symptoms of mania, including initiation to locomotor activity, activity and exploration, and anger (see [25]).

1.3. The BAS and Romantic Love

People experiencing romantic love display a range of cognitions, emotions, and behaviors suggestive of heightened BAS activity. These include increased reward valuation, willingness to expend effort to gain reward, heightened initial hedonic response to success in the form of learning deficits, and lack of satiety in response to success (see [25]).

People experiencing romantic love demonstrate an increased reward valuation of the loved one. The loved one takes on a "special meaning" [26] (p. 32). The perception of the loved one changes, and idealization ensues, as does the belief that the loved one is the "perfect romantic partner" [10] (p. 391) for them and that their loved one satisfies their preferred standards of physical attractiveness [27] (p. 395). The loved one becomes the most important person in their life.

People experiencing romantic love appear to demonstrate a willingness to expend effort to gain reward. Romantic lovers often engage in courtship (see [6] for a review of the costs and benefits of courtship among people experiencing romantic love), which involves a series of signals and behaviors that serve as a means of assessing potential partner quality and willingness to invest in a relationship [28,29]. People experiencing romantic love are also willing to reorder daily priorities, make themselves available to their loved one, and take steps to make themselves desirable to their loved one by changing their "clothing, mannerisms, habits, or values" [26] (p. 33).

Some people experiencing romantic love may demonstrate some aspects of heightened initial hedonic response to success in the form of learning deficits. The most cogent example of this is the instances of obsessive pursuit (usually committed by men), which occur in the absence of rewarding interaction from the loved one. Men, in particular, but not exclusively, have a tendency to misinterpret politeness or friendliness for sexual interest from potential sexual partners (see [30] for review). Such a false positive bias is potentially present in people experiencing romantic love and can result in repeated attempts by an individual to court a loved one despite there being obvious indications that such efforts will be fruitless. That both females and males can be subject to ineffective courting demonstrates the potent motivational effect romantic love can have on both sexes. This is one BAS sensitivity component that warrants further investigation in people experiencing romantic love.

People experiencing romantic love demonstrate a lack of satiety in response to success. For example, even when an individual in love feels emotionally close to their loved one, there can be a desire to be even closer. A sense of avolition and uncontrollability is a feature of romantic love [26] (p. 33). This is evidenced by an individual reordering their daily activities to spend increasingly long periods with their loved one and, in the modern environment, the obsessive monitoring of social media pages of the loved one. More generally, people experiencing romantic love experience prolonged affect, confidence, and increased energy over prolonged periods, as is indicated by the hypomanic symptoms found to be present in adolescents experiencing romantic love reported by Brand and colleagues [31].

1.4. Salience of Loved One-Related Stimuli and the BAS

There is evidence that when an individual is in love, the loved one takes on a special meaning [26]. This can be considered in terms of loved one-related stimuli having increased salience, probably as a result of oxytocin activity in one or more motivation pathways [32] (see also [33]). This has been demonstrated empirically in terms of memory and attention [34], as well as the heightened BAS sensitivity characteristics of romantic love detailed above. Because the BAS is situated within a motivational system, we believe that this salience of the loved one and loved one-related stimuli means the BAS probably responds in a particularly sensitive manner to loved one-related stimuli.

This heightened salience of loved one-related stimuli among individuals experiencing romantic love suggests that BAS sensitivity, somewhat analogous to anxiety (see [35]), may exist in a trait and state form. General BAS sensitivity may be relatively stable and influence behavior over the life course in a consistent manner. This is a type of trait BAS sensitivity. There are also periods when the BAS may become particularly sensitive, such as during a manic episode (see [25]), or in relation to a particular person, such as in circumstances of romantic love. This is a type of state of BAS sensitivity. The foci of the current studies are this state of BAS sensitivity that is characteristic of romantic love.

1.5. The BAS Scale

One common measure of BAS sensitivity is the BAS Scale [36], which includes three subscales: reward responsiveness, drive, and fun-seeking. The BAS Scale was originally validated by Carver and White (1994) in conjunction with items assessing the behavioral inhibition system (BIS) using exploratory factor analysis, Cronbach's alpha (reliability), and correlation scores with other related measures (convergent validity). The analysis found four factors explained the BIS/BAS Scale: (i) BIS, (ii) BAS reward responsiveness, (iii) BAS drive, and (vi) BAS fun-seeking. More recently, efforts using confirmatory factor analysis have been undertaken to confirm the reliability of the BAS Scale (e.g., [37–44]) and a single factor (two-factor BIS/BAS Scale) has been suggested (e.g., [38,39,43]) with some degree of support [38,43].

The reward-responsiveness subscale assesses the tendency to respond to rewards with energy and enthusiasm, the drive subscale assesses motivation to pursue goals, and the fun-seeking subscale assesses the tendency to pursue positive experiences without regard to potential threats or costs [36] (see [25] for a summary of findings in relation to BAS Scale subscales and bipolar disorder). It seems feasible that all three subscales could contribute to aspects of romantic love, as the BAS responds to loved one-related stimuli.

1.6. The Current Studies

This is the first attempt to investigate the Behavioral Activation System and romantic love. As a result, we undertake preliminary work to shed light on the relationships between these two constructs. We amended the BAS Scale to assess *BAS Sensitivity to a Loved One* (BAS-SLO; described below). In Study 1, we validate the BAS-SLO Scale. This was a necessary step in developing an initial understanding of the relationship between the behavioral activation system and romantic love. We used confirmatory factor analysis to assess the suitability of three factor structures: (i) a one-factor model; (ii) a three-factor, 13-item structure; and (iii) a three-factor, 12-item structure. We determined that a three-factor, 12-item structure possessed the best goodness of fit. We calculated Cronbach's alphas to test internal reliability and correlated subscales with a related measure to assess convergent validity for this structure. In Study 2, we tested the hypothesis that the BAS-SLO Scale will be positively associated with the intensity of romantic love. Findings are considered within an evolutionary framework, which helps elucidate the mechanisms and evolutionary history of romantic love.

2. Study 1: Validating the BAS-SLO Scale

2.1. Materials and Methods

2.1.1. Participants

Participants were 1556 English-speaking young adults who self-identified as being in love taken from the Romantic Love Survey 2022 [45]. Appendix A presents the characteristics of participants used in Study 1 and the country of residence of participants. We use the majority of the ideas for sample characteristics reporting from Bode and Kowal [7].

2.1.2. Measures

The Behavioral Activation System Sensitivity to a Loved One (BAS-SLO) Scale was created by amending each item of the BAS Scale to relate to an individual's loved one or relationship with their loved one. Participants were asked, "Indicate how much the following applies to you". Responses were scored on a four-point scale (1 = very true for me; 4 = very false for me). Scores for each item are reverse coded, and subscale scores are summed. Table 1 presents the original BAS Scale items and the BAS-SLO Scale items for each subscale.

We also used the Passionate Love Scale—30 (PLS-30) to assess the convergent validity of the BAS-SLO scale. The PLS-30 is a 30-item measure of the cognitive, emotional, and behavioral characteristics of romantic love. Each item records scores by assessing agreement with statements on a nine-point Likert scale (1 = not at all true; 9 = definitely true). It is the most commonly used measure of romantic love in biological studies of romantic love [7]. Cronbach's alpha for the PLS-30 in this sample was 0.944.

Table 1. Original BAS Scale items and the equivalent BAS-SLO Scale items.

Item	BAS Scale Items	BAS-SLO Scale Items
Reward responsiveness subscale		
1	When I'm doing well at something, I love to keep at it.	When I'm doing well at something my partner values, I love to keep at it
2	When I get something I want, I feel excited and energized	When my partner tells me they love me, I feel excited and energized
3	When I see an opportunity for something I like, I get excited right away	When I see an opportunity to spend time with my partner, I get excited right away
4	When good things happen to me, it affects me strongly	When good things happen to my partner, it affects me strongly
5	It would excite me to win a contest	It would excite me for my partner and me to win a contest
Drive subscale		
1	I go out of my way to get things I want	I go out of my way to maintain my relationship with my partner
2	When I want something, I usually go all-out to get it	When it comes to maintaining my relationship with my partner, I usually go all-out
3	If I see a chance to get something I want, I move on it right away	If I see a chance to strengthen my relationship with my partner, I move on it straight away
4	When I go after something, I use a "no holds barred" approach	When it comes to maintaining my relationship with my partner, I use a "no holds barred" approach
Fun-seeking subscale		
1	I'm always willing to try something new if I think it will be fun	I'm always willing to try new things with my partner if I think it will be fun
2	I will often do things for no other reason than that they might be fun	I will often do things with my partner for no other reason than they are fun
3	I often act on the spur of the moment	I often act on the spur of the moment with my partner
4	I crave excitement and new sensations	I crave excitement and new sensations with my partner

2.1.3. Procedure

We conducted a confirmatory factor analysis (CFA) on the 13 items of the BAS-SLO Scale using techniques/suggestions from a guidance paper [46]) and predicted a three-factor solution in line with the original BAS Scale factor structure [36]. A CFA using a one-factor solution was also conducted, as there is some literature suggesting that the BAS can be explained by a single factor [38,39,43]. At the suggestion of one reviewer, following an initial round of peer review, we then conducted another three-factor CFA of 11 items from the proposed BAS-SLO (removing two poorly loaded items; reward responsiveness item 5 and fun-seeking item 3).

A weighted least square mean and variance adjusted (WLSMV) method of confirmatory factor analysis was used as the data were ordinal [47]. The comparative fit index (CFI), standardized root-mean-square error of approximation (RMSEA), and standardized root-mean-square residual (SRMR) were used to assess the appropriateness of all three models in accordance with common practice (see [46]).

The following criteria, based on work by Hu and Bentler [48] and the model CFA example by Knetka and Runyon [46], were used to assess the adequacy of the model: CFI > 0.95 (although 0.90 is required to ensure mis-specified models are not deemed acceptable), RMSEA < 0.06, and SRMR < 0.08. Internal reliability was assessed by calculating Cronbach's alpha for each BAS-SLO subscale. Values of >0.70 were considered acceptable (see [49]). We assessed convergent validity by correlating BAS-SLO Scale subscales (i.e., reward responsiveness, drive, and fun-seeking) with the PLS-30 and the amended HCL-32. Factor loadings, covariances, and goodness of fit indices were calculated using the Lavaan package for R version 4.2.2 in R Studio. The CFA diagram was created in AMOS version 26. Convergent validity analyses were conducted using SPSS version 27.

2.2. Results

No items from the BAS-SLO were missing data. Two cases were missing data for the PLS-30. These two cases were not included in the correlation analysis. Table 2 presents the means, standard deviations, skewness statistics, and kurtosis statistics for the 13 items of the BAS-SLO. Most of the data were moderately skewed, but this was deemed acceptable as the robust maximum likelihood method has been shown to be robust against violations of normality (see [47]).

Table 2. Means, standard deviations, skewness statistics, and kurtosis statistics for BAS-SLO Scale items in Study 1.

	M	SD	Skewness	Kurtosis
R1	3.58	0.56	−0.92	0.08
R2	3.67	0.55	−1.59	2.21
R3	3.56	0.62	−1.23	0.94
R4	3.57	0.64	−1.42	1.86
R5	3.56	0.66	−1.37	1.29
D1	3.21	0.77	−0.80	0.30
D2	3.12	0.76	−0.65	0.24
D3	3.37	0.71	−0.98	0.74
D4	2.84	0.78	−0.23	−0.039
F1	3.62	0.57	−1.33	1.55
F2	3.42	0.70	−1.00	0.44
F3	3.06	0.73	−0.36	−0.34
F4	3.34	0.69	−0.67	−0.22

R = Reward responsiveness subscale; D = Drive subscale; F = Fun-seeking subscale.

2.2.1. Three-Factor, 13-Item Model

Results from the three-factor 13-item CFA indicated that, in our sample, the model had adequate but not good psychometric properties (see Appendix B for a summary table of goodness of fit statistics for all models). CFI was 0.944, indicating an acceptable (but not quite good) fit. RMSEA was 0.055, indicating good fit. SRMR was 0.041, indicating good fit. Factor loadings ranged from 0.44 to 0.80, with the majority above 0.60 (see Appendix C), suggesting that the factors explained most of the items reasonably (but not very) well. Factors correlated with each other from 0.40 (drive and fun-seeking) to 0.66 (reward responsiveness and fun-seeking), suggesting the discriminate validity was acceptable. Two items (R5 and F3) loaded poorly onto the reward responsiveness and fun-seeking factors (0.44 and 0.52), respectively. Appendix C presents the results of the three-factor, 13-item CFA.

2.2.2. One-Factor, 13-Item Model

Results from the one-factor, 13-item CFA indicated that, in our sample, the model had very poor psychometric properties. CFI was 0.709, indicating very poor fit. RMSEA was 0.121, indicating very poor fit. SRMR was 0.086, indicating poor fit. Because this model had very poor fit, we do not report further on the results.

2.2.3. Three-Factor, 11-Item Model

Because R5 and F3 loaded substantially lower than all the other items in the three-factor, 13-item CFA, we removed these items and ran another three-factor CFA, this time with 11 items. Results indicated that, in our sample, the three-factor, 11-item model had good psychometric properties, but loadings were not generally improved from the three-factor, 13-item CFA. CFI was 0.966, indicating good fit. RMSEA was 0.048, indicating good fit. SRMR was 0.037, indicating good fit. Factor loadings ranged from 0.55 to 0.80, with the majority above 0.60 (see Figure 1), suggesting that the factors explained most of the items reasonably (but not very) well. Factors correlated with each other from 0.40 (drive and fun-seeking) to 0.68 (reward responsiveness and fun-seeking), suggesting the discriminate validity was acceptable. Figure 1 presents the results of the three-factor, 11-item CFA.

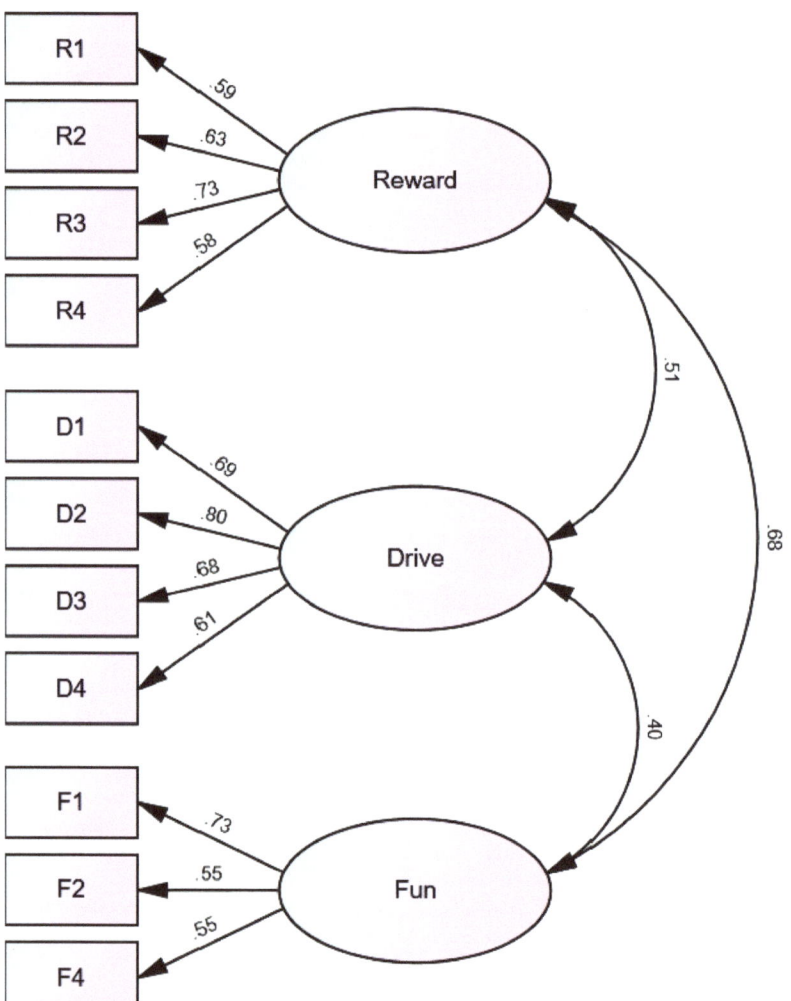

Figure 1. Results of the three-factor, 11-item CFA model for the BAS-SLO Scale. Note: Survey items (for description, see Table 3) are represented by rectangles, and latent factors are represented by ovals. Reward = reward responsiveness; Drive = drive; Fun = fun-seeking. The numbers above the one-directional arrows connecting factors to items represent standardized factor loadings. The numbers to the right of the bi-directional arrows connecting factors represent correlations between the factors.

Table 3. Correlations among each BAS-SLO Scale subscale and the PLS-30 in Study 1.

BAS-SLO Scale Subscales	PLS-30
Reward	0.560 ***
Drive	0.418 ***
Fun-seeking	0.358 ***

$n = 1554$; *** $p < 0.001$.

Cronbach's alpha for the three-factor, 11-item BAS-SLO Scale was 0.725 for reward responsiveness, indicating acceptable internal reliability; 0.786 for drive, indicating acceptable internal reliability; and 0.629 for fun-seeking, indicating marginally questionable internal reliability. Cronbach's alphas for all subscales aligned closely with those of the original BAS subscales (reward responsiveness = 0.73, drive = 0.76, fun-seeking = 0.66; [36]) and with subsequent studies (e.g., [37,39]).

Convergent validity was assessed by correlating each of the BAS-SLO Scale subscales with the PLS-30. We anticipated that each BAS-SLO Scale subscale would correlate highly with the PLS-30. Table 3 presents the correlations between the BAS-SLO Scale subscales and the PLS-30. PLS-30 had a large association with reward responsiveness and a medium association with drive and fun-seeking. This suggests good convergent validity.

2.3. Discussion

Study 1 reported three CFAs of the BAS-SLO Scale. A three-factor model for the BAS-SLO Scale with 11 items that aligned with the three factors of the original BAS Scale (reward responsiveness, drive, and fun-seeking) was deemed to be an appropriate model by CFA, as well as the reliability and convergent validity analyses. This is especially the case when considered in light of the psychometric properties of the original BAS Scale and subsequent studies indicating a three-factor model of the BAS Scale utilizing confirmatory factor analysis (e.g., [42–44]). Indices of fit generally supported the notion of an acceptable model with good fit. Factor loadings were lower than would be ideal, suggesting the factors did not explain the data well. Correlations among the factors suggest the discriminate validity of the BAS-SLO is moderately low. Internal reliability of the subscales ranged from marginal to acceptable. This is in line with alphas for these three subscales in previous studies [42–44]. Correlations between subscales of the BAS-SLO Scale and the PLS-30 were roughly as expected, suggesting good convergent validity. In sum, we think the BAS-SLO is a measure that could be used in studies investigating BAS sensitivity to a loved one and romantic love, as well as a range of other related phenomena. Appendix D presents the final items of the proposed BAS-SLO Scale.

3. Study 2: The BAS and Romantic Love
3.1. Materials and Methods
3.1.1. Participants

Participants were a subsample of study 1 participants, 812 English-speaking young adults who self-identified as being in love from the Romantic Love Survey 2022 [45]. Participants who had been in love for 23 months or less and scored above 130 on the PLS were included in the analysis. Two years is a likely period of time in which individuals experience early-stage romantic love rather than long-term romantic love (see [6]). Two cases were missing one data point, and these cases were removed. One intersex participant was removed. Appendix E presents the characteristics of participants used in Study 2 and the country of residence of the participants. We use the majority of the ideas for sample characteristics reporting from Bode and Kowal [7].

3.1.2. Measures

Behavioral Activation System sensitivity to a loved one was measured using the three subscales of the 11-item BAS-SLO Scale validated in Study 1. Intensity of romantic love was measured using the Passionate Love Scale (PLS-30; [10]; described in Study 1). *Sex* was measured using a simple question asking, "What is your biological sex?" Data were coded as 1 (female) or 2 (male). Some studies have suggested that females experience romantic love marginally more intensely than males [50,51]. Love in romantic relationships has been thought to follow a specific trajectory of intensity related to intimacy, passion, and commitment [52]. As such, the length of time an individual has been in love may be associated with the waxing or waning intensity of romantic love. *Months in love* was assessed by asking participants how long they had been in love with their loved one. Obsessive thinking is definitive of early-stage romantic love (see [10,53,54]) and one proposed biological component of romantic love [33]. It therefore follows that it may have a direct influence on the intensity of romantic love. Percent of time thinking about a loved one (*obsessive thinking*) was measured by asking participants, "What percentage of your waking hours do you spend thinking about the person you love?" Responses were on a scale from 0% to 100%. *Commitment* was measured by using five items from the TLS-15 commitment subscale [55] but with a nine-point scoring approach. Each item records scores by assessing agreement with statements ranging from 1 (not at all) to 9 (extremely). Romantic love is believed to serve as a commitment device [56,57] and, therefore, may have a direct association with the intensity of romantic love.

3.1.3. Procedure

To test the hypothesis that BAS sensitivity to a loved one would predict romantic love, we undertook a hierarchical linear regression whereby the BAS-SLO Scale predicted PLS-30. Step one included controls. Step 2 included controls and each of the three BAS-SLO Scale subscales.

3.2. Results

Table 4 reports the correlations among all variables used in Study 2 analyses and their descriptive statistics.

Table 4. Correlations among variables used in Study 2 and their descriptive statistics.

	Variable	1	2	3	4	5	6	7	8
1	Reward responsiveness	1	0.413 ***	0.465 ***	0.520 ***	−0.106 **	0.071 *	0.207 ***	0.450 ***
2	Drive		1	0.327 ***	0.468 ***	−0.048	0.099 **	0.308 ***	0.344 ***
3	Fun-seeking			1	0.340 ***	−0.087 *	0.035	0.121 ***	0.262 ***
4	PLS-30				1	−0.112 **	0.137 ***	0.465 ***	0.612 ***
5	Sex (male)					1	−0.064	−0.209 ***	−0.074 *
6	Months in love						1	0.063	0.232 ***
7	Obsessive thinking							1	0.330 ***
8	Commitment								1
	n					423			
	%					52.09			
	M	14.33	12.49	10.43	209.64		8.13	49.15	36.55
	SD	1.67	2.34	1.42	31.27		5.97	22.58	6.85

* $p < 0.05$; ** $p < 0.01$; *** $p < 0.001$.

Our hypothesis predicted that the BAS-SLO Scale would be positively associated with the intensity of romantic love. To test this hypothesis, we undertook a hierarchical linear regression whereby the BAS-SLO Scale predicted PLS-30 scores after controlling for sex, months in love, obsessive thinking, and commitment. All assumptions for linear regression were met. The hierarchical linear regression predicting the intensity of romantic love revealed that, at Step 1, control variables contributed significantly to the regression model, with $F(6, 805) = 166.987$ and $p < 0.001$, and accounted for 45.02% of the variance in intensity of romantic love. Adding the BAS-SLO Scale to the regression model (Step 2) explained an additional 8.89% of the variation in the intensity of romantic love, and this change in adjusted R^2 was significant; $F(3, 802) = 136.519$ and $p < 0.001$. Each individual BAS-SLO Scale subscale contributed significantly to the model (reward responsiveness,

$p < 0.001$; drive, $p < 0.001$; and fun-seeking, $p = 0.017$). Table 5 presents the regression statistics for this analysis.

Table 5. Hierarchical regression model of intensity of romantic love.

	R^2	Adjusted R^2	Adjusted R^2 Change	b	SE	β	t	p	95% CI Lower	95% CI Upper
Step 1	0.453 ***	0.450 ***								
Sex				−0.772	1.668	−0.012	−0.463	0.644	−4.046	2.502
Months in love				−0.013	0.140	−0.002	−0.090	0.928	−0.288	0.263
Obsessive thinking				0.405	0.039	0.292	10.392	<0.001	0.328	0.481
Commitment				2.353	0.129	0.516	18.212	<0.001	2.099	2.607
Step 2	0.543 ***	0.539 ***	0.089 ***							
Sex				0.152	1.534	0.002	0.099	0.921	−2.860	3.164
Months in love				0.019	0.129	0.004	0.147	0.883	−0.234	0.272
Obsessive thinking				0.339	0.037	0.245	9.252	<0.001	0.267	0.410
Commitment				1.667	0.131	0.365	12.733	<0.001	1.410	1.924
Reward responsiveness				3.898	0.561	0.209	6.951	<0.001	2.797	4.999
Drive				2.131	0.370	0.159	5.753	<0.001	1.404	2.858
Fun-seeking				1.438	0.601	0.065	2.391	0.017	0.257	2.618

$n = 812$; *** $p < 0.001$.

3.3. Discussion

Study 2 used the BAS-SLO Scale to examine the associations between the BAS sensitivity to a loved one and the intensity of romantic love in young adults experiencing romantic love for less than two years. We hypothesized that the BAS sensitivity to a loved one would be positively associated with the intensity of romantic love. Our hypothesis was confirmed. The BAS-SLO Scale explained 8.89% of the variance in the intensity of romantic love (measured by the PLS-30), confirming our hypothesis. This amounts to a medium effect [58] of BAS sensitivity to a loved one on the intensity of romantic love. All three subscales contributed significantly to the model, and this suggests that the BAS plays a role in romantic love. That all three subscales contributed to the model raises the question as to whether each subscale contributes to specific components that characterize the intensity of romantic love in the PLS-30.

The findings of Study 2 are important because they demonstrate that the BAS-SLO Scale may be useful in investigating romantic love and provide the first evidence that the BAS plays a role in romantic love. The findings suggest that future studies may be able to identify the unique components of romantic love caused by the BAS and its state of sensitivity to a loved one. Future studies could use the BAS-SLO Scale to predict individual features of the intensity of romantic love. The use of the BAS-SLO Scale could also potentially be extended to investigate aspects of established pair bonds and relationships characterized by pair bond maintenance and not characterized by the presence of pair bond formation and romantic love (see [33]). Further, the BAS-SLO Scale's use could be combined with fMRI analyses to identify the neurobiological components of the BAS and their contribution to romantic love.

This study is not without limitations, however. The sample is constituted entirely of young adults in the first two years of romantic love. As a result, the sample is neither representative of the entirety of the human population who experiences romantic love nor the entire spectrum of romantic love (see [7] for issues of generalizability). Further, the analysis was undertaken on a subsample of that used to validate the Scale in Study 1. This limits the implications of the findings, given that the Scale may possess different properties in a different sample. Nonetheless, the study has demonstrated the potential usefulness of the BAS-SLO Scale and provided the first evidence that the BAS plays a role in romantic love.

4. General Discussion

This article presents the first direct evidence of the relationships between BAS sensitivity and romantic love. Study 1 demonstrated that it is possible to measure BAS sensitivity to a loved one. Study 2 demonstrated that this means of measurement can be useful in empirical studies investigating the relationship between the BAS and romantic love. Combined, these two studies suggest that BAS sensitivity to a loved one is a real phenomenon and that the state of romantic love is probably associated with BAS sensitivity to a loved one. This has implications for understanding the mechanisms and evolutionary history of romantic love (see [59]).

The reason the BAS can be particularly sensitive to a loved one may relate to the concept of salience. Froemke and Young [32] have suggested that oxytocin acts on motivation pathways to increase the salience of specific social stimuli. In humans, this may take place in the ventral tegmental area (VTA). The VTA is consistently implicated in fMRI studies of people experiencing romantic love (see [6,60,61]). Although void of oxytocin receptors, the human VTA has been identified as the area in which oxytocin attaches salience to socially rewarding cues [62]. This increased salience probably results in further up-regulation of dopamine pathways, presumably including those that characterize the activity of the BAS. This supports Bode's [33] contention that the bonding attraction system in romantic love is characterized by both oxytocin and dopamine activity, among other factors.

Several studies have shed light on the neural structures associated with BAS sensitivity (assessed with the BAS Scale) in normal samples. BAS sensitivity has been associated with activity in the VTA–nucleus accumbens pathway and the orbitofrontal cortex [21], and BAS reward responsiveness has been associated with lateral prefrontal cortex, anterior cingulate cortex, and ventral striatum [22] in healthy samples. Interestingly, BAS drive has been associated with less activity in the putamen, caudate, and thalamus, and BAS reward responsiveness has been associated with increased activity in the left precentral gyrus in response to different intensities of infant cries among mothers [23]. Variation in regional gray matter volume in the ventromedial prefrontal cortex and inferior parietal lobule has also been associated with BAS Scale scores [24]. There is also evidence that reward network glutamate levels contribute to individual differences in BAS reward responsiveness [63]. These structures generally overlap with those found in romantic love (see [6]).

Knowledge about the neural structures associated with BAS sensitivity, their overlap with the structures associated with romantic love, and now, a means of measuring BAS sensitivity to a loved one provide the means of measuring specific bio-psychological mechanisms that likely contribute to romantic love. Functional magnetic resonance imaging studies can begin to isolate the specific contribution of the BAS to the intensity of romantic love or specific features of romantic love. The implications of the studies reported in this article extend beyond a better understanding of the mechanisms of romantic love. They also provide insights into the evolutionary history of romantic love.

The findings support the notion that romantic love evolved by using pre-existing neural mechanisms (see [6]). The BAS is evolutionarily old, and romantic love made use of this system in a novel way. Instead of increasing general sensitivity, it generates a salience of a particular social stimulus (the loved one), which in turn increases sensitivity to the loved one. This increased salience is possibly the same mechanism that results in increased sensitivity among a plethora of other mechanisms. For example, evidence that lovers have an attentional and memory bias towards loved one-related stimuli [34] suggests that the stimuli possess greater importance or value than other stimuli. This is not the result of state changes to the attentional or memory system but rather the result of increased salience of loved one-related stimuli. This is a simple and elegant way of recruiting cognitive, emotional, and behavioral efforts in response to stimuli that have been identified at the input to be of great importance. This salience presumably required an internal schema of the loved one, an assessment of stimuli to identify their concordance, and then the application of increased value or weight to those stimuli. The concepts of salience and sensitivity are fundamental to a better understanding of the mechanisms of romantic love.

This process of increasing salience is probably at the core and very beginning of the evolution of romantic love and may be associated with the left VTA [61]. Mutation permitted the increased valuation of particular social stimuli, and that was possibly the first step in its evolutionary history. The particular features of romantic love, and perhaps some of its functions, such as pair bonding, may have evolved long after this initial step. Courtship attraction, which is also associated with an increased salience of social stimuli (see [33]), and sexual desire probably become intertwined with romantic love over the following generations. This is in line with previous suggestions that a precursor to contemporary romantic love emerged prior to the evolution of pair bonds [33,64].

The findings of these two studies also highlight the likelihood that BAS sensitivity exists in both a trait and state manner. The traditional BAS Scale assesses dispositional trait sensitivity, whereas the BAS-SLO Scale assesses what can be considered a type of state sensitivity. Parallels with anxiety may help to guide future researchers when elucidating these distinct but related phenomena. To better understand the similarities and differences between trait and state BAS sensitivity, it will be necessary to identify the role of trait sensitivity in romantic love.

5. Conclusions

This article reported two studies related to the behavioral activation system and romantic love. In Study 1, the BAS-SLO Scale was validated in a sample of 1556 partnered young adults experiencing romantic love. The validation determined that the characteristics of the BAS-SLO Scale were sufficient to justify its use in future psychological and imaging studies. In study 2, hierarchical linear regression was used to identify BAS-SLO Scale associations with the intensity of romantic love in a subsample of 812 partnered young adults experiencing romantic love for two years or less. The BAS-SLO Scale explained 8.89% of the variance in the intensity of romantic love. The findings shed light on one of the biopsychological mechanisms that contribute to romantic love and provide insights into the specific functions of regions associated with romantic love from fMRI studies. The BAS-SLO Scale should be used in future psychological and imaging studies.

Author Contributions: Conceptualization, A.B.; methodology, A.B. and P.S.K.; formal analysis, A.B.; data curation, A.B.; writing—original draft preparation, A.B.; writing—review and editing, P.S.K.; visualization, A.B.; supervision, P.S.K.; project administration, A.B. All authors have read and agreed to the published version of the manuscript.

Funding: This research received no external funding.

Institutional Review Board Statement: The collection of data used in these studies was approved by the Australian National University Human Research Ethics Committee (Protocol 2022/298).

Informed Consent Statement: Informed consent was obtained from all subjects involved in the study.

Data Availability Statement: The data and code used this study are available form authors upon request.

Acknowledgments: The authors thank Marta Kowal for providing useful comments on an earlier version of the manuscript.

Conflicts of Interest: The authors declare no conflict of interest.

Appendix A

Table A1. Study 1 sample characteristics.

	Range	Mean	SD	Median	n	%
Sample					1556	100.00
Female					814	52.31
Heterosexual					1142	73.39
Age	18.00, 25.00	22.44	1.83	23.00		
PLS-30 (mean item; 1–9)	1.93, 9.00	7.02	1.13	7.17		
TLS-Commitment (mean item; 1–9)	1.80, 9.00	7.57	1.34	7.80		
Time thinking (%)	1.00, 100.00	49.68	23.45	50.00		
Dating, not co-habiting					479	30.78
Committed, not co-habiting					715	45.95
Committed, co-habiting					314	20.18
Married or de facto					48	3.08
Years in love (0–10 or more)	0.00, 10.00	1.90	2.15	1.00		
Relationship duration (years)	0.00, 10.00	1.82	2.05	1.00		
Relationship satisfaction (1–5)	1.00, 5.00	4.25	0.78	4.00		
HCL-32 (0–32)	0.00, 28.00	16.38	4.91	17.00		
Having sex (no/yes)					1377	88.62
Sex times per week	0.00, 30.00	3.03	2.79	2.00		
>13 years of education					1352	86.89
Current student (no/yes)					1046	67.22
Not working					629	40.42
Less than full-time work					491	31.56
Full-time work					436	28.02
AQOL-4D (12–48)	12.00, 35.00	17.59	3.48	17.00		

PLS-30 = Passionate Love Scale (divided by number of items); TLS-Commitment = five items from the TLS-15 Commitment subscale [55] but using a nine-point response option (divided by number of items); Obsessive thinking = Percent of time thinking about loved one; HCL-32 = Amended Hypomanic Checklist—32; AQOL-4D = Assessment of Quality of Life—4D; A small number of data points are missing among these variables.

Table A2. Country of residence of Study 1 participants.

Country	n	%
South Africa	182	11.70
Poland	136	8.74
Mexico	115	7.39
Portugal	111	7.13
Italy	110	7.07
UK and NI	109	7.01
Greece	93	5.98
USA	91	5.85
Spain	90	5.78
Germany	76	4.88
Hungary	67	4.31
Netherlands	67	4.31
Canada	43	2.76
Chile	36	2.31
France	31	1.99
Czech Republic	23	1.48
Slovenia	23	1.48
Australia	20	1.29
Belgium	20	1.29
Estonia	18	1.16
Latvia	18	1.16
Rest of sample	77	4.95

Rest of sample = Finland, Sweden, Austria, Ireland, Israel, New Zealand, Switzerland, Denmark, Japan, Norway, Luxembourg, South Korea.

Appendix B

Table A3. Fit indices for one-factor and three-factor models of the BAS-SLO Scale in a sample of 1556 young adults self-reporting romantic love.

	CFI	RMSEA	SRMR
Criteria	>0.950 (0.900)	<0.060	<0.080
One-factor model	0.709	0.121	0.086
Three-factor model (13 items)	0.944	0.055	0.041
Three-factor model (11 items)	0.966	0.048	0.037

Appendix C

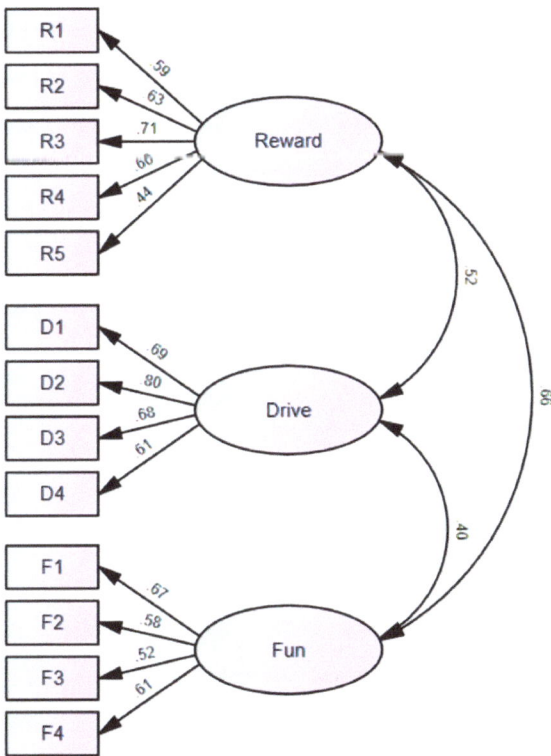

Figure A1. Results of the three-factor, 13-item CFA model for the BAS-SLO Scale. Note: Survey items (for description, see Table 3) are represented by rectangles, and latent factors are represented by ovals. Reward = reward responsiveness; Drive = drive; Fun = fun-seeking. The numbers above the one-directional arrows connecting factors to items represent standardized factor loadings. The numbers to the right of the bi-directional arrows connecting factors represent correlations between the factors.

Appendix D

Table A4. Final items of the proposed BAS-SLO Scale.

Item	BAS Scale Items	BAS-SLO Scale Items
Reward responsiveness subscale		
1	When I'm doing well at something, I love to keep at it.	When I'm doing well at something my partner values, I love to keep at it
2	When I get something I want, I feel excited and energized	When my partner tells me they love me, I feel excited and energized
3	When I see an opportunity for something I like, I get excited right away	When I see an opportunity to spend time with my partner, I get excited right away
4	When good things happen to me, it affects me strongly	When good things happen to my partner, it affects me strongly
Drive subscale		
1	I go out of my way to get things I want	I go out of my way to maintain my relationship with my partner
2	When I want something, I usually go all-out to get it	When it comes to maintaining my relationship with my partner, I usually go all-out
3	If I see a chance to get something I want, I move on it right away	If I see a chance to strengthen my relationship with my partner, I move on it straight away
4	When I go after something, I use a "no holds barred" approach	When it comes to maintaining my relationship with my partner, I use a "no holds barred" approach
Fun-seeking subscale		
1	I'm always willing to try something new if I think it will be fun	I'm always willing to try new things with my partner if I think it will be fun
2	I will often do things for no other reason than that they might be fun	I will often do things with my partner for no other reason than they are fun
3	I crave excitement and new sensations	I crave excitement and new sensations with my partner

Appendix E

Table A5. Study 2 sample characteristics.

	Range	Mean	SD	Median	n	%
Sample					812	100.00
Female					389	47.91
Heterosexual					592	72.91
Age	18.00, 25.00	22.16	1.86	22.00		
PLS-30 (mean item; 1–9)	4.37, 9.00	6.99	1.04	7.10		
TLS-Commitment (mean item; 1–9)	2.00, 9.00	1.22	1.37	7.60		
Time thinking (%)	2.00, 100.00	49.10	22.58	49.00		
Dating, not co-habiting					358	44.09
Committed, not co-habiting					373	45.94
Committed, co-habiting					75	9.24
Married or de facto					6	0.74
Months in love (0–23)						
Relationship satisfaction (1–5)	1.00, 5.00	4.18	0.78	4.00		
HCL-32 (0–32)	0.00, 28.00	16.35	4.79	17.00		
Having sex (no/yes)					722	89.04
Sex times per week	0.00, 20.00	3.21	2.87	3.00		

Table A5. *Cont.*

	Range	Mean	SD	Median	n	%
>13 years of education					693	85.34
Current student (no/yes)					569	70.07
Not working					355	43.72
Less than full-time work					275	33.87
Full-time work					182	22.41
AQOL-4D (12–48)	12.00, 35.00	17.55	3.47	17.00		

PLS-30 = Passionate Love Scale (divided by number of items); TLS-Commitment = five items from the TLS-15 Commitment subscale [55] but using a nine-point response option (divided by number of items); Obsessive thinking = Percent of time thinking about loved one; HCL-32 = Amended Hypomanic Checklist—32; AQOL-4D = Assessment of Quality of Life—4D; A small number of data points are missing among these variables.

Table A6. Country of residence of Study 2 participants.

Country	n	%
South Africa	101	12.44
Poland	73	8.99
UK and NI	59	7.27
Portugal	57	7.02
Mexico	56	6.90
Greece	51	6.28
Germany	50	6.16
Spain	49	6.03
Italy	47	5.79
USA	39	4.80
Hungary	38	4.68
The Netherlands	31	3.82
Canada	22	2.71
Chile	22	2.71
France	16	1.97
Slovenia	14	1.72
Estonia	11	1.35
Australia	10	1.23
Czech Republic	10	1.23
Latvia	9	1.11
Austria	8	0.99
Rest of sample	39	4.80

Rest of sample = Finland, Ireland, Israel, New Zealand, Belgium, Sweden, Switzerland, Japan, South Korea, Denmark, Luxembourg, Norway.

References

1. Rusu, M.S. Theorising love in sociological thought: Classical contributions to a sociology of love. *J. Class. Sociol.* **2017**, *18*, 3–20. [CrossRef]
2. de Rougemont, D. *Love in the Western World*; Princeton University Press: Princeton, NJ, USA, 1983.
3. Jankowiak, W.R. (Ed.) *Romantic Passion: A Universal Experience?* Columbia University Press: New York, NY, USA, 1995.
4. Hatfield, E.; Walster, G.W. *A New Look at Love*, 1985 ed.; University Press of America: Lanham, MD, USA, 1985.
5. Karandashev, V. *Cultural Typologies of Love*; Springer: Cham, Switzerland, 2022. [CrossRef]
6. Bode, A.; Kushnick, G. Proximate and Ultimate Perspectives on Romantic Love. *Front. Psychol.* **2021**, *12*, 1088. [CrossRef]
7. Bode, A.; Kowal, M. Toward consistent reporting of sample characteristics in studies investigating the biological mechanisms of romantic love. *Front. Psychol.* **2023**, *14*, 983419. [CrossRef] [PubMed]
8. Feybesse, C.; Hatfield, E. Passionate Love. In *The New Psychology of Love*, 2nd ed.; Sternberg, R.J., Sternberg, K., Eds.; Cambridge University Press: Cambridge, UK, 2019.
9. Jankowiak, W.R. (Ed.) *Intimacies: Love and Sex Across Cultures*; Columbia University Press: New York, NY, USA, 2008.
10. Hatfield, E.; Sprecher, S. Measuring passionate love in intimate relationships. *J. Adolesc.* **1986**, *9*, 383–410. [CrossRef]
11. Karandashev, V. *Romantic Love in Cultural Contexts*; Springer: Berlin/Heidelberg, Germany, 2017.
12. Karandashev, V. *Cross-Cultural Perspectives on the Experience and Expression of Love*; Springer Nature: Cham, Switzerland, 2019.
13. Tennov, D. *Love and Limerence: The Experience of Being in Love*; Stein & Day: New York, NY, USA, 1979.
14. Bringle, R.G.; Winnick, T.; Rydell, R.J. The Prevalence and Nature of Unrequited Love. *SAGE Open* **2013**, *3*, 2158244013492160. [CrossRef]

15. O'Leary, K.D.; Acevedo, B.P.; Aron, A.; Huddy, L.; Mashek, D. Is Long-Term Love More Than A Rare Phenomenon? If So, What Are Its Correlates? *Soc. Psychol. Personal. Sci.* **2011**, *3*, 241–249. [CrossRef]
16. Acevedo, B.P.; Aron, A. Does a Long-Term Relationship Kill Romantic Love? *Rev. Gen. Psychol.* **2009**, *13*, 59–65. [CrossRef]
17. Sheets, V.L. Passion for life: Self-expansion and passionate love across the life span. *J. Soc. Pers. Relatsh.* **2013**, *31*, 958–974. [CrossRef]
18. Cacioppo, S.; Bianchi-Demicheli, F.; Hatfield, E.; Rapson, R.L. Social Neuroscience of Love. *Clin. Neuropsychiatry* **2012**, *9*, 3–13.
19. Song, H.W.; Zou, Z.L.; Kou, J.; Liu, Y.; Yang, L.Z.; Zilverstand, A.; Uquillas, F.D.; Zhang, X.C. Love-related changes in the brain: A resting-state functional magnetic resonance imaging study. *Front. Hum. Neurosci.* **2015**, *9*, 13. [CrossRef]
20. Wang, C.; Song, S.S.; Uquillas, F.D.; Zilverstand, A.; Song, H.W.; Chen, H.; Zou, Z.L. Altered brain network organization in romantic love as measured with resting-state fMRI and graph theory. *Brain Imaging Behav.* **2020**, *14*, 2771–2784. [CrossRef] [PubMed]
21. Wang, J.X.; Zhuang, J.Y.; Fu, L.; Lei, Q.; Fan, M.; Zhang, W. How ovarian hormones influence the behavioral activation and inhibition system through the dopamine pathway. *PLoS ONE* **2020**, *15*, e0237032. [CrossRef] [PubMed]
22. Fuentes-Claramonte, P.; Ávila, C.; Rodríguez-Pujadas, A.; Ventura-Campos, N.; Bustamante, J.C.; Costumero, V.; Rosell-Negre, P.; Barrós-Loscertales, A. Reward sensitivity modulates brain activity in the prefrontal cortex, ACC and striatum during task switching. *PLoS ONE* **2015**, *10*, e0123073. [CrossRef] [PubMed]
23. Montoya, J.L.; Landi, N.; Kober, H.; Worhunsky, P.D.; Rutherford, H.J.; Mencl, W.E.; Mayes, L.C.; Potenza, M.N. Regional brain responses in nulliparous women to emotional infant stimuli. *PLoS ONE* **2012**, *7*, e36270. [CrossRef]
24. Li, Y.; Qiao, L.; Sun, J.; Wei, D.; Li, W.; Qiu, J.; Zhang, Q.; Shi, H. Gender-specific neuroanatomical basis of behavioral inhibition/approach systems (BIS/BAS) in a large sample of young adults: A voxel-based morphometric investigation. *Behav. Brain Res.* **2014**, *274*, 400–408. [CrossRef]
25. Johnson, S.L.; Edge, M.D.; Holmes, M.K.; Carver, C.S. The behavioral activation system and mania. *Annu. Rev. Clin. Psychol.* **2012**, *8*, 243–267. [CrossRef]
26. Fisher, H.E. Lust, attraction, and attachment in mammalian reproduction. *Hum. Nat. -Interdiscip. Biosoc. Perspect.* **1998**, *9*, 23–52. [CrossRef]
27. Hendrick, C.; Hendrick, S. A theory and method of love. *J. Pers. Soc. Psychol.* **1986**, *50*, 392–402. [CrossRef]
28. Trivers, R.L. Parental investment and sexual selection. In *Sexual Selection and the Descent of Man*; Campbell, B., Ed.; Aldine: Chicago, IL, USA, 1972; pp. 136–179.
29. Wachtmeister, C.-A.; Enquist, M. The evolution of courtship rituals in monogamous species. *Behav. Ecol.* **2000**, *11*, 405–410. [CrossRef]
30. Farris, C.; Treat, T.A.; Viken, R.J.; McFall, R.M. Sexual coercion and the misperception of sexual intent. *Clin. Psychol. Rev.* **2008**, *28*, 48–66. [CrossRef]
31. Brand, S.; Luethi, M.; von Planta, A.; Hatzinger, M.; Holsboer-Trachsler, E. Romantic love, hypomania, and sleep pattern in adolescents. *J. Adolesc. Health* **2007**, *41*, 69–76. [CrossRef] [PubMed]
32. Froemke, R.; Young, L. Oxytocin, Neural Plasticity, and Social Behavior. *Annu. Rev. Neurosci.* **2021**, *44*, 359–381. [CrossRef] [PubMed]
33. Bode, A. Romantic love evolved by co-opting mother-infant bonding. *Front. Psychol.* **2023**, *14*, 1176067. [CrossRef] [PubMed]
34. Langeslag, S.; Olivier, J.; Köhlen, M.; Nijs, I.; Van Strien, J. Increased attention and memory for beloved-related information during infatuation: Behavioral and electrophysiological data. *Soc. Cogn. Affect. Neurosci.* **2015**, *10*, 136–144. [CrossRef]
35. Spielberger, C.D.; Gorsuch, R.L.; Lushene, R.E. *Manual for the State-Trait Anxiety Inventory (Self-Evaluation Questionanire)*; COnsulting Psychologists Press: Palo Alto, CA, USA, 1970.
36. Carver, C.S.; White, T.L. Behavioral inhibition, behavioral activation, and affective responses to impending reward and punishment: The BIS/BAS Scales. *J. Pers. Soc. Psychol.* **1994**, *67*, 319–333. [CrossRef]
37. Moreira, D.; Almeida, F.; Pinto, M.; Segarra, P.; Barbosa, F. Data concerning the psychometric properties of the Behavioral Inhibition/Behavioral Activation Scales for the Portuguese population. *Psychol. Assess.* **2015**, *27*, 1117–1122. [CrossRef]
38. Maack, D.J.; Ebesutani, C. A re-examination of the BIS/BAS scales: Evidence for BIS and BAS as unidimensional scales. *Int. J. Methods Psychiatr. Res.* **2018**, *27*, e1612. [CrossRef]
39. Cogswell, A.; Alloy, L.B.; van Dulmen, M.H.M.; Fresco, D.M. A psychometric evaluation of behavioral inhibition and approach self-report measures. *Personal. Individ. Differ.* **2006**, *40*, 1649–1658. [CrossRef]
40. Xu, M.; Wang, J.; Jin, Z.; Xia, L.; Lian, Q.; Huyang, S.; Wu, D. The Behavioral Inhibition System/Behavioral Activation System Scales: Measurement Invariance Across Gender in Chinese University Students. *Front. Psychol.* **2021**, *12*, 681753. [CrossRef]
41. Che, Q.; Yang, P.; Gao, H.; Liu, M.; Zhang, J.; Cai, T. Application of the Chinese Version of the BIS/BAS Scales in Participants With a Substance Use Disorder: An Analysis of Psychometric Properties and Comparison With Community Residents. *Front. Psychol.* **2020**, *11*, 912. [CrossRef]
42. Campbell-Sills, L.; Liverant, G.I.; Brown, T.A. Psychometric evaluation of the behavioral inhibition/behavioral activation scales in a large sample of outpatients with anxiety and mood disorders. *Psychol. Assess.* **2004**, *16*, 244–254. [CrossRef]
43. Jorm, A.F.; Christensen, H.; Henderson, A.S.; Jacomb, P.A.; Korten, A.E.; Rodgers, B. Using the BIS/BAS scales to measure behavioural inhibition and behavioural activation: Factor structure, validity and norms in a large community sample. *Personal. Individ. Differ.* **1999**, *26*, 49–58. [CrossRef]

44. Heubeck, B.G.; Wilkinson, R.B.; Cologon, J. A second look at Carver and White's (1994) BIS/BAS scales. *Personal. Individ. Differ.* **1998**, *25*, 785–800. [CrossRef]
45. Bode, A.; Kavanagh, P.S. *Romantic Love Survey 2022*, 3rd ed.; UNC Dataverse: Chapel Hill, NC, USA, 2022. [CrossRef]
46. Knekta, E.; Runyon, C.; Eddy, S. One Size Doesn't Fit All: Using Factor Analysis to Gather Validity Evidence When Using Surveys in Your Research. *CBE Life Sci. Educ.* **2019**, *18*, rm1. [CrossRef]
47. Li, C.-H. Confirmatory factor analysis with ordinal data: Comparing robust maximum likelihood and diagonally weighted least squares. *Behav. Res. Methods* **2016**, *48*, 936–949. [CrossRef]
48. Hu, L.T.; Bentler, P.M. Cutoff criteria for fit indexes in covariance structure analysis: Conventional criteria versus new alternatives. *Struct. Equ. Model. A Multidiscip. J.* **1999**, *6*, 1–55. [CrossRef]
49. Tavakol, M.; Dennick, R. Making sense of Cronbach's alpha. *Int. J. Med. Educ.* **2011**, *2*, 53–55. [CrossRef]
50. Cannas Aghedu, F.; Veneziani, C.A.; Manari, T.; Feybesse, C.; Bisiacchi, P.S. Assessing passionate love: Italian validation of the PLS (reduced version). *Sex. Relatsh. Ther.* **2018**, *35*, 77–88. [CrossRef]
51. Hendrick, S.S.; Hendrick, C. Gender differences and similarities in sex and love. *Pers. Relat.* **1995**, *2*, 55–65. [CrossRef]
52. Sternberg, R.J. A triangular theory of love. *Psychol. Rev.* **1986**, *93*, 119–135. [CrossRef]
53. Brand, S.; Foell, S.; Bajoghli, H.; Keshavarzi, Z.; Kalak, N.; Gerber, M.; Schmidt, N.B.; Norton, P.J.; Holsboer-Trachsler, E. "Tell me, how bright your hypomania is, and I tell you, if you are happily in love!"-Among young adults in love, bright side hypomania is related to reduced depression and anxiety, and better sleep quality. *Int. J. Psychiat. Clin.* **2015**, *19*, 24–31. [CrossRef] [PubMed]
54. Langeslag, S.J.E.; van der Veen, F.M.; Fekkes, D. Blood Levels of Serotonin Are Differentially Affected by Romantic Love in Men and Women. *J. Psychophysiol.* **2012**, *26*, 92–98. [CrossRef]
55. Kowal, M.; Sorokowski, P.; Dinić, B.M.; Pisanski, K.; Gjoneska, B.; Frederick, D.A.; Pfuhl, G.; Milfont, T.L.; Bode, A.; Aguilar, L.; et al. Validation of the Short Version (TLS-15) of the Triangular Love Scale (TLS-45) across 37 Languages. *Arch. Sex. Behav.* **2023**, 1–19. [CrossRef] [PubMed]
56. Frank, R.H. *Passion within Reason: The Strategic Role of the Emotions*; Norton: New York, NY, USA, 1988.
57. Buss, D.M. The evolution of love in humans. In *The New Psychology of Love*, 2nd ed.; Sternberg, R.J., Sternberg, K., Eds.; Cambridge University Press: Cambridge, UK, 2019.
58. Cohen, J. *Statistical Power Analysis for the Behavioral Sciences*; Academic Press: Cambridge, MA, USA, 2013.
59. Zietsch, B.P.; Sidari, M.J.; Murphy, S.C.; Sherlock, J.M.; Lee, A.J. For the good of evolutionary psychology, let's reunite proximate and ultimate explanations. *Evol. Hum. Behav.* **2020**, *42*, 76–78. [CrossRef]
60. Xu, X.M.; Weng, X.C.; Aron, A. The mesolimbic dopamine pathway and romantic love. In *Brain Mapping: An Encyclopedic Reference*; Toga, A.W., Mesulam, M.M., Kastner, S., Eds.; Elsevier: Oxford, UK, 2015.
61. Shih, H.-C.; Kuo, M.-E.; Wu, C.W.; Chao, Y.-P.; Huang, H.-W.; Huang, C.-M. The Neurobiological Basis of Love: A Meta-Analysis of Human Functional Neuroimaging Studies of Maternal and Passionate Love. *Brain Sci.* **2022**, *12*, 830. [CrossRef] [PubMed]
62. Groppe, S.E.; Gossen, A.; Rademacher, L.; Hahn, A.; Westphal, L.; Gründer, G.; Spreckelmeyer, K.N. Oxytocin influences processing of socially relevant cues in the ventral tegmental area of the human brain. *Biol. Psychiatry* **2013**, *74*, 172–179. [CrossRef]
63. Sydnor, V.J.; Larsen, B.; Kohler, C.; Crow, A.J.D.; Rush, S.L.; Calkins, M.E.; Gur, R.C.; Gur, R.E.; Ruparel, K.; Kable, J.W.; et al. Diminished reward responsiveness is associated with lower reward network GluCEST: An ultra-high field glutamate imaging study. *Mol. Psychiatry* **2021**, *26*, 2137–2147. [CrossRef]
64. Fisher, H.E. *Anatomy of Love: A Natural History of Mating, Marriage, and Why We Stray*, 2nd ed.; W. W. Norton & Company: New York, NY, USA, 2016.

Disclaimer/Publisher's Note: The statements, opinions and data contained in all publications are solely those of the individual author(s) and contributor(s) and not of MDPI and/or the editor(s). MDPI and/or the editor(s) disclaim responsibility for any injury to people or property resulting from any ideas, methods, instructions or products referred to in the content.

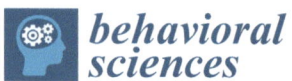
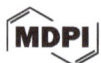

Article

Development and Preliminary Validation of the Lovebird Scale

Sara Cloonan [1,*], Lara Ault [2], Karen L. Weihs [3] and Richard D. Lane [3]

1. Department of Psychology, University of Georgia, Athens, GA 30605, USA
2. Department of Social Sciences, Saint Leo University, Saint Leo, FL 33574, USA; lara.ault@saintleo.edu
3. Department of Psychiatry, College of Medicine, University of Arizona, Tucson, AZ 85721, USA; weihs@psychiatry.arizona.edu (K.L.W.); lane@psychiatry.arizona.edu (R.D.L.)

* Correspondence: sara.cloonan@uga.edu

Abstract: The term "lovebirds" is often used to describe the loving behaviors and interactions between two romantic partners, but what specific processes distinguish these flourishing lovebird relationships from other committed but "numbed" relationships? The present study aimed to address this knowledge gap through the development and preliminary validation of the Lovebird Scale. The Lovebird Scale describes the thoughts, feelings, behaviors, and habits that constitute and maintain relationship flourishing, which in turn could promote aspects of individual flourishing such as positive affect. We conducted three studies using data collected from 996 English-speaking U.S. adults (64.2% Female, M = 39.2 years old) who reported being in a romantic relationship for at least six months (M = 11.2 years). In Study 1, we conducted an exploratory factor analysis to determine the underlying factor structure. In Study 2, confirmatory factor analyses revealed a three-factor model nested within a higher-order factor representing lovebird relationships. In Study 3, we cross-validated the higher-order structure, examined the construct validity of the scale, and explored associations between the Lovebird Scale and affective state. Finally, we discuss how the Lovebird Scale contributes to the growing field of positive relationship science as well as conceptual and clinical implications of the scale.

Keywords: romantic relationships; relationship quality; romantic love; lovebirds; psychometrics

Citation: Cloonan, S.; Ault, L.; Weihs, K.L.; Lane, R.D. Development and Preliminary Validation of the Lovebird Scale. *Behav. Sci.* **2024**, *14*, 747. https://doi.org/10.3390/bs14090747

Academic Editors: Bianca P. Acevedo, Adam Bode and Jerrell Cassady

Received: 26 May 2024
Revised: 19 August 2024
Accepted: 24 August 2024
Published: 26 August 2024

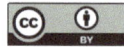

Copyright: © 2024 by the authors. Licensee MDPI, Basel, Switzerland. This article is an open access article distributed under the terms and conditions of the Creative Commons Attribution (CC BY) license (https:// creativecommons.org/licenses/by/ 4.0/).

1. Introduction

The importance of romantic relationships for health and well-being is well documented. Individuals in committed relationships tend to report better mental and physical health, engage in fewer risky behaviors, and have lower morbidity and mortality rates [1–4]. Merely being in a long-term committed relationship does not guarantee these benefits; rather, they are largely dependent on the quality of the relationship [3,5]. Thus, building and maintaining high relationship quality over time appear key to attaining the benefits of being in a romantic relationship. In order to do this, however, there is a need to (1) identify the properties that constitute and maintain such high-quality relationships and (2) determine how these properties contribute to aspects of individual health and well-being.

Previous research has primarily focused on the presence (or absence) of negative processes that diminish relationship quality largely because these negative processes tend to have a greater impact on relationship stability and health outcomes [6,7]. For example, Gottman [8] found it takes five positive behaviors to counterbalance the impact of one negative behavior on participants' moods during relationship conflict. While understanding the consequences of negative relationship processes has helped illustrate the importance of romantic relationships for health and well-being, this focus paints an incomplete picture of relationship functioning. Instead, an absence of dysfunction may mean an absence of pain but not the presence of positive benefits [9]. Fincham and Beach (2010) [7] have referred to functioning relationships that lack such rewards as "numbed" relationships. While these numbed relationships may be long-lasting, partners' commitment might be motivated by a desire to avoid relationship dissolution rather than a desire to approach relationship maintenance [9]. Beyond screening for low-satisfied couples, however, there is also a need to delineate between those who are moderately satisfied but numbed and those who are highly satisfied with their relationships. Differentiating between these types of relationships is key to understanding how to facilitate optimal relationship functioning rather than preventing relationship suffering.

To address this, recent work has emphasized the construct of *relationship flourishing*. At the individual level, flourishing is characterized by high levels of positive emotion and psychosocial functioning [10]; similarly, relationship flourishing aims to capture the positive relationship processes that contribute to "a sense that their life as a couple is a life well lived" [7]. These processes can include, but are not limited to, emotional connection, partner support, forgiveness, acceptance, trust, respect, positive affect, satisfaction, commitment, and love [7]. Over the past decade, scholars have developed several models to further our understanding of relationship flourishing. For example, the Strong Relationality Model of Relationship Flourishing (SRM) is centered on the idea that "Ethical Responsiveness" (i.e., viewing one's partner as an "Other" versus an object) motivates partners to engage in pro-relationship behaviors called "Responsible Actions" (e.g., gratitude, support, affection), which then facilitates other forms of "Relational-Connectivity" (e.g., intimacy, belongingness, mutual friendship) [11]. Wood, et al. [12] provide empirical support for the SRM in their longitudinal study, finding that perceived partner support mediated the impact of individual stress on gratitude–recognition (i.e., "Responsible Actions") 12 months later, which then resulted in greater intimacy (i.e., "Relational-Connectivity") between partners at 24 months. In addition to relational-connectivity, Galovan, et al. [13] also highlight the important role of dispositional virtues (e.g., viewing one's partner as being "other-centered" versus "self-centered", humble, compassionate, and positive), ethical behaviors (e.g., making time for one another, performing random acts of kindness for each other), and a greater focus on "we" rather than "I" in creating and maintaining flourishing relationships. In sum, these findings show that there is more to relationship quality than just perceptions of satisfaction, particularly within flourishing relationships [13–15].

The emphasis on negative relationship processes that, until recently, has dominated the literature has largely influenced the way we assess relationship quality [7,15]. Specifically, existing measures tend to operationalize relationship quality as a unidimensional construct with a single bipolar dimension ranging from extremely satisfied to extremely dissatisfied [7,16]. While previous research has justified the "conceptual simplicity" of existing scales to prevent misinterpretation and ambiguity [16], it is also possible that the global, unidimensional approach to measuring relationship quality fails to capture the intricacies of relationships that contribute to relationship flourishing [15]. However, several measures targeting aspects of flourishing relationships have been published in recent years. The Relationship Flourishing Scale (RFS) takes a eudemonic rather than hedonic approach to measuring relationship quality by assessing the degree of meaning, personal growth, relational giving, and goal sharing individuals derive from their relationship [15]. The Relational-Connectivity Scale (RCS) is based on the Strong Relationality Model of Relationship Flourishing (SRM) and aims to evaluate couples' sense of belonging, mutual friendship, and intimacy [13]. While both measures offer valuable insight into specific facets of relationship flourishing, they are missing domains needed to assess relationship flourishing holistically, such as relational savoring, physical intimacy, responsiveness, self-disclosure, and positive affectivity. Thus, describing the specific behaviors, interactions, and feelings that contribute to the development and maintenance of long-lasting, flourishing relationships is key to improving both relational and individual well-being.

The present research aims to add to the field of relationship science through the development and validation of a multidimensional, self-report measure of relationship flourishing called the Lovebird Scale. We use the term "lovebirds" as it is often used colloquially to describe extremely affectionate and long-lasting romantic couples who are "in love" with each other, as opposed to just having loving feelings towards one another.

Further, the term lovebirds captures the feelings of closeness and warmth in everyday interactions between partners that reinforce and further deepen their love for each other. Thus, the Lovebird Scale aims to bridge the gap between lay and academic understandings of lovebirds and relationship flourishing by developing a multifaceted scale that captures the specific behaviors, cognitions, and feelings that contribute to flourishing relationships, which differ from other long-term committed but numbed relationships. Further, the Lovebird Scale addresses key domains identified by previous scales (e.g., RFS, RCS) in addition to other constructs, such as savoring and responsiveness, to provide a broader understanding of relationship flourishing.

A secondary goal of this study is to examine positive and negative affectivity of individuals in flourishing relationships using the newly developed Lovebird Scale. Previous research has shown that flourishing individuals experience more positive affect than negative affect at a ratio of approximately 3:1 [17,18]; however, few studies have examined positive and negative affectivity within the context of flourishing relationships [7]. To address this, we hypothesized that the Lovebird Scale would be associated with more positive affect (PA) and less negative affect (NA). Further, we expected the Lovebird Scale to predict affective state above and beyond existing measures of relationship quality.

Through this research, we hope to further our understanding of what constitutes long-lasting, flourishing lovebird relationships as well as what makes them distinct from other committed but numbed relationships. Moreover, with a distinct measure of "above average" relationship quality, researchers could examine how lovebirds' conflict resolution strategies, communication styles, and physical and emotional health may differ from those who are merely satisfied with their relationship.

2. Study 1

2.1. Materials and Methods

2.1.1. Item Generation

Items on the initial Lovebird Scale were developed based on unstructured qualitative interviews with long-term romantic couples who described themselves as being lovebirds. Couples were recruited using convenience sampling from the community surrounding a public university in the Southwest United States. While unstructured interviews are more time-consuming and, thus, limit the number of interviews that can be conducted, an important strength of them is that participants are allowed to use their own words to describe their relationship and why they consider themselves to be lovebirds. The initial set of lovebird items were generated based on constructs identified in previous studies (e.g., goal sharing, mutual friendship, responsible actions, and intimacy) and on the themes and quotes taken from the interviews (e.g., prioritizing each other's happiness, the "little things" their partner does for them, physical intimacy, and respect). To help distinguish lovebird relationships from other types of relationships, we developed another set of items aiming to capture committed but numbed relationships. In the present research, numbed relationships were characterized as those in which partners may be satisfied with their relationship but are not positively engaged as robustly as those in lovebird relationships (See Galovan, Carroll, Schramm, Leonhardt, Zuluaga, McKenadel and Oleksuik [13] description of "satisfied but less connected" relationships or Fincham and Beach's (2010) [7] description of numbed relationships). Individuals in numbed relationships may not consider themselves to be deeply "in love" with each other and may be motivated to stay together for reasons other than their love for each other (e.g., financial reasons, children/dependents).

This first iteration of the Lovebird Scale contained 74 items, which were then reviewed by a panel of four relationship experts that included faculty members and clinicians from the psychology and psychiatry departments at a public university in the Southwest United States, who then excluded items that were redundant or were ambiguously written. The remaining 49 items formed the initial Lovebird Scale that was tested in Study 1. The participants were instructed to read each statement and choose the most appropriate response using a 7-point Likert scale ranging from 1 (*Strongly disagree*) to 7 (*Strongly agree*), keeping their current partner and relationship in mind.

2.1.2. Participants and Procedure

Recruitment and data collection for Study 1 occurred in June 2021. Participants were recruited via CloudResearch [19]. Participants needed to be at least 18 years old and currently involved in a romantic relationship for at least six months. Individuals who met the eligibility criteria and passed CloudResearch data security measures (i.e., ReCAPTCHA) were invited to complete an online Qualtrics survey (approximately 10 min) about romantic relationships. All participants provided electronic consent and were offered a monetary incentive for their participation. An institutional review board at a small, private Southeastern university reviewed and approved all aspects of this study.

A total of 552 participants completed Study 1. Twelve participants were excluded prior to analyses because they had missing data, reported a relationship length less than six months, or reported low relationship satisfaction. [20,21]. We chose to exclude participants with low relationship satisfaction because the goal of the scale is to differentiate between individuals in two types of satisfied relationships: those who may be in moderately satisfied but numbed relationships versus those in highly satisfied lovebird relationships. Low relationship satisfaction was defined as Relationship Assessment Scale (RAS) scores more than three standard deviations below the sample mean (i.e., total RAS scores < 11.08). The final analytic sample used for the EFA included $N = 540$. This resulted in an observation-to-item ratio of approximately 11, meeting previous recommendations for EFAs (between 5 and 10 observations per item) [22]. The participants were 39.9 years old ($SD = 13.2$), 60.6% female, 80.0% white, and 85.0% heterosexual. A total of 67.6% of the participants were married, and 91.3% currently lived with their partner. Their current relationship duration was 11.4 years ($SD = 10.8$ years) (see Table S1).

2.1.3. Measures

In addition to the Lovebird Scale, the participants completed several measures of relationship quality as well as a demographic questionnaire that assessed age, biological sex, gender identity, racial/ethnic background, sexual orientation, and relationship length. Descriptive statistics and reliabilities for all scales used in Study 1 are in Table 1.

Relationship Assessment Scale

Relationship satisfaction was measured using the Relationship Assessment Scale (RAS), a 7-item scale designed to assess global relationship satisfaction [20]. Example items include "How well does your partner meet your needs?" and "How much do you love your partner?". Cronbach's alpha was reported to be $\alpha = 0.86$ in the original sample [20].

Mutual Psychological Development Questionnaire

Perceived mutuality between partners was measured using the Mutual Psychological Development Questionnaire (MPDQ) [23]. The MPDQ is a 22-item self-report measure in which participants rate their own experience as well as perceptions of their partner's experience when discussing something of importance to themselves or to their partner using a 6-point Likert scale. Example items include "be receptive" and "try to understand" for the self-subscale, and "respect point of view" and "see the humor in things" for the partner subscale. The MPDQ has excellent internal consistency ($\alpha = 0.92$ for spouse/partner), test–retest reliability ($\alpha = 0.90$), and construct validity [23].

Relationship Prototypes

We also included two investigator-developed relationship prototypes that described typical lovebird and numbed relationships to ensure that our conceptualization of lovebird and numbed relationships were being accurately captured by the Lovebird Scale. Each prototype consisted of approximately the same word count and semantic structure

(M = 165.5 words). A sliding scale from 1 to 100 indicated how accurately each prototype described their current relationship. Both relationship prototypes can be found in Appendix B.

Table 1. Descriptive statistics and collections for Study 1 variables [1].

Variable	1	2	3	4	5	6	7	8
1. Mutuality	--							
2. Romance	0.72 ***	--						
3. Disconnect	−0.59 ***	−0.56 ***	--					
4. RAS	0.76 ***	0.69 ***	−0.71 ***	--				
5. MPDQ Self	0.57 ***	0.57 ***	−0.69 ***	0.64 ***	--			
6. MPDQ Partner	0.74 ***	0.60 ***	−0.65 ***	0.72 ***	0.69 ***	--		
7. Lovebird Prototype	0.72 ***	0.68 ***	−0.57 ***	0.81 ***	0.52 ***	0.65 ***	--	
8. Numbed Prototype	−0.28 ***	−0.35 ***	0.48 ***	−0.30 ***	−0.31 ***	−0.32 ***	−0.26 ***	--
M	5.50	5.48	2.93	28.9	4.77	4.51	75.8	46.3
SD	0.9	1.0	1.3	5.5	0.7	0.9	24.2	33.2
Range	5.15	4.80	6.00	23.0	3.60	4.44	100.0	100.0
Cronbach's a	0.93	0.89	0.86	0.90	0.87	0.88	--	--

[1] N = 540. RAS = Relationship Assessment Scale; MPDQ = Mutual Psychological Development Questionnaire. *** p < 0.001.

2.1.4. Statistical Analyses

Data were analyzed using R Studio (version 2022.12.0+353) [Posit 24,R Core 25]). We conducted an exploratory factor analysis (EFA) using principal axis factoring (PAF) estimation with promax rotation to determine the underlying factor structure of the initial 49-item Lovebird Scale. Factorability of the data was determined using inter-item correlations (<0.80), the Kaiser–Meyer–Olkin (KMO) measure of sampling adequacy (>0.50), and the Bartlett's test of sphericity (p < 0.05) [24]. We conducted a parallel analysis using the EFAtools R package to determine the appropriate number of factors to be extracted from the data [25]. The criteria to determine which items should be eliminated were (a) items with factor loadings less than 0.40; (b) items with cross-loadings greater than 0.20; (c) items with communalities less than 0.20; and (d) conceptual fit [24]. Cronbach's alphas were also calculated to assess internal consistency, with values $\geq$ 0.70 considered acceptable [26]. Bivariate Pearson's correlations were used to assess the preliminary convergent validity of the Lovebird Scale. Statistical significance for all analyses was set at the α = 0.05 level.

2.2. Results

The results from the KMO measure of sampling adequacy (0.97) and the Bartlett's test of sphericity (χ^2(1128) = 16,423.08, p < 0.001) suggested that an EFA was appropriate for the data. All 49 items had at least one inter-item correlation greater than 0.30, and no inter-item correlation pairs were greater than 0.80, further supporting the factorability of the data. Based on the results from the parallel analysis and Scree plot, we first tested a five-factor EFA solution, which explained 43% of the variance in the data. A three-factor solution yielded three distinct factors that had at least three items with factor loadings greater than 0.40 that also did not highly load onto the other factors. Thus, we decided to proceed with a three-factor solution. We removed items with low factor loadings or multiple high cross-loadings in a stepwise fashion, reevaluating the three-factor structure after each step, leaving 31 items. The final three-factor solution explained 46% of the variance in the items (Table 2).

Table 2. Results from the exploratory factor analysis in Study 1 [1].

Item	Factor Loadings		
	LB-M	LB-R	LB-D
6. I trust my partner completely and I can tell my partner anything.	0.70		
10. My partner never intentionally insults me, puts me down, or makes me feel bad.	0.82		
12. My partner and I have recurring problems that we can't get past.	−0.55		0.37
13. We are each other's best friend.	0.57	0.32	
33. We are very kind to each other.	0.78		
38. My partner accepts every part of me, even the things I dislike about myself.	0.69		
41. My partner and I respect each other's opinions, even when we don't agree with each other.	0.73		
44. My partner and I fit well together.	0.61	0.25	
45. I support my partner in their goals and aspirations, and they do the same for me.	0.58		
47. I can talk to my partner about anything, even if it is a difficult conversation.	0.86		
48. I don't have to sacrifice aspects of myself to keep my partner happy.	0.76		
1. When I hear certain songs, I think of how much I love my partner.		0.64	
4. All of life's ups and downs seem pretty insignificant compared to the love that we share.		0.54	
5. Our sex life is deeply satisfying.		0.69	
17. Sometimes when I'm alone I find myself thinking about how much I love my partner.		0.70	
18. The more time we spend together the more I enjoy my partner's company.	0.27	0.55	
19. We share a seamless continuum of compassionate and erotic love.		0.76	
22. I find my partner extremely physically attractive.	−0.21	0.70	
24. I often find myself thinking about special things I can do to make my partner happy.		0.68	
30. Touching is natural and fundamental to our relationship.		0.53	
37. My partner and I go through life savoring moments together.	0.31	0.52	
20. I am easily attracted to others when I am away from home.			0.77
27. When I see lovey-dovey couples I think they are unrealistic or out of touch.			0.54
31. We stay together for external reasons such as marriage vows and children, more than because of our enjoyment of being together.	−0.23		0.54
32. I often think about former lovers.			0.87
36. Although I love my partner, I would not say that I am currently "in love".			0.66
46. I feel like I need space after we spend a lot of time together.			0.60
14. My partner and I know how to make each other laugh, even on our bad days.	0.46	0.29	
26. We don't have to do anything in particular to thoroughly enjoy being together.	0.44		
34. I am more myself when I am alone than when I am with my partner.	−0.27		0.49
49. There are things about my partner that I wish I could change	−0.25		0.40

[1] N = 540. LB-M = Lovebird Scale—Mutuality subscale; LB-R = Lovebird Scale—Romance subscale; LB-D = Lovebird Scale—Disconnect subscale. Factor loadings were estimated using principal axis factoring with a Promax rotation. Factor loadings less than 0.20 were omitted from the table for clarity purposes.

Factor 1 was labeled "Mutuality", Factor 2 was labeled "Romance", and Factor 3 was labeled "Disconnect". The Mutuality subscale captured the pro-relationship behaviors and social interactions that signal trust, acceptance, respect, and support. The Romance subscale reflected the behavioral and cognitive processes that facilitate feelings of love and passion between partners, such as physical intimacy and relational savoring. The Disconnect subscale included items that represented indifference and/or ambivalence towards the relationship. All three factors demonstrated high internal consistency ($\alpha = 0.86$ to 0.93) and were significantly correlated with each other ($p < 0.001$). Bivariate correlations between the Lovebird Scale, relationship prototypes, and existing measures of relationship quality (RAS and MPDQ) provided preliminary evidence for the convergent validity of the scale. A summary of these correlations can be found in Table 1. We further examined the three-factor structure using confirmatory factor analyses in Study 2.

3. Study 2

3.1. Materials and Methods

3.1.1. Participants and Procedure

Recruitment and data collection for Study 2 occurred in October 2021 using the same method and eligibility criteria as Study 1. Those who had not participated in Study 1 were invited to complete an online Qualtrics survey (approximately 15 min) about romantic relationships. All aspects of this study were IRB approved. All participants provided electronic consent prior to participation and were offered a monetary incentive for their participation.

A total of 223 participants completed Study 2. Removal of participants due to the exclusion criteria described in Study 1 resulted in a final analyzed sample of $N = 215$. The participants were 38.7 years old ($SD = 11.6$), 67% female, 84.7% white, and 86% heterosexual. A total of 61.4% of the participants were married, and 91.6% currently lived with their partner. The participants reported being in their current relationship for an average of 10.5 years ($SD = 12.7$ years). A summary of sample characteristics for Study 2 can be found in Table S1.

3.1.2. Measures

In addition to the Lovebird Scale, RAS, MPDQ, relationship prototypes, and demographic questionnaire, the participants completed several other measures of relationship quality. Descriptive statistics and reliabilities for all scales used in Study 2 can be found in Table 3.

Perceived Relationship Quality Components Inventory

The Perceived Relationship Quality Components Inventory (PRQC) is an 18-item measure of relationship quality containing six subscales: Satisfaction ("How satisfied are you with your relationship?"), Commitment ("How committed are you to your relationship?"), Intimacy ("How connected are you to your partner?"), Trust ("How much can you count on your partner?"), Passion ("How passionate is your relationship?"), and Love ("How much do you love your partner?"). The PRQC has demonstrated high internal consistency ($\alpha = 0.78$ to 0.96) in previous research [14].

Relationship Quality Scale

The Relationship Quality Scale (RQS) is a brief, 9-item measure of relationship quality that was developed using a diverse sample of individuals representing over 60 countries. Participants are asked to rate their degree of agreement with various statements regarding their current relationship. Example items include "This is the relationship I have always dreamed of" and "I think of my partner as my soulmate". The RQS has demonstrated high internal consistency ($\alpha = 0.89$) in previous research [27].

Table 3. Descriptive statistics and correlations for Study 2 variables [1].

Variable	1	2	3	4	5	6	7	8	9	10	11	12	13	14	15	16
1.Mutuality	—															
2.Romance	0.77 ***	—														
3.Disconnect	−0.71 ***	−0.69 ***	—													
4.Lovebird Composite	0.93 ***	0.88 ***	−0.89 ***	—												
5.RAS	0.83 ***	0.67 ***	−0.75 ***	0.84 ***	—											
6.MPDQ Self	0.69 ***	0.63 ***	−0.68 ***	0.75 ***	0.63 ***	—										
7.MPDQ Partner	0.79 ***	0.64 ***	−0.69 ***	0.79 ***	0.73 ***	0.76 ***	—									
8.PRQC Satisfaction	0.84 ***	0.72 ***	−0.71 ***	0.84 ***	0.89 ***	0.59 ***	0.72 ***	—								
9.PRQC Commitment	0.60 ***	0.62 ***	−0.58 ***	0.66 ***	0.62 ***	0.46 ***	0.45 ***	0.64 ***	—							
10.PRQC Intimacy	0.74 ***	0.79 ***	−0.67 ***	0.80 ***	0.79 ***	0.60 ***	0.65 ***	0.82 ***	0.55 ***	—						
11.PRQC Trust	0.74 ***	0.55 ***	−0.56 ***	0.69 ***	0.73 ***	0.49 ***	0.59 ***	0.74 ***	0.49 ***	0.59 ***	—					
12.PRQC Passion	0.46 ***	0.67 ***	−0.45 ***	0.56 ***	0.51 ***	0.44 ***	0.47 ***	0.58 ***	0.35 ***	0.72 ***	0.36 ***	—				
13.PRQC Love	0.73 ***	0.81 ***	−0.66 ***	0.80 ***	0.69 ***	0.59 ***	0.59 ***	0.72 ***	0.75 ***	0.74 ***	0.57 ***	0.52 ***	—			
14.RQS	0.86 ***	0.79 ***	−0.78 ***	0.90 ***	0.87 ***	0.67 ***	0.74 ***	0.87 ***	0.69 ***	0.79 ***	0.72 ***	0.54 ***	0.80 ***	—		
15.Lovebird Prototype	0.75 ***	0.73 ***	−0.68 ***	0.79 ***	0.77 ***	0.60 ***	0.62 ***	0.77 ***	0.56 ***	0.74 ***	0.54 ***	0.54 ***	0.75 ***	0.79 ***	—	
16.Numbed Prototype	−0.41 ***	−0.44 ***	0.60 ***	−0.54 ***	−0.46 ***	−0.44 ***	−0.45 ***	−0.45 ***	−0.27 ***	−0.45 ***	−0.32 ***	−0.42 ***	−0.40 ***	−0.49 ***	−0.40 ***	—
M	5.68	5.71	2.85	5.74	29.3	4.73	4.53	5.91	6.54	5.30	6.20	4.74	6.32	37.0	77.3	43.6
SD	1.1	0.9	1.3	1.0	5.2	0.7	0.9	1.2	0.9	1.3	1.1	1.7	1.1	6.6	26.8	37.9
Range	4.80	4.88	6.00	4.96	22.0	3.00	4.00	5.00	5.00	6.30	5.00	6.00	5.00	29.0	100	100
Cronbach's α	0.92	0.87	0.87	0.95	0.90	0.86	0.89	0.96	0.95	0.39	0.89	0.93	0.92	0.92	—	—

[1] $N = 215$. RAS = Relationship Assessment Scale; MPDQ = Mutual Psychological Development Questionnaire; PRQC = Perceived Relationship Quality Components Inventory; RQS = Relationship Quality Scale. *** $p < 0.001$.

3.1.3. Statistical Analyses

Data were analyzed using R Studio (version 2022.12.0+353) [Posit 24, R Core 25]. We conducted a series of confirmatory factor analyses (CFAs) with robust maximum likelihood estimation (MLR) using the R package *lavaan*, version 0.6-18 [28]. We first tested the model proposed by the EFA in Study 1, followed by a one-factor model and an orthogonal model to examine any improvements in model fit. Factor variances were fixed to 1, and factor loadings were allowed to be freely estimated. Consistent with previous recommendations, overall model fit was evaluated using the following model fit indices: root-mean-square error of approximation (RMSEA) ≤ 0.06, comparative fit index (CFI) ≥ 0.90, standardized root-mean-square residual (SRMR) ≤ 0.08, and chi-square/degrees of freedom ratio (χ^2/df) ≤ 3 [24,29,30]. We consulted modification indices to determine if there were any empirically and/or theoretically reasonable modifications that could be made to improve overall model fit. Once the best fitting model was identified, we examined a higher-order model in which the subscales of the Lovebird Scale were nested within a second-order factor representing lovebird relationships globally. Cronbach's alphas were also calculated to assess internal consistency, with values ≥ 0.70 considered acceptable [26]. We tested the convergent validity of the Lovebird Scale by examining bivariate Pearson's correlations. Statistical significance for all analyses was set at the $\alpha = 0.05$ level.

3.2. Results

The results from the CFA on the EFA model were modest ($\chi^2(431) = 875.9$, $p < 0.001$; $\chi^2/df = 2.03$; CFI = 0.857; SRMR = 0.062; RMSEA = 0.069, 95% CI [0.063, 0.075], $p < 0.001$) but significantly better than the orthogonal ($\chi^2(434) = 1223.4$, $p < 0.001$; $\chi^2/df = 2.82$; CFI = 0.737; SRMR = 0.316 RMSEA = 0.092, 95% CI [0.087, 0.097], $p < 0.001$) and single-factor models ($\chi^2(434) = 1002.3$, $p < 0.001$; $\chi^2/df = 2.82$; CFI = 0.811; SRMR = 0.078; RMSEA = 0.078, 95% CI [0.072, 0.084], $p < 0.001$), supporting a multidimensional model with correlated factors. Based on modification indices, we made several revisions to the original EFA model in an incremental fashion: item 12 ("My partner and I have recurring problems that we can't get past") was moved from Mutuality to Disconnect, item 37 ("My partner and I go through life savoring moments together") was moved from Romance to Mutuality, and item 13 ("We are each other's best friend") was moved from Mutuality to Romance; item 14 ("My partner and I know how to make each other laugh, even on our bad days") was removed from the model due to high cross-loadings on Mutuality and Romance; and items 4, 19, 26, and 27 were removed from the model due to low loadings on their assigned factors. The revised 26-item model produced acceptable model fit statistics ($\chi^2(296) = 485.6$, $p < 0.001$; $\chi^2/df = 1.64$; CFI = 0.925; SRMR = 0.055; RMSEA = 0.055, 95% CI [0.047, 0.062], $p = 0.162$). Standardized regression weights ranged from 0.556 to 0.882 ($p < .001$), and all item variances were positive (i.e., no Heywood cases). Based on these results, we retained 26 items for the final Lovebird Scale (Appendix A). The three subscales exhibited high internal consistency, with Cronbach alphas ranging from 0.87 to 0.92.

To account for high inter-factor correlations, we tested a higher-order model in which the three factors were nested within one higher order factor representing lovebird relationships (Figure 1). Although model fit indices for the higher-order model in this sample were slightly less than those of the original three-factor model and the recommended cut-offs, they were still in an acceptable range [30]. Moreover, the higher-order Lovebird factor accounted for a large portion of the variance among the first-order factors, with R^2 values ranging from 0.746 to 0.871. The higher-order Lovebird factor also had high internal consistency, with a Cronbach's alpha of 0.95.

Convergent validity for the revised Lovebird Scale was tested using correlations with the relationship prototypes and existing measures of relationship quality (RAS, MPDQ, PRQC, and RQS). All correlations for the three subscales were statistically significant ($p < 0.001$) and in the expected direction. Composite lovebird scores were created by reverse scoring items on the Disconnect subscale and then calculating the average of all three subscales. As expected, the composite lovebird scores were significantly and positively correlated with the RAS, MPDQ, PRQC, and RQS ($p < 0.001$). A summary of correlations between all Study 2 variables can be found in Table 3. We cross-validated the higher-order model and investigated the construct validity in Study 3.

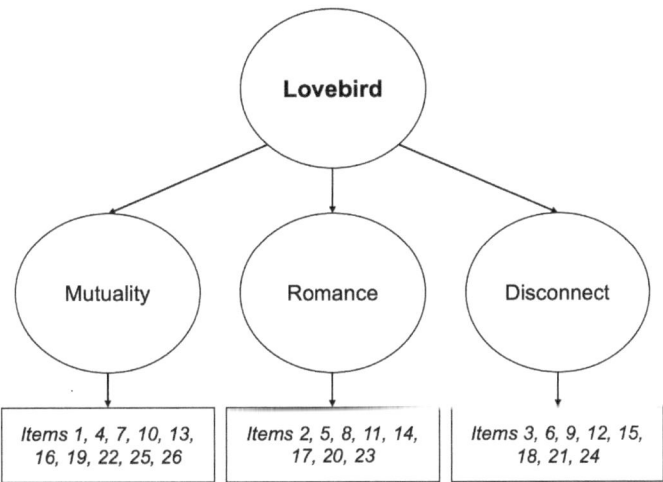

Figure 1. Higher-order factor structure of the Lovebird Scale. Item numbers are based on those listed in the final version of the Lovebird Scale found in Appendix A.

4. Study 3
4.1. Materials and Methods
4.1.1. Participants and Procedure

Recruitment and data collection for Study 3 occurred in December 2021 using the same method and eligibility criteria as Study 1. Those who had not participated in Study 1 or 2 were invited to complete an online Qualtrics survey (approximately 30 min) about romantic relationships. Institutional review board approval, collection of electronic consent, and a monetary incentive were identical to Studies 1 and 2. A total of 252 participants completed Study 3. Eleven participants were removed based on the exclusion criteria described in Study 1 and/or scored over the sample mean Infrequency score ($M = 1.1$), resulting in a final analytic sample of $N = 241$. On average, the participants were 39.1 years old ($SD = 10.2$), 69.7% female, 83% white, and 86.7% heterosexual. Seventy percent of the participants were married, and 92.9% currently lived with their partner. The participants reported being in their current relationship for an average of 11.7 years ($SD = 11.2$ years). A summary of sample characteristics for Study 3 can be found in Table S1.

4.1.2. Measures

In addition to the Lovebird Scale, RAS, MPDQ, relationship prototypes, and demographics questionnaire, the participants completed several other measures of relationship quality, attachment style, and affective state. Since the survey for Study 3 was longer than the first two surveys, we also included a six-item attention check measure (Infrequency Scale). Descriptive statistics and reliabilities for all scales used in Study 3 are in Table 4.

Dyadic Adjustment Scale

The Dyadic Adjustment Scale-32 (DAS-32) is a 32-item scale designed to assess relationship quality in cohabiting or married couples [31]. The DAS-32 consists of ordinal, Likert, and dichotomous scales, with total scores ranging from 0 to 151. The DAS-32 has also demonstrated acceptable internal consistency and construct validity in previous research ($\alpha = 0.58$ to 0.96; $M = 0.915$; 95% CI [0.906, 0.922]) [31,32].

Adult Attachment Scale

Anxious and avoidant attachment were measured using the revised 18-item Adult Attachment Scale (AAS). Statements describe varying degrees of comfort with closeness and intimacy as well as fear of rejection within close relationships [33]. The revised AAS has demonstrated acceptable reliability in previous research (α = 0.80 to 0.83) [33].

Positive and Negative Affect Schedule

Affective state was measured using the Positive and Negative Affect Schedule (PANAS), a 20-item self-report measure containing 10 items representing PA (e.g., "Enthusiastic", "Attentive") and 10 items representing NA (e.g., "Irritable", "Upset") [34]. Participants are asked to indicate the extent to which they have felt each affective state over the past week. The PANAS has also demonstrated high internal consistency in previous research (PA α = 0.89, 95% CI [0.88–0.90]; NA α = 0.85, 95% CI [0.84–0.87]) [35].

Infrequency Scale (Attention Check)

Previous research suggests including attention check measures in online surveys to ensure participants are paying attention to the questions and are answering honestly [36]. Thus, a brief, 6-item Infrequency Scale was also included in the assessment battery as an attention check measure. Example items include "I enjoy visiting London, Wisconsin" and "I once rode my bicycle from New York City to San Diego". Participants who scored over the sample mean Infrequency score (M = 1.1) were removed prior to analysis.

4.1.3. Statistical Analyses

Data were analyzed with the statistical package and methods used in Study 2. We conducted confirmatory factor analyses (CFA) with robust maximum likelihood estimation (MLR) using the R package *lavaan* [28]. Model fit and internal consistency were evaluated using the same criteria used in Study 2. We tested the convergent validity of the Lovebird Scale by examining bivariate Pearson correlations with existing measures of relationship quality (RAS, MPDQ, DAS-32). We used the Fronell–Larcker criterion to assess discriminant validity, which states that the square root of the average variance extracted (AVE) of each latent variable must be greater than the correlation between the latent variable and other constructs, in this case, attachment style. Finally, we tested the incremental validity of the Lovebird Scale by estimating a series of regression models where both the Lovebird Scale, RAS, and DAS-32 were entered as simultaneous predictors of PA and NA. Statistical significance for all analyses was set at the α = 0.05 level.

4.2. Results

The higher-order model demonstrated acceptable model fit in our cross-validation analyses, although slightly lower than those observed in Study 2 ($\chi^2(296)$ = 616.64, p < 0.001; χ^2/df = 2.08; CFI = 0.885; SRMR = 0.061; RMSEA = 0.067, 95% CI [0.060, 0.074], p < 0.001). Standardized regression weights ranged from 0.469 to 0.833 (p < 0.001). The higher-order Lovebird factor accounted for a large portion of the variance among the first-order factors, with R^2 values ranging from 0.818 to 0.845. The three subscales exhibited high internal consistency, with Cronbach alphas ranging from 0.85 to 0.92. The higher-order Lovebird factor also had high internal consistency, with a Cronbach's alpha of 0.94.

We tested the convergent validity of the Lovebird Scale by examining correlations with the relationship prototypes and existing measures of relationship quality (RAS, MPDQ, and DAS-32). All correlations were statistically significant (p < 0.05) and in the expected direction. Correlations between composite lovebird scores and existing relationship quality measures ranged from 0.50 to 0.86, with the smallest correlation being with the DAS Consensus subscale and largest correlation being with the RAS and DAS Satisfaction subscale. A summary of correlations between all Study 3 variables can be found in Table 4.

Table 4. Descriptive statistics and correlations for Study 3 variables [1].

Variable	1	2	3	4	5	6	7	8	9	10	11	12	13	14
1.Mutuality	—													
2.Romance	0.72 ***	—												
3.Disconnect	−0.70 ***	−0.66 ***	—											
4.Lovebird Composite	0.92 ***	0.86 ***	−0.89 ***	—										
5.RAS	0.82 ***	0.70 ***	−0.78 ***	0.86 ***	—									
6.MPDQ Self	0.60 ***	0.65 ***	−0.61 ***	0.69 ***	0.58 ***	—								
7.MPDQ Partner	0.73 ***	0.64 ***	−0.70 ***	0.78 ***	0.67 ***	0.74 ***	—							
8.DAS-32	0.70 ***	0.63 ***	−0.67 ***	0.75 ***	0.69 ***	0.59 ***	0.67 ***	—						
9.AAS Anxiety	−0.23 **	−0.13 *	0.34 ***	−0.28 ***	−0.28 ***	−0.35 ***	−0.35 ***	−0.29 ***	—					
10.AAS Avoidant	−0.18 **	−0.17 **	0.17 **	−0.20 **	−0.18 **	−0.34 ***	−0.27 ***	−0.24 ***	0.46 ***	—				
11.PANAS Positive	0.20 **	0.34 ***	−0.18 **	0.25 ***	0.21 ***	0.38 ***	0.26 **	0.20 **	−0.36 ***	−0.44 ***	—			
12.PANAS Negative	−0.08	−0.05	0.21 **	−0.14 *	−0.13	−0.25 ***	−0.20 **	−0.23 ***	0.45 ***	0.46 ***	−0.31 ***	—		
13.Lovebird Prototype	0.76 ***	0.74 ***	−0.71 ***	0.79 ***	0.84 ***	0.48 ***	0.61 ***	0.64 ***	−0.32 ***	−0.21 ***	0.23 ***	−0.11	—	
14.Numbed Prototype	−0.24 ***	−0.35 ***	0.42 ***	−0.37 ***	−0.32 ***	−0.30 ***	−0.28 ***	−0.32 ***	0.18 **	−0.06	−0.14 *	0.05	−0.32 ***	—
M	5.75	5.73	2.83	5.78	29.6	4.72	4.55	111.3	2.76	2.72	33.1	17.9	77.9	47.9
SD	1.0	0.9	1.2	1.0	5.2	0.7	0.8	22.0	1.0	0.8	7.9	7.6	24.0	39.4
Range	4.00	3.62	5.12	4.00	23.0	3.45	3.78	100.0	4.00	3.92	38.0	35.0	100.0	100.0
Cronbach's α	0.92	0.85	0.86	0.94	0.91	0.86	0.88	0.95	0.88	0.90	0.92	0.93	—	—

[1] $N = 241$. RAS = Relationship Assessment Scale; MPDQ = Mutual Psychological Development Questionnaire; DAS = Dyadic Adjustment Scale—Total; AAS = Adult Attachment Scale; PANAS = Positive and Negative Affect Schedule. * $p < 0.05$; ** $p < 0.01$; *** $p < 0.001$.

We assessed discriminant validity using the Fronell–Larcker criterion. We first computed the AVE for the three subscales and the higher-order Lovebird factor, which ranged from 0.43 to 0.55. We then calculated the square root of each AVE and compared them with correlations with the AAS Anxiety and Avoidant subscales. We observed small but statistically significant correlations ($p < 0.05$) between the three Lovebird subscales, composite lovebird scores, and the AAS subscales, all in the expected directions. Importantly, these correlations were smaller than the square root of the AVE for each latent variable, providing initial evidence for the discriminant validity of the Lovebird Scale.

Prior to our tests of incremental validity, we examined associations between the Lovebird Scale and both PANAS subscales. As expected, composite lovebird scores, Mutuality, and Romance were significantly associated with greater PA ($p < 0.01$). Disconnect was significantly correlated with less PA and more NA ($p < 0.05$). Surprisingly, neither Mutuality nor Romance were significantly correlated with NA, but there was a small negative correlation between composite lovebird and NA ($r = -0.14$, $p < 0.05$). We then tested the incremental validity of the Lovebird Scale by regressing both PANAS subscales on composite lovebird scores while controlling for the RAS and DAS-32. The Lovebird Scale emerged as a significant and unique predictor of PA above and beyond the RAS and DAS-32 but not NA. In both sets of models, composite lovebird scores were positively associated to PA (RAS model: $\beta = 2.86$, $p = 0.007$; DAS-32 model: $\beta = 2.28$, $p = 0.005$). Composite lovebird scores were not significantly associated to NA when controlling for the RAS and DAS-32 (RAS model: $\beta = -0.91$, $p = 0.392$; DAS-32 model: $\beta = 0.19$, $p = 0.809$).

5. Discussion

The field of relationship science is increasingly striving to understand what contributes to optimal relationship functioning as opposed to dysfunction [7,15]. The results of the three studies reported here provide preliminary evidence for the construct validity of the Lovebird Scale, a new domain-specific measure of optimal relationship function. Its development is an important step for understanding the key factors that contribute to long-lasting, flourishing relationships, including the various behavioral, cognitive, and affective processes that occur within such relationships.

5.1. Psychometric Properties of the Lovebird Scale

We conducted three studies to develop and validate the Lovebird Scale using data collected from three independent samples comprised of approximately one-thousand individuals in long-term (i.e., ≥ 6 months) romantic relationships. Mutuality, Romance, and Disconnect were the factors that resulted from the exploratory and confirmatory factor analyses conducted in Studies 1 and 2. We also tested a higher-order factor structure with the three subscales nested within one overarching lovebird factor, consistent with the idea that relationship quality is a multidimensional construct with several semi-independent domains that contribute to overall relationship quality [14]. The overarching lovebird factor and the three moderately correlated subscales nested within it surpassed standard Cronbach's alpha criteria (≥ 0.70) across all three studies, supporting the internal consistency of the scale. The Lovebird Scale also exhibited good convergent validity in all three studies, as observed through correlations with existing measures of relationship quality.

Mutuality within intimate relationships has previously been defined as the "modes of social interaction that facilitate participation in and growth through the relationship" [23]. In line with this definition, the Mutuality subscale within the Lovebird Scale captures the behaviors and interactions that reflect trust, respect, and responsiveness between partners. Mutuality may also facilitate authenticity and goal sharing, two key processes associated with relationship flourishing [11,37].

The Romance subscale captures the behavioral and cognitive processes that facilitate love and passion between partners, namely physical intimacy and savoring. Our findings suggest that physical intimacy may help foster lovebird relationships by increasing emotional intimacy, passion, and feelings of love between partners. Indeed, both sexual intimacy and physical touch have been found to play a vital role in relationship functioning and maintenance [38–41]. The Romance subscale also measures instances of relational savoring within lovebird relationships, which has been shown to buffer the negative effects of relationship stressors on relationship satisfaction, especially for those in highly satisfied couples [42–45].

The Disconnect subscale is comprised of items that reflect ambivalence and indifference within the relationship, all of which are characteristic of numbed relationships [7]. The Disconnect subscale also illustrates how the absence of positive relationship processes may lead to disaffection, a leading cause of relationship distress and dissolution characterized by a gradual decline in love and increase in feelings of indifference towards one's partner [46].

Mutuality, Romance, and composite lovebird scores were also associated with less insecure attachment, demonstrating satisfactory discriminant validity [47]. The Disconnect subscale was positively associated with both insecure attachment dimensions. This is not surprising, as we would expect individuals in lovebird couples to exhibit characteristics of secure attachment, such as engaging in constructive interactions (e.g., ability to discuss problems or insecurities), reporting greater feelings of connectedness, and experiencing less general conflict [47]. However, since we did not explicitly measure secure attachment in our study, more research is needed to confirm this.

5.2. Affective Experiences in Lovebird Relationships

We also examined the association of the Lovebird Scale with affective state, which is a central tenet of individual flourishing [17,18]. Both lovebird subscales were positively associated with PA. Romance was more strongly associated with PA than Mutuality, which suggests that taking time to think about and enjoy one's partner appears to be an important mechanism for increasing PA. This makes sense, given that savoring is a self-regulatory process used to generate positive emotions [43–45]. Physical intimacy has also been linked to more PA and less NA [48]. Thus, physical intimacy may enhance feelings of closeness between partners, which in turn promotes greater PA within lovebird relationships. Furthermore, composite lovebird scores emerged as significant and unique predictors of PA, above and beyond existing measures of relationship quality (RAS and DAS-32), thereby providing preliminary evidence for the incremental validity of the Lovebird Scale. This finding suggests that the Lovebird Scale may offer additional insight into positive affectivity within romantic relationships over existing measures.

The Disconnect subscale was associated with lower PA and greater NA. This is unsurprising, given that the aspects of numbed relationships, such as ambivalence and relational distancing, have been associated with greater NA [49–51]. Further, Gottman's research also revealed that some couples do not engage in negative, hostile behavior during conflict; rather, they behave in a more detached way, experiencing very little PA during conflict interactions. Though these relationships may last longer than the "disastrous" relationships, the lack of PA within them is more likely to result in relationship dissolution over time [52].

Interestingly, composite lovebird scores were not a unique predictor of NA when accounting for RAS and DAS-32 scores. These results suggest that existing relationship quality scales may be better at tapping into the negative affectivity within relationships than the Lovebird Scale. While surprising, there are several possible explanations for this finding. First, it is possible that people in lovebird relationships may value and validate whatever the partner is feeling, whether it is positive or negative, and there is no particular emphasis on making sure the other person does not experience NA. Second, even though they may experience NA, the higher levels of PA reported in lovebird relationships may "cancel out" the negative emotions to some degree [8]. Couples will inevitably experience NA during conflict; however, highly satisfied couples do not enter these states as often, and when they do, they are able to escape more easily [52]. Third, it is possible that the time to recovery for a given level of NA may be shorter in lovebird relationships. Although there is evidence to suggest that social sharing can lead to momentary increases in NA [53], one study found that sharing daily hassles predicted short- and long-term increases in closeness in romantic partners [54]. However, since there was no significant association in the current sample, we cannot rule out the possibility it was missed with this sample size. Similarly, Fowers, Laurenceau, Penfield, Cohen, Lang, Owenz and Pasipanodya [15] also found that the RFS was a better predictor of positive relationship processes but was less sensitive to measures of relationship distress than existing measures of relationship quality since these previous scales were primarily focused on identifying relationship dysfunction rather than relationship flourishing [7,15,16]. Thus, it should not be surprising that the Lovebird Scale was not a unique predictor of NA in the present study. Future research should examine the types of loving and other positive feelings that characterize lovebird versus numbed relationships, such as being in love, as well as being happy, satisfied, and warm. Longitudinal or daily experience studies can also track this ratio over time to determine how it relates to temporal changes in relationship flourishing.

5.3. Theoretical and Conceptual Implications

The Lovebird Scale adds to the growing field of positive relationship science, which emphasizes the role of positive relationship processes that contribute to relationship health and flourishing rather than the presence or absence of negative relationship processes [7]. Second, the Lovebird Scale advances the science of love by operationalizing the construct of "optimal" romantic relationships, going beyond broad ratings of relationship satisfaction to distinguish between lovebirds and other types of committed but numbed relationships. As recent research has noted, there is more to relationship quality than varying degrees of satisfaction, and this is reflected through the development of other measures of relationship flourishing, such as the Relationship Flourishing Scale and the Relational-Connectivity Scale. However, what sets the Lovebird Scale apart from these other measures is that it assesses constructs that are measured by each of those scales as well as includes other relevant domains of relationship flourishing, such as physical intimacy, relational savoring, and responsiveness. Additionally, while any couple may take the Lovebird Scale, the initial scale creation and validation were based on the notion of an extraordinary love for each other. By restricting the range of likely responses by screening for high satisfaction, we were able to more finely distinguish nuances in the items.

Finally, we examined associations between the Lovebird Scale and affective state, which, to our knowledge, has not been addressed by existing relationship flourishing measures. In their paper, Fincham and Beach [7] argue that understanding relationship flourishing requires consideration of positive and negative affectivity and, more specifically, what ratio is needed to create a positivity offset. Continuing to measure affective state within lovebird relationships will provide valuable insight into the everyday affective experiences of flourishing relationships. Further, we argue that the higher levels of PA observed in lovebird relationships occurs because there is a positive feedback loop of love within the couple that, in turn, enables each partner to thrive as both individuals and a relationship partner. In line with theories such as the find-remind-and-bind theory of gratitude [55] and the broaden-and-build theory of positive emotions [56], this positive feedback loop within the couple contributes to both higher levels of relationship quality on the dyad level as well as greater PA on the individual level. More research is needed to demonstrate this positive feedback loop as well as the hypothesized individual thriving of individuals in a lovebird relationship. Longitudinal studies may also help elucidate how the maintenance of lovebird relationships promotes sustained PA over time.

5.4. Clinical Implications

In addition to these conceptual implications, the present research has implications for practitioners as well. To date, many relationship interventions have targeted negative processes (e.g., maladaptive communication patterns, conflict resolution) that lead to poor relationship outcomes [57]. The study of lovebird relationships can improve existing couples' interventions and inspire novel interventions, particularly as it relates to everyday interactions within relationships. Bradbury and Bodenmann [57] argue that there is a need to systematically assess couples' ability to create, share, and capitalize on positive experiences to determine the best treatment plan for a given couple. The Lovebird Scale would be particularly useful for this, as it aims to capture the behaviors, thoughts, and feelings that contribute to positive relationship experiences in everyday life. For example, if relationship partners report low scores on the Romance subscale, practitioners may recommend interventions that focus on increasing relational savoring or intimacy [43], whereas low scores on the Mutuality subscale may indicate a need to focus on improving communication and increasing trust between partners through behavioral couple therapy approaches [57]. Research on the affective experiences of lovebird relationships would also be useful for developing emotion-focused couple therapy interventions that address both the way lovebirds manage their own emotions as well as the way they manage each other's emotions. In sum, incorporating the Lovebird Scale into clinical and therapeutic settings has the potential to improve practitioners' ability help couples overcome acute conflict or reinvigorate relationships that are trending towards committed but numbed relationships.

5.5. Limitations and Future Directions

There are several limitations of the present study that should be addressed. First, self-report questionnaires are subject to various biases, such as response bias, social desirability, and positive sentiment override, which refers to when an individual's perception of specific aspects of the relationship are influenced by their general feelings about the relationship [58]. Second, the cross-sectional nature of this study limits our ability to draw conclusions regarding causality. For example, since data were only collected at one time point, the findings may not reflect relationship quality over time and may be influenced by temporal fluctuations in relationship quality for a given level of PA or NA. Experience sampling or daily diary studies may help illustrate temporal changes in ratings of lovebirdness or numbness, while longitudinal studies would be beneficial for understanding how lovebird relationships are developed and maintained over time. In-laboratory behavioral observations may also help illustrate how lovebird couples interact with each other and how the factors identified in the present research manifest themselves in these interactions. Third, this study only captures the experiences of one relationship partner. Future research should have both partners complete the scale, as this could highlight potential relationship issues if one partner believes they are lovebirds but the other does not.

Another limitation to consider is the study sample. The use of an online recruitment platform such as CloudResearch allowed for us to recruit individuals from across the U.S., but despite this, our sample was still primarily white, female, educated (i.e., bachelor's degree or higher), and heterosexual, which ultimately limits the generalizability of our findings to more diverse populations. In addition, given the use of online recruitment methods, there is always the possibility that "bots" completed the survey, which can impact the quality of the data [19]. While multiple steps were taken to address this limitation in the current research (i.e., use of data security measures), future research should aim to replicate these findings in different populations and use other forms of data collection to minimize the possibility of automated bot responses.

There are also limitations regarding the scale development process that should be addressed. First, it is possible that the results from the CFAs may have been underpowered due to the small sample size. While the sample sizes in this study met previous recommendations for factor analysis (i.e., greater than 200), other recommendations suggest using a ratio of 10+ per item [22,24]. The small sample sizes may also inflate the risk of Type 1 error and multicollinearity, further underscoring the need for larger sample sizes in future research. Second, because we excluded individuals with low relationship quality from the analyses, the non-normal distribution of the data could have affected the analyses. Third, several double-barreled items were included in the final iteration of the Lovebird Scale, which may have also contributed to the less-than-ideal model fit indices found in Studies 2 and 3. Future research should routinely examine the model fit of the Lovebird Scale in larger samples and propose modifications, as needed, to improve the reliability and validity of these scales in addition to using item response theory (IRT) methods instead of traditional factory analysis methods like those used in the present study.

A fourth methodological limitation to consider is the limited number of measures used to establish the construct validity of the Lovebird Scale. Future research should incorporate more measures of love and other measures relevant to the specific facets of lovebird relationships (e.g., Perceived Responsiveness and Insensitivity Scale, Passionate Love Scale, Eros Love Style Scale, Friendship-Based love Scale, etc.) to further examine the construct validity of the scale.

Another issue to consider is the discriminant and incremental validity of the scale, given that the Lovebird Scale subscales displayed similar correlations with existing measures of relationship quality and affective state. One area for future investigation could be the construct of shared reality, which has been linked to various positive relationship processes such as feeling known and understanding others [59]. We would expect global lovebird scores to correlate more strongly with shared reality compared to existing measures of relationship satisfaction given the Lovebird Scale's emphasis on thoughts and behaviors that facilitate loving feelings and other positive affective states between partners. We were also not able to fully demonstrate the incremental validity of the Lovebird Scale. Future studies should include existing measures of relationship flourishing, such as the RFS and RCS, to establish the incremental validity of the Lovebird Scale, particularly when it comes to assessing both overall relationship quality as well as affective state.

Future research should also aim to determine if certain behaviors (as measured by self-report or through behavioral coding) are more strongly associated with one subscale over the others. For example, we might expect that individuals who score higher on the Romance subscale display a higher frequency of affectionate touch behaviors or report a greater degree of closeness with their partner, while those who score higher on the Mutuality subscale may report more responsiveness and use more constructive communication styles when discussing a marital conflict. Those who score high on the Disconnect subscale, thus being in more of a numbed relationship, might report feeling less authentic and use less constructive communication styles when discussing a conflict (e.g., stonewalling). Understanding these subscale-specific nuances could be helpful for answering future research questions, such as how specific relationship dynamics, as captured by the Lovebird Scale, predict mental and physical health outcomes in couples. It would also be interesting to examine how the subscales of the Lovebird Scale differ as a function of a relationship length, as this may help differentiate the various subscales from each other given the moderate-to-high correlations between them. Indeed, previous studies have found that the association between various aspects of love (companionate, passionate, romantic) differ among short- and long-term couples [60].

6. Conclusions

Despite the methodological limitations mentioned above, the present study provides preliminary evidence for the reliability and construct validity of the Lovebird Scale, a novel assessment of relationship quality that aims to bridge the gap between lay and academic understandings of lovebirds and relationship flourishing by developing a multifaceted scale that captures the specific behaviors, cognitions, and feelings that contribute to flourishing relationships, which differ from other long-term committed but numbed relationships. The Lovebird Scale offers a holistic assessment of romantic relationships by incorporating dimensions that are not fully captured by existing measures and integrating multiple facets, such as romance, mutuality, and disconnection, into a single scale, which allows for a more nuanced exploration of relationship well-being. Furthermore, the Lovebird Scale may also be a useful tool for delineating between those who are moderately satisfied but numbed and those who are highly satisfied with their relationships. By focusing on the factors that contribute to relationship flourishing, researchers and practitioners may be better able to design and implement interventions to help couples not only address issues with relationship functioning but also promote more meaningful, flourishing relationships.

Supplementary Materials: The following information can be downloaded at https://www.mdpi.com/article/10.3390/bs14090747/s1, Table S1: Sample characteristics for Studies 1–3.

Author Contributions: Conceptualization, S.C., K.L.W. and R.D.L.; methodology, S.C., K.L.W. and R.D.L.; formal analysis, S.C.; investigation, S.C.; data curation, S.C.; writing—original draft preparation, S.C.; writing—review and editing, S.C., L.A., K.L.W. and R.D.L.; supervision, L.A., K.L.W. and R.D.L. All authors have read and agreed to the published version of the manuscript.

Funding: This research received no external funding.

Institutional Review Board Statement: This study was conducted in accordance with the Declaration of Helsinki and approved by the Institutional Review Board of Saint Leo University (approved on 26 April 2021).

Informed Consent Statement: Informed consent was obtained from all subjects involved in this study.

Data Availability Statement: All data and analysis code have been made publicly available at the "APA Journal Articles: Data and Related Resources" Open Science Framework repository and can be accessed at https://osf.io/3p69f/. This study's design and its analysis were not pre-registered. A pre-print of this manuscript can be accessed at https://psyarxiv.com/zavkf.

Conflicts of Interest: The authors declare no conflicts of interest.

Appendix A. The Lovebird Scale

Instructions: You have been asked to complete this questionnaire because you are currently involved in a committed long-term romantic relationship. Please answer the following questions about your relationship using the scale below.

1 = Strongly disagree; 2 = Disagree; 3 = Disagree somewhat; 4 = Neither agree nor disagree; 5 = Agree somewhat; 6 = Agree; 7 = Strongly agree

1. I trust my partner completely and I can tell my partner anything. (m)
2. When I hear certain songs, I think of how much I love my partner. (r)
3. I am easily attracted to others when I am away from home. (d)
4. My partner never intentionally insults me, puts me down, or makes me feel bad. (m)
5. Our sex life is deeply satisfying. (r)
6. We stay together for external reasons such as marriage vows and children, more than because of our enjoyment of being together. (d)
7. We are very kind to each other. (m)
8. Sometimes when I'm alone I find myself thinking about how much I love my partner. (r)
9. I often think about former lovers. (d)
10. My partner accepts every part of me, even the things I dislike about myself. (m)
11. The more time we spend together the more I enjoy my partner's company. (r)
12. Although I love my partner, I would not say that I am currently "in love". (d)
13. My partner and I respect each other's opinions, even when we don't agree with each other. (m)
14. I find my partner extremely physically attractive. (r)
15. I feel like I need space after we spend a lot of time together. (d)
16. My partner and I fit well together. (m)
17. I often find myself thinking about special things I can do to make my partner happy. (r)
18. I am more myself when I am alone than when I am with my partner. (d)
19. I support my partner in their goals and aspirations, and they do the same for me. (m)
20. Touching is natural and fundamental to our relationship. (r)
21. There are things about my partner that I wish I could change. (d)
22. I can talk to my partner about anything, even if it is a difficult conversation. (m)
23. We are each other's best friend. (r)
24. My partner and I have recurring problems that we can't get past. (d)
25. I don't have to sacrifice aspects of myself to keep my partner happy. (m)
26. My partner and I go through life savoring moments together. (m)

Mutuality = items 1, 4, 7, 10, 13, 16, 19, 22, 25, 26
Romance = items 2, 5, 8, 11, 14, 17, 20, 23
Disconnect = items 3, 6, 9, 12, 15, 18, 21, 24

Scoring: Subscale scores are calculated by taking the average of each set of items. Composite lovebird scores are calculated by first reverse-scoring items on the Disconnect subscale and then taking the average of all items in the scale.

Appendix B. Relationship Prototypes

Instructions: Please read the statement below and use the sliding scale to indicate how accurately it describes your relationship.

Extremely inaccurate (0) -------- Extremely accurate (100)

Appendix B.1. Relationship Prototype 1 (Lovebird Prototype; 164 Words)

You are in love with your partner and feel that you have found "the love of your life", a real soul mate. You thoroughly enjoy being together, and you connect on multiple levels—intellectually, emotionally, and sexually. You frequently tell one another that you love each other. You do everything you can to make each other happy. No relationship is perfect, but you are able to work things out when things go off track because you are able to communicate clearly and respectfully. Keeping this relationship going in a very positive manner does not require a lot of work. You feel that you are experiencing the best that life has to offer and feel very fortunate to be in this relationship. You think the world would be a better place if other couples got along as well as the two of you do.

Appendix B.2. Relationship Prototype 1 (Numbed Prototype; 167 Words)

You chose to be with your partner for very good reasons, and the two of you are committed to each other for the long term. You respect one another and have worked out a way to have a life together that on the whole is successful. There are many things that you like and even admire about your partner, but there are also some things that bother you a lot, and they are not likely to change. You find yourself attracted to other people and even think about them occasionally but do not take any actions because you are committed to the relationship and don't want to destabilize it. Relationships can be a lot of work, but all things considered, they are worth it. Two people may initially have a lot of passion for one another, but eventually, that goes away and is replaced by other ways of staying connected. Overall, people shouldn't rely exclusively on one person for their happiness, so a well-rounded life is essential.

References

1. Braithwaite, S.R.; Delevi, R.; Fincham, F.D. Romantic relationships and the physical and mental health of college students. *Pers. Relatsh.* **2010**, *17*, 1–12. [CrossRef]
2. Dush, C.M.K.; Amato, P.R. Consequences of relationship status and quality for subjective well-being. *J. Soc. Pers. Relatsh.* **2005**, *22*, 607–627. [CrossRef]
3. Holt-Lunstad, J.; Birmingham, W.; Jones, B.Q. Is there something unique about marriage? The relative impact of marital status, relationship quality, and network social support on ambulatory blood pressure and mental health. *Ann. Behav. Med.* **2008**, *35*, 239–244. [CrossRef] [PubMed]
4. Robles, T.F.; Slatcher, R.B.; Trombello, J.M.; McGinn, M.M. Marital quality and health: A meta-analytic review. *Psychol. Bull.* **2014**, *140*, 140–187. [CrossRef]
5. Roberson, P.N.E.; Norona, J.C.; Lenger, K.A.; Olmstead, S.B. How do relationship stability and quality affect wellbeing?: Romantic relationship trajectories, depressive symptoms, and life satisfaction across 30 years. *J. Child Fam. Stud.* **2018**, *27*, 2171–2184. [CrossRef]
6. Braithwaite, S.R.; Holt-Lunstad, J. Romantic relationships and mental health. *Curr. Opin. Psychol.* **2017**, *13*, 120–125. [CrossRef]
7. Fincham, F.D.; Beach, S.R.H. Of Memes and Marriage: Toward a Positive Relationship Science. *J. Fam. Theory Rev.* **2010**, *2*, 4–24. [CrossRef]
8. Gottman, J. *What Predicts Divorce? The Relationship between Marital Processes and Marital Outcomes*; Psychology Press: New York, NY, USA, 1994.
9. Strachman, A.; Gable, S.L. Approach and avoidance relationship commitment. *Motiv. Emot.* **2006**, *30*, 117–126. [CrossRef]

10. Keyes, C.L.M. The mental health continuum: From languishing to flourishing in life. *J. Health Soc. Behav.* **2002**, *43*, 207–222. [CrossRef]
11. Galovan, A.M.; Schramm, D.G. Strong relationality and ethical responsiveness: A framework and conceptual model for family science. *J. Fam. Theory Rev.* **2018**, *10*, 199–218. [CrossRef]
12. Wood, N.D.; Fife, S.T.; Parnell, K.J.; Ross, D.B. Answering the ethical call of the other: A test of the Strong Relationality Model of Relationship Flourishing. *J. Marital Fam. Ther.* **2022**, *49*, 186–204. [CrossRef]
13. Galovan, A.M.; Carroll, J.S.; Schramm, D.G.; Leonhardt, N.D.; Zuluaga, J.; McKenadel, S.E.M.; Oleksuik, M.R. Satisfaction or connectivity?: Implications from the strong relationality model of flourishing couple relationships. *J. Marital Fam. Ther.* **2021**, *48*, 883–907. [CrossRef]
14. Fletcher, G.J.O.; Simpson, J.A.; Thomas, G. The Measurement of Perceived Relationship Quality Components: A Confirmatory Factor Analytic Approach. *Personal. Soc. Psychol. Bull.* **2000**, *26*, 340–354. [CrossRef]
15. Fowers, B.J.; Laurenceau, J.-P.; Penfield, R.D.; Cohen, L.M.; Lang, S.F.; Owenz, M.B.; Pasipanodya, E. Enhancing relationship quality measurement: The development of the Relationship Flourishing Scale. *J. Fam. Psychol.* **2016**, *30*, 997–1007. [CrossRef]
16. Fincham, F.D.; Rogge, R. Understanding Relationship Quality: Theoretical Challenges and New Tools for Assessment. *J. Fam. Theory Rev.* **2010**, *2*, 227–242. [CrossRef]
17. Diehl, M.; Hay, E.L.; Berg, K.M. The ratio between positive and negative affect and flourishing mental health across adulthood. *Aging Ment. Health* **2011**, *15*, 882–893. [CrossRef] [PubMed]
18. Frederickson, B.L.; Losada, M.F. Positive affect and the complex dynamics of human flourishing. *Am. Psychol.* **2005**, *60*, 678–686. [CrossRef]
19. Litman, L.; Robinson, J.; Abberbock, T. TurkPrime.com: A versatile crowdsourcing data acquisition platform for the behavioral sciences. *Behav. Res. Methods* **2017**, *49*, 433–442. [CrossRef] [PubMed]
20. Hendrick, S.S. A Generic Measure of Relationship Satisfaction. *J. Marriage Fam.* **1988**, *50*, 93. [CrossRef]
21. Vaughn, M.; Baier, M.E.M. Reliability and validity of the relationship assessment scale. *Am. J. Fam. Ther.* **1999**, *27*, 137–147. [CrossRef]
22. Watkins, M.W. Exploratory Factor Analysis: A Guide to Best Practice. *J. Black Psychol.* **2018**, *44*, 219–246. [CrossRef]
23. Genero, N.P.; Miller, J.B.; Surrey, J.; Baldwin, L.M. Measuring perceived mutuality in close relationships: Validation of the Mutual Psychological Development Questionnaire. *J. Fam. Psychol.* **1992**, *6*, 36–48. [CrossRef]
24. Knekta, E.; Runyon, C.; Eddy, S. One Size Doesn't Fit All: Using Factor Analysis to Gather Validity Evidence When Using Surveys in Your Research. *CBE Life Sci. Educ.* **2019**, *18*, rm1. [CrossRef] [PubMed]
25. Steiner, M.; Grieder, S. EFAtools: An R package with fast and flexible implementations of exploratory factor analysis tools. *J. Open Source Softw.* **2020**, *5*, 2521. [CrossRef]
26. Hair, J.F.; Black, B.; Black, W.C.; Babin, B.J.; Anderson, R.E. *Multivariate Data Analysis: A Global Perspective*, 7th ed.; Pearson Education: London, UK, 2010.
27. Chonody, J.M.; Gabb, J.; Killian, M.; Dunk-West, P. Measuring Relationship Quality in an International Study. *Res. Soc. Work Pract.* **2018**, *28*, 920–930. [CrossRef]
28. Rosseel, Y. lavaan: An R package for structural equation modeling. *J. Stat. Softw.* **2012**, *48*, 1–36. [CrossRef]
29. Kline, R.B. *Principles and Practice of Structural Equation Modeling*, 4th ed.; The Guilford Press: New York, NY, USA, 2016.
30. Hu, L.-T.; Bentler, P.M. Cutoff criteria for fit indexes in covariance structure analysis: Conventional criteria versus new alternatives. *Struct. Equ. Model.* **1999**, *6*, 1–55. [CrossRef]
31. Spanier, G.B. Measuring Dyadic Adjustment: New Scales for Assessing the Quality of Marriage and Similar Dyads. *J. Marriage Fam.* **1976**, *38*, 15. [CrossRef]
32. Graham, J.M.; Liu, Y.J.; Jeziorski, J.L. The Daydic Adjustment Scale: A reliability generalization meta-analysis. *J. Marriage Fam.* **2006**, *68*, 701–717. [CrossRef]
33. Collins, N.L. Working models of attachment: Implications for explanation, emotion, and behavior. *J. Personal. Soc. Psychol.* **1996**, *71*, 810–832. [CrossRef]
34. Watson, D.; Clark, L.A.; Tellegen, A. Development and validation of brief measures of positive and negative affect: The PANAS scales. *J. Personal. Soc. Psychol.* **1988**, *54*, 1063–1070. [CrossRef] [PubMed]
35. Crawford, J.R.; Henry, J.D. The Positive and Negative Affect Schedule (PANAS): Construct validity, measurement properties and normative data in a large non-clinical sample. *Br. J. Clin. Psychol.* **2004**, *43*, 245–265. [CrossRef] [PubMed]
36. Berinsky, A.J.; Margolis, M.F.; Sances, M.W. Separating the Shirkers from the Workers? Making Sure Respondents Pay Attention on Self-Administered Surveys. *Am. J. Political Sci.* **2014**, *58*, 739–753. [CrossRef]
37. Fowers, B.J.; Owenz, M.B. A eudaimonic theory of marital quality. *J. Fam. Theory Rev.* **2010**, *2*, 334–352. [CrossRef]
38. Hesse, C.; Mikkelson, A.C. Affection deprivation in romantic relationships. *Comun. Q.* **2017**, *65*, 20–38. [CrossRef]
39. Muise, A.; Maxwell, J.A.; Impett, E.A. What theories and methods from relationship research can contribute to sex research. *J. Sex Res.* **2018**, *55*, 540–562. [CrossRef]
40. Debrot, A.; Schoebi, D.; Perrez, M.; Horn, A.B. Touch as an interpersonal emotion regulation process in couples' daily lives: The mediating role of psychological intimacy. *Personal. Soc. Psychol. Bull.* **2013**, *39*, 1373–1385. [CrossRef]
41. Wagner, S.A.; Mattson, R.E.; Davila, J.; Johnson, M.D.; Cameron, N.M. Touch me just enough: The intersection of adult attachment, intimate touch, and marital satisfaction. *J. Soc. Pers. Relatsh.* **2020**, *37*, 1945–1967. [CrossRef]

42. Borelli, J.L.; Rasmussen, H.F.; Burkhart, M.L.; Sbarra, D.A. Relational savoring in long-distance relationships. *J. Soc. Pers. Relatsh.* **2015**, *32*, 1083–1108. [CrossRef]
43. Borelli, J.L.; Smiley, P.A.; Kerr, M.L.; Hong, K.; Hecht, H.K.; Blackard, M.B.; Falasiri, E.; Cervantes, B.R.; Bond, D.K. Relational savoring: An attachment-based approach to promoting interpersonal flourishing. *Psychotherapy* **2020**, *57*, 340–351. [CrossRef]
44. Costa-Ramalho, S.; Marques-Pinto, A.; Ribeiro, M.T.; Pereira, C.R. Savoring positive events in couple life: Impacts on relationship quality and dyadic adjustment. *Fam. Sci.* **2015**, *6*, 170–180. [CrossRef]
45. Lenger, K.A.; Gordon, C.L. To have and to savor: Examining associations between savoring and relationship satisfaction. *Couple Fam. Psychol. Res. Pract.* **2019**, *8*, 1–9. [CrossRef]
46. Abbasi, I.S.; Alghamdi, N.G. Polarized couples in therapy: Recognizing indifference as the opposite of love. *J. Sex Marital Ther.* **2017**, *43*, 40–48. [CrossRef]
47. Li, T.; Chan, D.K.S. How anxious and avoidant attachment affect romantic relationship quality differently: A meta-analytic review. *Eur. J. Soc. Psychol.* **2012**, *42*, 406–419. [CrossRef]
48. Debrot, A.; Meuwly, N.; Muise, A.; Impett, E.A.; Schoebi, D. More than just sex: Affection mediates the association between sexual activity and well-being. *Personal. Soc. Psychol. Bull.* **2017**, *43*, 287–299. [CrossRef] [PubMed]
49. Harasymchuk, C.; Fehr, B. Development of a prototype-based measure of relational boredom. *Pers. Relatsh.* **2012**, *19*, 162–181. [CrossRef]
50. Holt-Lunstad, J.; Uchino, B.N. Social Ambivalence and Disease (SAD): A theoretical model aimed at understanding the health implications of ambivalent relationships. *Perspect. Psychol. Sci.* **2019**, *14*, 941–966. [CrossRef] [PubMed]
51. Ross, K.M.; Rook, K.; Winczewski, L.; Collins, N.; Schetter, C.D. Close relationships and health: The interactive effect of positive and negative aspects. *Soc. Personal. Psychol. Compass* **2019**, *13*, e12468. [CrossRef]
52. Gottman, J.; Gottman, J. The natural principles of love. *J. Fam. Theory Rev.* **2017**, *9*, 7–26. [CrossRef]
53. Rimé, B.; Bouchat, P.; Paquot, L.; Giglio, L. Intrapersonal, interpersonal, and social sharing outcomes of the social sharing of emotion. *Curr. Opin. Psychol.* **2020**, *31*, 127–134. [CrossRef]
54. Rauers, A.; Riediger, M. Ease of mind or ties that bind? Costs and benefits of disclosing daily hassles in partnerships. *Soc. Psychol. Personal. Sci.* **2023**, *14*, 551–561. [CrossRef]
55. Algoe, S.B. Find, Remind, and Bind: The functions of gratitude in everyday relationships. *Soc. Personal. Psychol. Compass* **2012**, *6*, 455–469. [CrossRef]
56. Frederickson, B.L. The broaden-and-build theory of positive emotions. *Philos. Trans. R. Soc. Lond. Ser. B Biol. Sci.* **2004**, *359*, 1367–1378. [CrossRef] [PubMed]
57. Bradbury, T.N.; Bodenmann, G. Interventions for couples. *Annu. Rev. Clin. Psychol.* **2020**, *16*, 99–123. [CrossRef] [PubMed]
58. Weiss, R.L. Cognitive and strategic interventions in behavioral marital therapy. In *Marital Interaction: Analysis and Modification*; Hahlweg, K., Jacobson, N.S., Eds.; Guilford: New York, NY, USA, 1984; pp. 337–355.
59. Andersen, S.M.; Przybylinski, E. Shared reality in interpersonal relationships. *Curr. Opin. Psychol.* **2018**, *23*, 42–46. [CrossRef]
60. Acevedo, B.P.; Aron, A. Does a long-term relationship kill romantic love? *Rev. Gen. Psychol.* **2009**, *13*, 59–65. [CrossRef]

Disclaimer/Publisher's Note: The statements, opinions and data contained in all publications are solely those of the individual author(s) and contributor(s) and not of MDPI and/or the editor(s). MDPI and/or the editor(s) disclaim responsibility for any injury to people or property resulting from any ideas, methods, instructions or products referred to in the content.

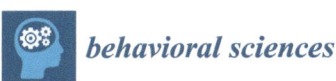

Article

Emerging Love: A Subjective Exploration of Romantic Bonds in Early Adulthood Within the South Korean Context

Seo Jung Shin [†], Ji Seong Yi [†] and Song Yi Lee *

Department of Counselling and Coaching, Dongguk University-Seoul, 30, Pildong-ro 1 gil, Jung-gu, Seoul 04620, Republic of Korea; tjwjd620822@gmail.com (S.J.S.)
* Correspondence: songyilee@dongguk.edu; Tel.: +82-10-6357-7310
[†] These authors contributed equally to this work.

Abstract: This study examines and categorises subjective perceptions of love among individuals in their twenties and thirties, offering insights into their viewpoints during early adulthood. The study employed the Q methodology, suitable for analysing subjective perceptions such as perspectives, thoughts, beliefs, and attitudes. It included 23 participants selected through purposive sampling from the 2030 generation residing in South Korea, with 40 statements constructed for the research. The findings revealed four types. Type 1, 'Love Healing', experiences psychological wellbeing through love. Type 2, 'Love Anxious', longs for true love but is anxious. Type 3, 'Love Myself', expresses hope for healthy love through self-awareness. Type 4, 'Love Mate', seeks to maintain psychological love while pursuing independence. This research also explores similarities and differences between existing adult attachment and love types, highlighting the need for practical support tailored to each type. These insights may serve as a foundation for developing coaching and counselling services that help individuals in their twenties and thirties cultivate healthy love and mature into their authentic selves.

Keywords: early adulthood; romantic love; types of love; attachment; adults' attachment; Q methodology

1. Introduction

Human growth occurs through relationships. It signifies the ability to adapt to society through ongoing interactions with others in various environmental conditions, leading individuals to make choices about their behaviours and lives accordingly. Interactions in human relationships provide psychological stability and self-esteem, which are essential for forming one's identity [1] and fostering empathy to understand others. While relationships and interactions hold significant meaning at all developmental stages, Erikson [2] suggests that individuals develop their identities by sharing trust and intimacy with others and forming new relationships in early adulthood. If one fails in this process, they may experience feelings of isolation and alienation, which can negatively affect relationships throughout adulthood. Therefore, forming intimate relationships is an important psychosocial developmental task in early adulthood.

In particular, Erikson [2] posited that romantic experiences during early adulthood play a crucial role in developing identity and intimacy. Early adulthood is when individuals establish their sense of identity and form intimate connections through romantic relationships, and the experiences of love during this time significantly impact development throughout adulthood and beyond [3]. The formation of intimacy deepens interpersonal relationships and is an essential process for creating bonds based on trust. One establishes trust through repeated positive interactions and sensitive responsiveness to each other's needs, serving as a crucial factor in deepening intimacy within relationships [4]. Psychologist Bowlby [5], who explained the importance of emotional bonds with others, proposed the attachment theory, which many scholars have since expanded. Attachment is the process through which a child develops a sense of trust and security, enabling them to explore

Citation: Shin, S.J.; Yi, J.S.; Lee, S.Y. Emerging Love: A Subjective Exploration of Romantic Bonds in Early Adulthood Within the South Korean Context. *Behav. Sci.* **2024**, *14*, 1135. https://doi.org/10.3390/bs14121135

Academic Editors: Bianca P. Acevedo and Adam Bode

Received: 27 September 2024
Revised: 24 November 2024
Accepted: 25 November 2024
Published: 26 November 2024

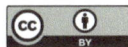

Copyright: © 2024 by the authors. Licensee MDPI, Basel, Switzerland. This article is an open access article distributed under the terms and conditions of the Creative Commons Attribution (CC BY) license (https://creativecommons.org/licenses/by/4.0/).

the world gradually. This sense of emotional safety arises when the primary caregiver consistently responds and provides warm, nurturing care [6]. South Korean society still regards dating and marriage as significant social norms. Consequently, one often associates romantic experiences with an individual's social accomplishment and successful transition into stable adulthood. In the Korean context, strong social stigmas around failure in dating or marriage may exert additional psychological pressure on individuals. Such societal expectations can influence personal attachment formation and emotional development [7].

These attachment experiences also impact interpersonal relationships in adulthood, with emotional and behavioural patterns in romantic relationships often sharing similar characteristics to those observed in parent–child relationships [8]. This stance implies that children who form stable attachments with their parents are more likely to develop healthy interpersonal relationships as adults. The family-centred culture and emphasis on relational harmony in South Korea reveal unique attachment patterns within the Korean context. In addition to the relationship with the primary caregiver, emotional bonds within Korean society and familial harmony contribute to the formation of secure attachment. Individuals with secure attachment tend to exhibit healthier emotional interactions in relationships with parents, friends, and romantic partners [9]. The attachment formed during adolescence continues to impact adulthood. Adolescent attachment is a crucial predictor of resilience in adulthood, specifically the ability to cope effectively with stress and adversity [10]. Additionally, the type of attachment established during adolescence influences the formation of trust and emotional bonds in adult relationships, playing a significant role in creating predictability in interpersonal interactions [11].

Scholars have provided different categorisations for the concept of adult attachment, which refers to the patterns of child attachment proposed by Bowlby [5] in the context of adult romantic relationships. For example, Hazan and Shaver [12] identified three types of attachment—secure, anxious, and avoidant—while Bartholomew and Horowitz [13] distinguished four types based on the dimensions of self-awareness and other awareness: secure—viewing oneself and others positively and maintaining close relationships; preoccupied—holding a negative self-view and excessively depending on others in relationships; dismissing—evaluating oneself positively but avoiding intimacy due to a lack of trust in others; and fearful—negatively assessing oneself and others, desiring close relationships while simultaneously fearing them (Figure 1) [13]. Thus, the attachment formed during adolescence, similar to the attachment relationships established with primary caregivers in childhood, also influences interpersonal relationships in adulthood.

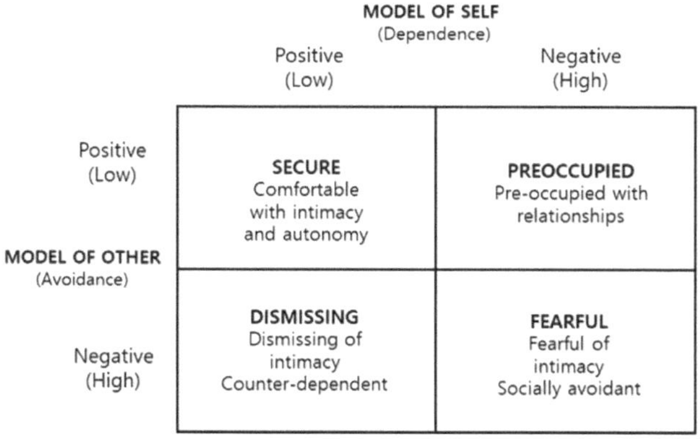

Figure 1. Model of adult attachment [13].

Recently, the term 'love and life balance' ('러라밸' in Korean) has gained popularity in Korean society, following the concept of 'work and life balance'. This new term emphasises the importance of maintaining a balance between love and life, indicating that love should not interfere with one's daily routine. Amid economic challenges and social changes, South Korea's millennial generation demonstrates a growing preference for selective and pragmatic relationships that align with individual needs. This generation increasingly forms relationships in a goal-oriented and practical manner, less constrained by traditional social expectations [14]. This phenomenon reflects a social trend that prioritises personal convenience; however, it contrasts with the significant role that interpersonal relationships play in providing emotional support and overall satisfaction in their lives. The stress experienced in interpersonal relationships is closely related to the academic stress of college students in early adulthood, which impacts their overall academic life [15]. Furthermore, higher interpersonal skills positively influence adaptation to college life, and social support greatly assists students in adjusting to new environments [16]. Thus, it is evident that interpersonal relationships are a significant concern during early adulthood and an essential element of overall life satisfaction.

In 2022, the Korea Population, Health, and Welfare Association conducted an online survey involving 1047 unmarried young individuals to assess the status of non-married youth. The survey revealed insights into their dating experiences, non-dating experiences, perceptions of sexuality, and sexual experiences. According to the findings, 65% of young people reported non-dating, with 70% of this group voluntarily non-dating. This generation is beginning to experience a non-dating trend beyond being unmarried [17]. Kim et al. [18] noted an increasing number of individuals who struggle to express their emotions and feel burdened by the overwhelming social pressure to be happy amidst anxiety and concern. This situation has led many to seek emotional proxies as they have nowhere to express their feelings [19]. Thus, they desire to experience romance through media or framed observational entertainment programs instead of through real-life romantic relationships.

Examining love in early adulthood through social phenomena reveals a significant gap between reality and actual desires. The various issues from this disparity affect early adulthood and demonstrate a cyclical interconnectedness with societal problems. Psychoanalyst and social psychologist Fromm [20] posited that contemporary society presents a paradoxical situation where individuals must fulfil the existential task of self-realisation amidst an incessant flow of competition. Fromm argued that modern individuals have become increasingly distant from aspects of the self to the extent that they may forget their identities. This argument has a close link to the realities of South Korean society, reflecting a phenomenon where individuals may lose themselves and experience identity erosion amid intense competition and pressures for achievement. As people strive to meet external expectations in areas like entrance exams and employment, opportunities for self-actualisation diminish, leading to a growing sense of emotional emptiness [21]. He emphasised that understanding love is essential for recovery. Furthermore, he asserted that the only way to realise spontaneity, which is the source of one's inherent personality and a happy life without sacrificing the self, is through love.

Fromm [20] articulated that love involves connecting with the other by giving everything, including joy, interest, knowledge, sorrow, and even life itself, thereby enriching their existence and allowing oneself to feel alive within that connection. He posited that individuals discover each other's true selves through such love and evolve into more mature human beings. Hatfield and Sprecher [22] defined love as a combination of human emotions and elements of behaviour, cognition, and affection, reflecting our actions, beliefs, and feelings. Further, existential psychologist May [23] defined love as 'delight in the presence of the other person and an affirming of his value and development as much as one's own' (p. 182), highlighting the importance of acquisitive and compassionate love towards those different from oneself. People in Eastern cultures often express love discreetly and keep it within rather than display it openly to others, in line with cultural tendencies. Historical records across cultures reveal that humans have consistently sought to pursue and preserve love. While expressions of love may vary between Eastern and Western cultures, the fundamental essence of love remains unchanged [24].

Since the 1990s, the study of love has emerged as a significant area of research within social psychology. Sternberg is a prominent scholar who conceptualised and studied love, culminating in the Triangular Theory of Love, which classifies love's components into intimacy, passion, and commitment. Canadian psychologist John Alan Lee [25] proposed the Colour Wheel Theory of Love, categorising love into six distinct types and outlining the characteristics of each type. Within this framework, the primary categories include eros (passionate love), ludus (playful love), and storge (companionate love), further subdividing into three subgroups: mania (possessive love), agape (selfless love), and pragma (pragmatic love).

Love can be a crucial element in personal growth and transformation, especially in early adulthood. The significance of love becomes even more profound as one matures into adulthood. Erikson [26] posited that experiencing an appropriate balance of isolation and intimacy can facilitate the development of the mature self-capacity known as 'love'. He further emphasised that romantic experiences of love provide opportunities for individuals to discover new facets of themselves and are vital in uncovering their true identities. Fredrickson [27] argues that romantic love enhances positive emotions, serving as a critical factor in building psychological resources. Similarly, Levinson [28] notes that romantic experiences during early adulthood are fundamental for self-understanding and relationship development, which contribute to forming a mature sense of self.

In summary, forming intimate relationships and experiencing love during early adulthood is necessary for the development of personal identity and intimacy, which, in turn, positively influences self-esteem. Consequently, love is the root of human existence. It is crucial in growth activities aimed at pursuing an ideal self-image and significantly influences the satisfaction or frustration of psychological needs [29].

A review of previous studies on love indicates that researchers have explored love and romantic relationships among university students in South Korea. One narrative study investigated male and female university students' perceptions of the definition of love, revealing that both groups commonly perceive love as a 'feeling' [30]. University students tend to accept love as a desired emotional experience that can make their existence more meaningful. In contrast to this desire for existential meaning through love, recent studies on university students' views on marriage have shown a significant decline in positive perceptions of marriage [31]. Furthermore, examining the relationship between attitudes towards marriage and types of love indicated that those with positive or evolving values regarding marriage tend to exhibit a strong inclination towards 'eros' (passionate love). An in-depth interview study by Oh and Park [32] on university students' relationships and happiness revealed that pursuing only one type of love can hinder the recognition of happiness. This finding suggests that a diverse range of love types is essential for sustaining healthy and enduring love. Thus, previous research underscores the necessity for a detailed investigation into perceptions of love in early adulthood.

Although studies have used Sternberg's three components of love [33–35], they primarily conducted quantitative research. Choi [36] researched the components of love based on the Enneagram personality types and suggested that love manifests through individuals' psychological dimensions, which gives rise to various attitudes and types of love. This finding also highlights the need for qualitative research grounded in in-depth approaches. In addition, Choi and Jun [37] emphasised the necessity of qualitative exploration concerning how one perceives love from an essential perspective.

For several years, the study of love as a subjective experience has been a topic of interest in psychology [38]. Studies have partially addressed how individuals perceive love in early adulthood [39–42]; however, few studies in this field have deeply analysed subjective perceptions of love from diverse perspectives. This lack suggests that psychological inquiry into how individuals uniquely perceive the meaning and experience of love is still evolving. Therefore, this study utilises the Q methodology to categorise and examine the characteristics of subjective perceptions of love among individuals in early adulthood. The findings serve as a foundation for developing coaching and counselling services that facilitate healthy expressions of love and contribute to the mature growth of authentic self-identity in early adulthood.

The research questions (RQs) for this study are as follows:

RQ1. What are the types of perceptions regarding love in early adulthood among South Koreans?

RQ2. What are the characteristics of each perception type regarding love in early adulthood among South Koreans?

2. Study Method

2.1. Research Procedure

The Q methodology is a research method developed by William Stephenson in the 1930s [43]. In research, generalisation is typically associated with statistical inference based on large samples, assuming that the findings apply to an entire population. However, the Q methodology emphasises subjectivity rather than data quantification and focuses on developing theories [44]. The core of Q methodology lies in exploring the correlations among individuals regarding a specific topic and categorising and interpreting these individuals' perspectives [45,46]. Generalising the research findings to the entire population is not a concern to Q-methodologists; rather, they focus on identifying individuals' subjective patterns of thought. The belief is that these patterns exist within the population from which the researcher draws the sample [47]. The Q sample assumes that such patterns only exist within the group. In other words, 'When we discover that X has blue eyes, we can argue that there may be others with blue eyes like X, but we cannot claim that everyone else has blue eyes' [48]. It involves quantifying individuals' subjective tendencies or values and interpreting the resulting categorised types [49]. Thus, the Q methodology is an objective and practical research approach suitable for understanding the cognitive structures underlying individuals' subjective perspectives [50].

Consequently, this study uses the Q methodology to categorise perceptions of love in early adulthood and discern the meanings associated with each type. The research process involves the following steps: constructing the Q sample, assembling the Q sample from the Q population, selecting the P sample, and classifying the Q sample through the P sample, followed by data analysis. We conducted this study after receiving approval from the Dongguk University Institutional Review Board (IRB no. DUIRB202308-22) following the procedure illustrated in Figure 2.

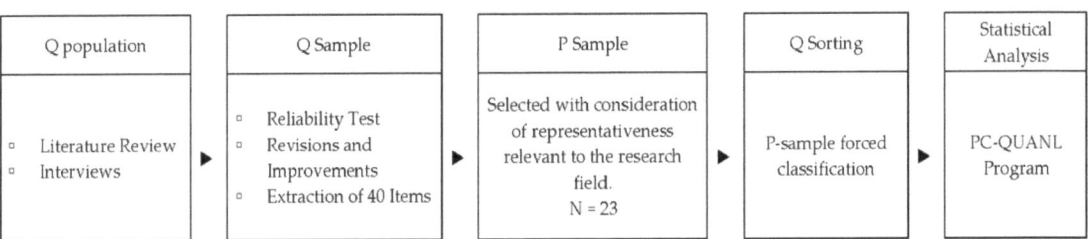

Figure 2. Q methodology steps.

2.1.1. Organisation of Q Population

In the Q methodology context, the population consists of all possible subjective statements that individuals can express. We can categorise subjective statements as messages, concepts, ideas, or communicable expressions [51]. The Q population refers to a collection of items related to the research topic gathered to study individuals' subjective characteristics within a culture [46]. In this study, prior to forming the population, we collected a Q population to examine perceptions of love in early adulthood by reviewing 11 academic theses and journal articles with keywords such as 'perception of love in early adulthood', 'love in early adulthood', and 'perceptions of love'. The titles are as follows. 'The Relationship Between Romantic Attachment, Self-Esteem, and Types of Love' [52], 'A Study on the Conceptual and Developmental Understanding of Love in Adulthood' [53], 'A Study on College Students' Types of Love and Sexual Attitudes' [54], 'The Impact of the Importance of Basic Psychological Needs and Gender Differences on the Components of Love: A Study on Romantic Partners' [55], 'An Exploratory Study on the Attitudes Towards Love in Unmarried Adult Males: Focusing on Gender Discriminatory Perceptions and Gender Role Conflicts' [56], 'A Study on Theater Therapy for Understanding Love' [29], 'Types of Love, Self-Esteem, Trust, and Relationship Satisfaction in Early Adulthood' [57], 'A Study on the Elements of Love Perceived by College Students' [37], 'Measuring Passionate Love in Intimate Relationships' [22], 'Dating Apps: Towards Post-Romantic Love in Digital Societies' [58], and 'Love and Relationship Satisfaction as a Function of Romantic Relationship Stages' [59].

Additionally, we secured 93 statements through internet search engines such as Google, Naver, and Daum. Following this, we conducted semi-structured interviews with four individuals: one male and one female in their twenties, and one male and one female in their thirties. After explaining the purpose of the research and obtaining consent, we conducted the interviews using semi-structured questions, including 'What comes to mind when you think of love', 'What does love mean to you', 'What kind of love do you consider to be good love', 'Conversely, what kind of love do you think is not good', 'What aspects do you think are important regarding love', 'What experiences have you had related to love', and 'Finally, what else would you like to share about love'? Each interview lasted approximately 50 min, resulting in the addition of 49 statements. This study aimed to broadly explore the subjective perceptions and experiences of love held by early adulthood participants, focusing on their subjective perspectives on experiencing and interpreting love. Thus, we constructed 142 Q population items.

2.1.2. Selection of the Q Sample

The Q sample comprises extracted statements from the Q population, which participants use in Q sorting [46,60]. The Q sample underwent validity verification in this study across three distinct phases. We organised the 142 statements in an Excel file and categorised them based on their content, as follows: psychological state, attitude/method, reality, growth, element, benefit, and self-awareness. Subsequently, we classified the statements as positive, negative, or neutral. Through a thorough review of the organised statements, we modified and deleted statements to address redundancy and ambiguity, resulting in the final selection of 40 statements (Table 1). Following this, one individual in their twenties and one in their thirties assessed the appropriateness and comprehensibility of the statements. Finally, we conducted a pre-test with two experts familiar with the Q methodology. This process culminated in the final selection of 40 statements that effectively represent the Q population and exhibit high discriminative validity for the Q sample.

Table 1. Q statements and Z-scores of love types.

No	Q Statement	Love Healing Z-Scores	Love Anxious Z-Scores	Love Myself Z-Scores	Independent Love Z-Scores	Category
1	Comfort makes the process of love richer and more stable.	1.5	0.8	0.9	0.7	Psychological State
2	Though parting after love is sad, love is something you want to experience again.	0.5	−0.6	0.6	−0.5	Psychological State

Table 1. Cont.

No	Q Statement	Love Healing Z-Scores	Love Anxious Z-Scores	Love Myself Z-Scores	Independent Love Z-Scores	Category
3	I often feel fear or annoyance at the thought of forming relationships with others.	−0.1	0.9	−0.6	0.1	Psychological State
4	When I love, I feel jealousy.	0.1	0.6	0.3	−0.3	Psychological State
5	It seems that sharing everyday life with the one I love is happiness.	1.2	−0.3	0.5	0.9	Attitude/Method
6	Seeing my parents makes me not want to get married.	−1.4	−1.1	−0.5	−0.3	Reality
7	I am not sure if I will ever meet someone I truly love in my lifetime.	−1.3	1.5	−0.5	−2.0	Psychological State
8	Romance is important, but I want to focus more on my career and personal growth.	−0.8	0.7	0	0.7	Attitude/Method
9	The depth of love is proportional to the trust between partners.	1.5	−0.6	0.5	1.6	Psychological State
10	Pursuing shared hobbies or goals can strengthen the bond between partners.	0.8	0.9	−0.1	0.6	Attitude/Method
11	I want to have a healthy love, but I am not sure how to do it.	−0.7	1.4	−0.8	−1.3	Attitude/Method
12	I have not experienced true love yet.	−0.8	2.2	−1.7	−2.1	Attitude/Method
13	When I love, I learn the ability to care for others.	0.8	−0.3	1.7	0.4	Growth
14	I believe that helping each other grow is a sign of healthy love.	0.8	1.2	0.7	0.8	Growth
15	Having a loving partner helps provide psychological stability.	1.5	−0.2	−0.2	1.2	Psychological State
16	Not giving my heart deeply in a relationship is a way to protect myself.	−1.6	−0.5	1.2	−0.3	Psychological State
17	Love tends to create a sense of identification between each other.	−0.5	−1.2	−1.0	−0.3	Psychological State
18	I believe loving someone means seeing them as they are, without conditions.	0.6	0.1	−0.3	−0.7	Element
19	Love helps me forget the hardships of life.	1.2	−1.7	−0.6	−1.0	Benefit
20	Love is about gaining my closest friend.	1.3	0.5	1.3	0.1	Benefit

Table 1. *Cont.*

No	Q Statement	Love Healing Z-Scores	Love Anxious Z-Scores	Love Myself Z-Scores	Independent Love Z-Scores	Category
21	Good love is about overcoming challenging times together.	0.7	0.3	−0.2	0.6	Element
22	Love is the most important aspect of human relationships.	0.6	−0.4	−0.1	0.4	Attitude/Method
23	Love and marriage are separate.	−1.1	−1.0	−1.4	1.4	Attitude/Method
24	I believe that knowing myself well is essential for having good love.	0.9	0.3	2.4	2.1	Self-Awareness
25	If I do not like who I am when I am in love, I do not think it's a healthy love.	0	−0.4	1.4	−0.3	Self-Awareness
26	I feel reluctant to date someone who has experienced many romantic relationships.	−1.1	−0.9	−0.7	0.1	Attitude/Method
27	I prefer living with the person I love rather than getting married.	−1.5	0.8	−1.2	−0.3	Attitude/Method
28	I find that dating through apps is more comfortable than meeting in person.	−1.9	−2.1	−1.8	−2.2	Attitude/Method
29	A satisfying sex life is one of the important aspects of a romantic relationship.	0.2	0.7	0.3	0.7	Element
30	A good romantic relationship seems to involve resolving conflicts in a healthy way.	0.7	0.7	1.6	1.7	Attitude/Method
31	If I like who I am when I am in love, it is a good love.	0.5	1.2	0.9	−0.6	Self-Awareness
32	Love is about respecting myself and my partner just as we are.	1.2	1.1	1.2	1.0	Attitude/Method
33	Sometimes, love is expressed through self-sacrifice.	−0.1	−0.2	−0.3	0.4	Attitude/Method
34	Having more experience in dating can be helpful when in a relationship.	−0.5	−0.4	0.3	−0.1	Attitude/Method
35	At first, relationships may be based on emotional attraction, but later, continuous effort is needed.	0.8	0.2	0.1	0.2	Attitude/Method
36	It seems that who I fall in love with can change who I am.	−0.1	−0.2	0.2	−0.4	Self-Awareness
37	Balancing work and a romantic relationship feels overwhelming.	−0.9	−1.0	−1.6	−0.9	Reality

Table 1. Cont.

No	Q Statement	Love Healing Z-Scores	Love Anxious Z-Scores	Love Myself Z-Scores	Independent Love Z-Scores	Category
38	I want to focus more on self-development than on love.	−0.6	0.7	−0.9	0.2	Reality
39	It is sad to have to worry about money while in a relationship.	−1.0	−1.5	−0.3	−1.0	Reality
40	Love is something that people without worries (like employment or money) can pursue.	−1.5	−2.2	−1.5	−1.6	Reality

2.1.3. Composition of P Sample

The P sample refers to the research participants who classify the Q sample [61]. Since the Q methodology does not aim for demographic generalisation, the P sample's demographic representativeness is unnecessary [62]. Furthermore, the Q methodology addresses intraindividual rather than interindividual differences in significance, allowing for flexibility in the number of participants in the P sample. Consequently, a small sample size is preferred, with an appropriate number of participants being approximately 40 ± 20 [63]. Additionally, selecting participants relevant to the research topic is crucial to enhancing the study's quality [49]. Therefore, this study utilised purposive sampling to select 23 individuals as the P sample based on the research objectives.

2.1.4. Q Sample Sorting

Q sorting refers to how the P sample arranges statements from the Q sample in order of importance based on their perspectives [46]. The Q sorting task differs from commonly used quantitative scales in psychology, such as the Likert scale, as it measures individual preference differences [64]. The method of Q sorting involves participants reading each statement and categorising them according to a forced distribution method [65]. The P sample conducted Q sorting following the Q sorting procedure outlined by Kil et al. [49]; Figure 3 illustrates the Q distribution.

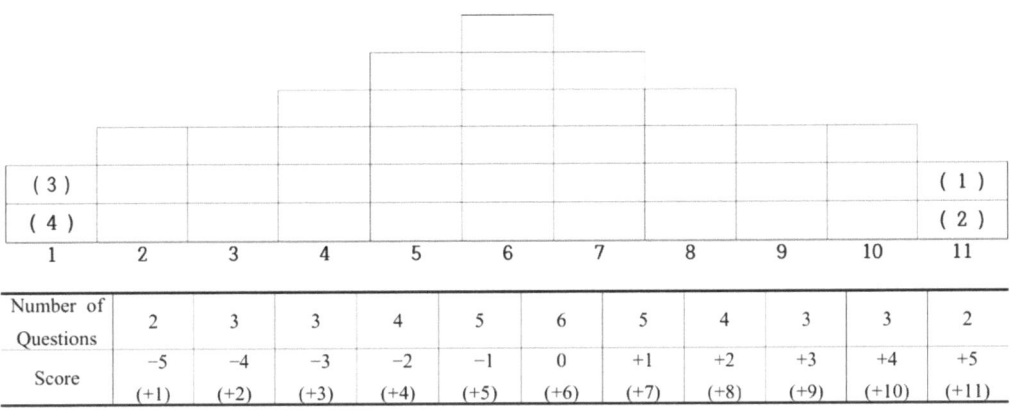

Figure 3. Q sorting distribution chart.

During Q sorting, we instructed research participants to place statements at either end of the spectrum based on their level of agreement, filling from the outer edges towards the centre while organising neutral statements. We guided participants to review the entire set and adjust the items in the Q grid. Finally, we asked them to provide reasons for the two statements with which they most agreed and disagreed. This opportunity allows for a detailed explanation of the participants' opinions and thoughts, which can be useful for factor interpretation in subsequent data analysis [46]. This study's P sample conducted Q sorting from 9 to 23 October 2023. To facilitate understanding of the Q sorting, we prepared an instructional document. Among the participants, we engaged seven face-to-face, while 16 participated remotely (via phone or video conference). The Q sorting took approximately 30 to 40 min for each participant, and we provided coffee coupons as a token of appreciation for their participation.

2.1.5. Data Analysis

The present study utilised the QUANL program, which maximises the variance explained for analysis [46]. After confirming the statement numbers of the Q sort distribution, we scored the collected data from 1 to 11 points and coded and entered the weighted values into the computer. Subsequently, we employed the PC-QUANAL program, a Q sorting data analysis tool, utilising principal component factor analysis as the Q factor analysis method. We determined the number of factors based on an eigenvalue threshold of 1.0000 or greater to ensure optimal classification of types. Additionally, we used Q statements with a Z-score greater than one to identify the characteristics of each type. Furthermore, by focusing on participants with high weights within each type, we identified the items with which the participants most agreed and disagreed and documented the reasons, serving as a reference for interpreting the characteristics of each type.

3. Study Results

3.1. Result Analysis

We categorised the results of the subjective exploratory research on romantic bonds in early adulthood into four types. Table 1 presents the Z-scores for each statement associated with each type, along with their categorisation based on the content of the statements. For the categorisation process, we documented and organized 142 statements collected from the Q population into an Excel file. We then classified these statements into 'psychological state', 'attitude/method', 'reality', 'growth', 'element', 'benefit', and 'self-awareness' based on their content. We further classified these statements into positive, negative, and neutral categories and selected the final 40 questions through a process of revision and elimination.

Table 2 summarises the results, revealing four distinct types. The eigenvalues for each type are as follows: Love Healing = 8.8730, Love Anxious = 1.8600, Love Myself = 1.5812, and Independent Love = 1.0124, with a cumulative variance of 0.5787.

Table 2. Eigenvalues and explanatory variances in the sorting of four love types.

Content	Love Healing	Love Anxious	Love Myself	Independent Love
Chosen eigenvalues	8.8730	1.8600	1.5648	1.0124
Total variance	0.3858	0.0809	0.0680	0.0440
Cumulative	0.3858	0.4667	0.5347	0.5787
Solution variance	0.6666	0.1397	0.1176	0.0761
Cumulative	0.6666	0.0864	0.9239	1.0000

The correlations among the four types are in Table 3. The correlation between Love Healing and Love Myself is the highest at 0.614, followed by 0.144 between Love Anxious and Independent Love. Notably, the Q methodology does not assume complete independence among factors but focuses on identifying factors. Therefore, researchers do not debate the significance of the correlation coefficients in the factor extraction process [46].

Table 3. Correlation coefficients between love types.

Type	Love Healing	Love Anxious	Love Myself	Independent Love
Love Healing	1.000	0.252	0.614	0.598
Love Anxious		1.000	0.248	0.144
Love Myself			1.000	0.573
Independent Love				1.000

Among the 23 participants, 11 comprised Type 1 (Love Healing), 3 were Type 2 (Love Anxious), 5 were Type 3 (Love Myself), and 4 were Type 4 (Independent Love). Supplementary Material Table S1 presents the demographic characteristics and factor weights of the four types.

3.2. Perception Type Characteristics

3.2.1. Type 1: Love Healing

Love Healing's characteristic is experiencing psychological well-being through love. The statements with which those in the Love Healing type agreed the most were 'Having a loving partner helps provide psychological stability' (Q15, $Z = 1.53$) and 'Comfort makes the process of love richer and more stable' (Q1, $Z = 1.51$). Conversely, the statements with the highest disagreement were 'I find that dating through apps is more comfortable than meeting in person' (Q28, $Z = -1.92$) and 'Not giving my heart deeply in a relationship is a way to protect myself' (Q16, $Z = -1.59$). Table 1 provides the representative statements and their Z sores for the Love Healing type.

In the Love Healing type, the statement with the highest difference from the average Z-scores of other types was Q19: 'Love helps me forget the hardships of life' (Diff. = 2.284). Conversely, the statement with the lowest difference was Q16: 'Not giving my heart deeply in a relationship is a way to protect myself' (Diff. = −1.730). The statements from this type that exhibited a Z-score difference of ±1.00 or greater compared to the averages of other types are in Supplementary Materials.

P23, a Love Healing participant, stated:

> I feel a sense of stability when I experience comfort, allowing me to reveal my true self. The same goes for my partner. As we accumulate such moments, respect and trust build together, creating a bond I can share with someone for a long time.

Similarly, P3 expressed:

> Having spent a long time with my current boyfriend, we have become close enough to discuss things I cannot share with my family or friends. I believe he will always be by my side, and it feels like I have found my closest friend in life.

Thus, those in the Love Healing category reflect positive emotions such as psychological stability, trust, and respect through love. They highlight the characteristics of inner growth through relationships. Based on these findings, we designated those in this category as the 'Love Healing' type because they experience psychological well-being through love.

3.2.2. Type 2: Love Anxious

While the Love Anxious type longs for true love, they are anxious about love. The statements with which the Love Anxious type agreed most were 'I have not experienced true love yet' (Q12, $Z = 2.25$) and 'I am not sure if I will ever meet someone I truly love in my lifetime' (Q7, $Z = 1.49$). Conversely, the statements with the lowest levels of agreement were 'Love is something that people without worries (like employment or money) can pursue' (Q40, $Z = -2.17$) and 'I find that dating through apps is more comfortable than meeting in person' (Q28, $Z = -2.07$). Table 1 provides the representative statements and their Z-scores for those in the Love Anxious category.

In the Love Anxious group, the statement with the highest difference in Z-scores compared to the means of other types is Q12, 'I have not experienced true love yet' (Diff. = 3.778). Conversely, the statement with the lowest difference is Q9, 'The degree of love is proportional to mutual trust' (Diff. = −1.788). The statements from this type that exhibit a Z-score difference of ±1.00 or more compared to the means of other types are in Supplementary Materials.

The participant with the highest factor weight in the Love Anxious category, P22, stated:

Since I have never experienced love, I am unsure what love is or even if it exists. Therefore, I have a strong desire to experience it. Moreover, I ponder what is necessary for love to endure. I believe it involves supporting each other's growth. The continuity of love is not about appearances or money but rather about encouraging each other's dreams and helping one another progress through those dreams. I believe that is what sustains love.

P8 expressed:

I think we cannot change people and that they remain the same. There is no perfect person, and I am not perfect either. Therefore, I believe love is about understanding and accepting myself and the other person as we are, which is why I chose this perspective.

In this way, those classified as Love Anxious recognise that healthy relationships involve mutual growth, understanding, and respect for one another, which they perceive as true love. They also exhibit feelings of anxiety regarding forming intimate relationships. Based on these characteristics, we designated those in this group as the 'Love Anxious' type because they long for true love, although they are anxious about it.

3.2.3. Type 3: Love Myself

Those in the Love Myself group express hope for healthy love through self-awareness. The statements with which those in the Love Myself category most agreed were 'I believe that knowing myself well is essential for having good love' (Q24, Z = 2.43) and 'When I love, I learn to care for others' (Q13, Z = 1.73). Conversely, the statements that received the lowest agreement were 'I find that dating through apps is more comfortable than meeting in person' (Q28, Z = −1.83) and 'I have not experienced true love yet' (Q12, Z = −1.70). Table 1 provides the representative statements and their Z-scores for those in this group.

In the Love Myself group, the statement with the highest difference in Z-score of at least ±1.00 compared to other types is Q16: 'Not giving my heart deeply in a relationship is a way to protect myself' (Diff. = 1.978). Conversely, the statement with the lowest difference is Q23: 'Love and marriage are separate' (Diff. = −0.213). The statements relating to this type's Z-score difference of at least ±1.00 compared to other types are in Supplementary Materials.

P7, with the highest factor weight among the Love Myself group, stated:

My partner feels like a mirror to me when I am in love. They bring out aspects of myself I was unaware of, and I sometimes have to confront traits I dislike. I believe that the extent to which I understand myself allows for healthy communication in relationships based on that self-awareness.

Similarly, P4 expressed:

To adjust and coordinate with any partner, I must clearly understand what I like, dislike and my goals. If I change depending on my partner, I might forget who I am at some point; therefore, I believe starting a relationship with a high level of self-awareness and self-esteem is essential.

Thus, those categorized as 'Love Myself' reflect a desire to maintain a healthy relationship through self-awareness. Based on these characteristics, we designated this type as 'Love Myself' because it expresses hope for healthy love through self-awareness.

3.2.4. Type 4: Independent Love

Those in the Independent Love group seek to maintain psychological love while pursuing independence. The statements with which this type most agreed were, 'I believe that knowing myself well is essential for having good love' (Q24, Z = 2.10) and 'A good romantic relationship seems to involve resolving conflicts in a healthy way' (Q30, Z = 1.66). Conversely, the statements with the lowest levels of agreement were 'I find that dating through apps is more comfortable than meeting in person' (Q28, Z = −2.16) and 'I have not experienced true love yet' (Q12, Z = −2.09). Table 1 provides the representative statements and their Z-scores for the Independent Love type.

Among those of the Independent Love type, the statement with the highest Z-score difference of ±1.00 compared to other types is 'Love and marriage are separate' (Q23, Diff. = 2.517), while the statement with the lowest Z-score difference is 'I have not experienced true love yet' (Q12, Diff. = −1.998). The statements in the Independent Love group that exhibit a Z-score difference of ±1.00 or more compared to the averages of other types are in Supplementary Materials.

P13, with the highest factor weight among those in the Independent Love group, stated:

> As I grow older, I often fear repeating past mistakes from previous relationships, even with someone I've known for a long time. Developing a new relationship requires careful communication and effort from the start, which can sometimes feel burdensome compared to the enjoyment of advancing the relationship. Consequently, I tend to consider whether the person is capable of understanding and whether we can connect meaningfully before contemplating the progression of our relationship.

In addition, P19 expressed, 'I believe I am who I am, and the other person is who they are. As we spend more time together and share experiences, respecting each other's true selves is essential to achieve harmony in the relationship'. Moreover, P21 remarked:

> I consider love a relationship based on sacrifice. When two individuals meet, they invest their time, money, emotions, and other resources for love. As the relationship deepens and evolves into genuine love, I feel a profound sense of commitment, akin to risking everything for that person. Therefore, sacrificing for my partner represents true love to me.

Thus, the Independent Love type reflects characteristics of maintaining psychological love while pursuing independence in personal life. Based on these characteristics, we designated Type 4 as the 'Independent Love' type because it seeks to maintain psychological love while pursuing independence.

3.3. Consensus Items

Consensus items refer to those statements with which all participants agree [66]. Rather than interpreting the characteristics of each type individually, consensus items allow for a comprehensive understanding of the overall traits across types through common statements. We identified 17 consensus items across the types described in Table 4.

Table 4. Consensus love items.

No	Statement	Z-Score
30	A good romantic relationship seems to involve resolving conflicts in a healthy way.	1.15
32	Love is about respecting myself and my partner just as we are.	1.11
1	Comfort makes the process of love richer and more stable.	0.98
14	I believe that helping each other grow is a sign of healthy love.	0.88
10	Pursuing shared hobbies or goals can strengthen the bond between partners.	0.53

Table 4. *Cont.*

No	Statement	Z-Score
29	A satisfying sex life is one of the important aspects of a romantic relationship.	0.48
21	Good love is about overcoming challenging times together.	0.36
35	At first, relationships may be based on emotional attraction, but later, continuous effort is needed.	0.32
4	When I love, I feel jealousy.	0.17
22	Love is the most important aspect of human relationships.	0.13
33	Sometimes, love is expressed through self-sacrifice.	−0.05
36	It seems that who I fall in love with can change who I am.	−0.13
34	Having more experience in dating can be helpful when in a relationship.	−0.16
17	Love tends to create a sense of identification between each other.	−0.75
37	Balancing work and a romantic relationship feels overwhelming.	−1.08
40	Love is something that people without worries (like employment or money) can pursue.	−1.68
28	I find that dating through apps is more comfortable than meeting in person.	−1.99

4. Discussion

This study explored the different types of love perceptions in early adulthood and examined each type's characteristics using the Q methodology, which is ideal for analysing subjective perceptions. Through Q factor analysis, we identified four types of subjective perceptions regarding love in early adulthood: Type 1 (the 'Love Healing' type) experiences psychological well-being through love, Type 2 (the 'Love Anxious' type) longs for true love but is anxious about love, Type 3 (the 'Love Myself' type) expresses hope for healthy love through self-awareness, and Type 4 (the 'Independent Love' type) seeks to maintain psychological love while pursuing independence.

The Love Healing type comprised 11 participants with characteristics of psychological well-being, such as positive emotions, attitudes towards life, and inner growth, which allowed them to accept themselves positively and form trusting, stable relationships with their partners. These characteristics align with Bartholomew and Horowitz's [13] 'secure attachment type', marked by high intimacy, comfort, and autonomy. This type corresponds to the 'secure' category of adult attachment styles. Individuals with secure attachment have a well-integrated sense of self-identity and high self-esteem. They also show high intimacy towards and trust in their loved ones, are open and flexible, and do not find self-disclosure difficult [12,13,67,68]. Due to their positive internal working models, these individuals consider being loved to be natural and express high satisfaction in relationships through the comfort and happiness of mutual trust. Additionally, Marrero-Quevedo and colleagues [69] reported a positive relationship between secure attachment and psychological well-being, which resonates with the characteristics of the Love Healing type.

The Love Healing type also reflects similarities with John Alan Lee's [25] love styles of eros (passionate love) and agape (selfless love). Frazier and Esterly [70] found that higher levels of passionate and selfless love positively correlated with relationship intimacy, commitment, passion, and satisfaction, while passionate love positively affected trust. This view aligns with the findings related to the Love Healing type. Sternberg's [71,72] Triangular Theory of Love systematically presents love as intimacy, passion, and commitment. Those in the Love Healing category demonstrate all three components, though with a stronger emphasis on intimacy and commitment. Madey and Rodgers [73] also reported that secure attachment relates to intimacy and commitment, a finding consistent with the findings in the Love Healing group.

The additional statements provided by participants in the Love Healing type reveal a shared perception that the key to love lies in 'acknowledging and accepting each other's differences while respecting and understanding the partner and oneself'. Participants emphasised the importance of effort in maintaining a loving relationship. For example, P6 said:

> As time goes by, there are fewer new things to discover about each other, and we could mistake this as love fading. Therefore, it is important to acknowledge and respect each other and to work on loving the familiar aspects even more.

Similarly, P10 said, 'I believe that maintaining the feelings of affection requires paying attention to the partner and treating them with care and affection, rather than neglecting them'. This emphasis on sustaining relationships through effort aligns with Bierhoff and Grau's [74] findings, which show that individuals with secure attachments tend to maintain long-term stable relationships. On the other hand, perceptions of passionate love, particularly the element of physical and sexual attraction highlighted in John Alan Lee's [25] passionate love and Sternberg's [71,72] passion component, were not prominent in the Love Healing type. De Munck et al. [75] suggested that the concept of romantic love might vary across cultures, indicating the need to explore whether these findings reflect characteristics of Korean culture.

We found that the Love Anxious type was characterised by a longing for true love accompanied by anxiety. Three participants in the P sample belong to this type. Love Anxious individuals perceived that they had not yet experienced genuine love, viewing a healthy love as one where both partners support each other's growth and maintain mutual respect. They also expected personal growth through love. However, they demonstrated a negative outlook on whether true love exists or whether they could experience it. Thus, they preferred cohabitation over marriage, a desire to focus more on self-development than love, and a sense of fear or reluctance to form close relationships. These characteristics reflect a longing for true love and anxiety about forming intimate connections, leading to avoidance behaviours.

This finding aligns with the fearful attachment style in Bartholomew and Horowitz's [13] model, which shows a mix of approach and avoidance tendencies. Hazan and Shaver's [12] three-category attachment theory originally classified the fearful style under the avoidant attachment style but later distinguished it as a separate category. People with avoidant attachments display similar traits. Bierhoff and Grau [74] noted that individuals with avoidant attachment struggle to accept their partners as they are, fear emotional closeness, and maintain emotional distance, making it difficult to fall in love or experience passionate love. These characteristics align with those of the Love Anxious type.

Unlike the Love Healing type, which aligned with John Alan Lee's [25] love types, the Love Anxious type did not correspond to any specific love style. However, Frazier and Esterly [70] found that relationships with higher levels of passionate and selfless love exhibited greater intimacy, passion, commitment, and satisfaction, which contrasts with the tendencies of the Love Anxious type. Additionally, previous research has reported that individuals with ambivalent or avoidant attachment styles display possessive love, characterised by strong jealousy and attachment [76], a trait not observed in the Love Anxious type.

Levy and Davis [77] reported an association between lower levels of anxiety and avoidant with higher levels of intimacy, passion, and commitment, as outlined in Sternberg's Triangular Theory of Love. In contrast, those in the Love Anxious group demonstrated low recognition of all three components. Supporting statements from Love Anxious participants include 'I have never experienced love, so I don't know what love is or whether it even exists' (P22), 'Though breakups are sad, I have never been in a relationship that made me want to fall in love again' (P10), and 'I don't want to spend the emotional energy required to meet new people, stay in touch, and think about them' (P8). However, positive experiences in forming stable relationships can transform attachment styles [78]. Therefore, providing educational and coaching programs to help individuals classified as Love Anxious develop their attachment style and experience fulfilling love relationships may be beneficial.

The Love Myself type exhibited characteristics associated with intimacy and commitment from Sternberg's [71,72] Triangular Theory of Love. Specifically, Love Myself individuals displayed a commitment to love through self-awareness, leading to a sense of connectedness in intimate relationships and a drive to sustain that love. One of the most notable features of those classified as Love Myself types is how individuals gain self-awareness through their relationship dynamics and their partners' reactions. Supporting statements from participants in this group include 'My partner feels like a mirror to me' (P7), 'I believe that knowing myself well helps me maintain balance and not be swayed, regardless of who I'm with' (P4), and 'Knowing myself well reduces the chances of projecting my dissatisfaction onto my partner' (P16). This result aligns with Cooley's [79] concept of the 'Looking-Glass Self', which emphasises that social interaction forms and continuously reshapes self-identity. This concept mirrors the Love Myself type's characteristic of recognising oneself through close, influential relationships with their partner.

Research shows that individuals in early adulthood (twenties to thirties) with a clearer self-perception, including subjective evaluations of their worth or competence, are better equipped for interpersonal competence [80]. Moreover, emotional clarity is essential in conveying one's needs, intentions, and desires to others while also recognising and responding to the intentions of others in interpersonal relationships [81]. Therefore, for individuals in the Love Myself group, who prioritise understanding their emotions and identifying their needs, coaching programs that enhance self-awareness and communication training for conflict resolution are necessary to foster healthy dialogue and relationship development.

The Independent Love type, the love mate type, seeks to maintain psychological love while pursuing independence in life. This type comprised four participants from the P sample. Although the Independent Love type shared the same statements of agreement and disagreement as those in the Love Myself group, the reasons behind their choices reveal significant differences. In those classified as Love Myself, self-awareness was a way to protect themselves in relationships, promoting a desire for healthy love. In contrast, those categorised in the Independent Love group demonstrated a focus on self over a partner—for example, 'If I keep adjusting to my partner, I will lose myself and adopt an unhealthy mindset' (P9), 'I am myself, and my partner is their self. I believe that relationships are built by sharing moments and building memories together, but it's important to respect each other's individuality. I am the main character in my life' (P19), and 'One of my priorities is knowing myself. I believe love is a relationship that requires sacrifice, but I see sacrificing for my partner as a sign of true love' (P21). These statements reflect self-awareness that centres on the individual rather than the partner.

Furthermore, while they perceive their romantic partner as special in their relationships, unlike friends, they recognise that deepening love often brings a sense of security but also requires sacrifices in one's life. Like those of the Love Myself type, individuals in the Independent Love group combine intimacy, which enhances emotional connection and social support, with commitment, which involves a willingness to sustain love through personal sacrifices [71,72]. However, unlike the Love Myself type, those in the Independent Love group emphasise that love requires sacrifice and commitment, but only if they can maintain their independence. Once they achieve psychological and social independence, they can commit to love, allowing them to form intimacy.

In this regard, the Independent Love type contrasts with the Love Myself type in that they do not necessarily see marriage as the ultimate goal of true love. While they find stability through deep relationships, they also desire mutual respect for their personal lives before reaching that point. This perspective aligns with previous studies on Korean youth's pursuit of independence, particularly in response to changing societal values and the instability of their personal and macro-level social environments [82–85]. Thus, the Independent Love type represents a mix of secure attachment, characterised by comfort in relationships and healthy conflict resolution, and dismissing attachment, marked by high self-esteem and strong independence [13]. In diagrammatic terms, we could position this type closer to the secure end of the attachment spectrum while retaining elements of dismissing attachment.

The consensus items included five statements with a standard score of ± 1 or higher across all types: 'A good romantic relationship seems to involve resolving conflicts in a healthy way' (Q30, $z = 1.15$), 'Love is about respecting myself and my partner just as we are (Q32, $z = 1.11$)', 'Balancing work and a romantic relationship feels overwhelming' (Q37, $z = -1.08$), 'Love is something that people without worries (like employment or money) can pursue' (Q40, z = −1.68), and 'I find that dating through apps is more comfortable than meeting in person' (Q28, z = −1.99).

A common feature across the four types is the emphasis on resolving conflicts in a healthy manner and respecting oneself and one's partner, suggesting that these individuals are contemplating the nature of true love. Lloyd [86] argued for the importance of resolving conflicts based on research findings that healthy conflict resolution leads to positive changes in relationship satisfaction for couples. Furthermore, rather than external conditions (such as employment, work life, or money) serving as negative factors in love, the findings suggest that love can help individuals overcome external difficulties.

This study identified the perception types of love in early adulthood and showed that young adults commonly grapple with the concept of true love and exhibit a consistent desire to improve for the sake of maintaining healthy relationships. Kang [87] revealed that young adults in South Korean society seek love and happiness despite various conflicts, striving to bridge the gap between romantic ideals and reality and pursuing self-reflective love through relationships with others. This viewpoint aligns with the findings of the present study. Despite these commonalities, it was evident that their perceptions of love varied significantly. Rather than categorising them into distinct adult attachment types, the findings revealed that while individuals exhibited characteristics from various attachment types, they more prominently expressed certain attachment styles.

5. Conclusions

This study analysed subjective perceptions of love in early adulthood within South Korean society using the Q methodology, identifying distinct perception types. The significance of this research lies in its pioneering use of Q methodology to classify perception types regarding love in early adulthood. Figure 4 illustrates a schematic representation of this study's four findings.

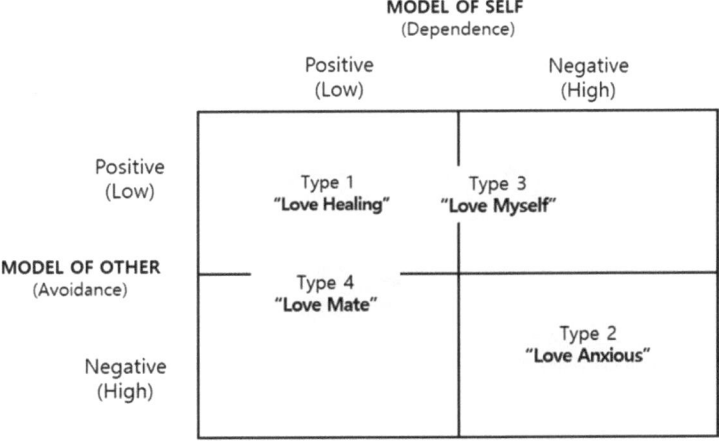

Figure 4. Love perception type model of early adulthood.

The study results indicated that the four perception types relate to Bartholomew and Horowitz's [13] adult attachment styles, revealing specific similarities and differences. The Love Healing type closely resembled the secure attachment style, while the Love Anxious type exhibited characteristics highly similar to the fearful style. The Love Myself type displayed traits of the preoccupied style, leaning towards the secure attachment style. Finally, the Independent Love type demonstrated features of the dismissing style, which is close to secure attachment. Additionally, we found the four perception types associated with John Alan Lee's six styles of love and Sternberg's triangular theory of love. The study also identified the key characteristics of each type.

The Love Healing type experienced psychological stability and positive emotions through love and sought inner growth via romantic relationships. In contrast, the Love Anxious type showed a yearning for true love, with a focus on mutual growth and a tendency towards anxiety. The third type, Love Myself, valued self-awareness and self-esteem as central to relationships, emphasising independence while pursuing mature and healthy love. Finally, the Independent Love type prioritised independence while maintaining emotional bonds, viewing love and marriage separately and valuing a balance between love and personal life. Kang [87] found no direct transfer of Western concepts of romantic love to South Korean society, even those that had evolved with distinct characteristics. He observed that young adults in Korea, facing economic difficulties and rapid social changes, tend to prefer more practical romantic relationships, blending ideals of romantic love with the reality of insecure, individualistic love. This perspective aligns with the characteristics of the Love Anxious and Independent Love types in the present study.

On the other hand, a commonality among all four types was the emphasis on psychological stability and growth through love. Participants shared a commitment to mutual understanding and respect, recognising the importance of relationships, a willingness to resolve conflicts in a healthy way, and the view that love is not a fleeting emotion but a significant element requiring continuous effort. These findings reflect South Korea's unique social norms, family-centredness, and emphasis on psychological stability, exhibiting a pattern distinct from that of Western societies. Confucianism from China has profoundly influenced South Korea, emphasising relational harmony, still viewing love and marriage as significant social tasks, and reinforcing traditional family structures [88]. In contrast, Western societies emphasise individual independence and self-realisation, placing greater importance on personal choice in love and marriage. Karandashev [89] notes that Western cultures prioritise protecting and maintaining the self-concept, while Eastern cultures, which emphasise interdependence, tend to use preventive strategies to sustain relationships. This tendency impacts romantic relationships, with Eastern cultures showing a correlation between individual change and relationship quality, a connection less relevant in Western contexts.

This study shows how individuals in early adulthood subjectively perceive love within the cultural context of South Korea, highlighting love's significant role in shaping self-identity and forming mature relationships. These findings may serve as foundational data for developing counselling and coaching services aimed at helping young adults in Korea experience positive and fulfilling love tailored to the characteristics of each identified type. Based on this study's findings, developing an enhanced love scale that incorporates existing love types and attachment styles for use in universities and field settings for young adults may be valuable in supporting personal growth through love. Finally, future research on the subjectivity of love during the transition to middle adulthood, based on this study, will deepen our understanding of how developmental processes and life transitions shape perceptions of love and attachment types. We expect this will be an expanded study offering profound insights into love during adult development.

6. Limitations

The limitations of this study and suggestions for future research are as follows. First, this study employed the Q methodology to examine the subjective perceptions of a small number of participants. While such a small sample size limits statistical generalizability, the Q methodology is designed to categorize subjective perceptions. Therefore, it was suitable for identifying perception types and characteristics regarding love in early adulthood. However, the findings of this study cannot be generalized. Future research should comprehensively investigate the factors influencing love in early adulthood, using quantitative methods to demonstrate how love facilitates personal growth. This would allow for a broader generalization of the findings.

Second, there is a limitation regarding whether the typological characteristics derived from Q methodology adequately reflect subjective perceptions of love. Therefore, we suggest qualitative research, such as interpretative phenomenological analysis, to explore each type's deeper internal perceptions and experiences regarding love in early adulthood.

Third, this study focuses on exploring perceptions of love within a specific age group in early adulthood. However, experiences of love may evolve as individuals between the ages of 20 and 40 encounter various life experiences and developmental tasks. Therefore, further research could help us understand how perceptions of love differ across ages. A comparative study across age groups, analysing differences in perceptions of love from ages 20 to 40, would help address this limitation. Such research could contribute to understanding the impact of romantic experiences, marital status, and changes in social roles on perceptions of love.

Fourth, this study did not adequately account for potential differences in perceptions of love based on gender. Despite possible variations in expectations and experiences of love by gender, the sample composition and analysis in this study did not allow for a clear explanation of these differences. Future research should explore perception differences by gender in greater detail.

Finally, this study focused on a sample restricted to South Korea, which does not fully account for cultural diversity. As perceptions and experiences of love may vary across cultural contexts, further research should explore love perceptions in other cultural settings. Such studies would enable an evaluation of the cultural universality of the findings and provide a broader understanding of perceptions of love.

Supplementary Materials: The following supporting information can be downloaded at: https://www.mdpi.com/article/10.3390/bs14121135/s1. Table S1. P Samples and Factor Weights by Love Type. Table S2. Statements of the Love Healing Type with a Z-Score Difference of at Least ±1.00 Compared to the Averages of Other Love Types. Table S3. Statements of the Love Anxious Type with a Z-Score Difference of at Least ±1.00 Compared to the Averages of Other Love Types. Table S4. Statements of the Love Myself Type with a Z-Score Difference of at Least ±1.00 Compared to the Averages of Other Love Types. Table S5. Statements of the Independent Love Type with a Z−Score Difference of at Least ±1.00 Compared to the Averages of Other Love Types.

Author Contributions: Conceptualisation, S.J.S., J.S.Y. and S.Y.L.; Data curation, S.Y.L.; Formal analysis, J.S.Y.; Investigation, S.J.S. and J.S.Y.; Methodology, S.J.S. and J.S.Y.; Resources, S.J.S.; Validation, S.Y.L.; Writing—original draft, S.J.S., J.S.Y. and S.Y.L.; Writing—review and editing, S.Y.L. All authors have read and agreed to the published version of the manuscript.

Funding: This research received no external funding.

Institutional Review Board Statement: The study was conducted in accordance with the Declaration of Helsinki and approved by the Institutional Review Board of Dongguk University (IRB no. DUIRB202308-22 and 30 August 2023).

Informed Consent Statement: We obtained informed consent from all subjects involved in the study.

Data Availability Statement: The datasets generated and/or analysed during the current study are not publicly available to preserve the anonymity of the respondents but are available from the corresponding author upon reasonable request.

Conflicts of Interest: The authors declare no conflicts of interest.

References

1. Seo, I.Y. Building relationships in the non-face-to-face era: Changes in human relations in the youth through the gaze of university students and qualitative exploration for empathy education. *Soc. Sci. Stud.* **2021**, *29*, 126–181.
2. Erikson, E.H. *Identity Youth and Crisis*, 7th ed.; WW Norton & Company: New York, NY, USA, 1968.
3. Han, S.-y.; Hong, H.-y. The study of the singles' love styles related to their self-esteem, relationship satisfaction, and trust. *Korean J. Interdiscip. Ther.* **2010**, *2*, 25–48.
4. Mikulincer, M.; Shaver, P.R.; Horesh, N. Attachment bases of emotion regulation and posttraumatic adjustment. In *Emotion Regulation in Couples and Families: Pathways to Dysfunction and Health*; American Psychological Association: Washington, DC, USA, 2006.
5. Bowlby, J. The nature of the child's tie to his mother, 1. *Int. J. Psychoanal.* **1958**, *39*, 350–373. [PubMed]
6. Bowlby, J.; Ainsworth, M.; Bretherton, I. The origins of attachment theory. *Dev. Psychol.* **1992**, *28*, 759–775.

7. An, S.; Lee, H.; Lee, J.; Kang, S. Social stigma of suicide in South Korea: A cultural perspective. *Death Stud.* **2022**, *47*, 259–267. [CrossRef]
8. Bode, A. Corrigendum: Romantic love evolved by co-opting mother–infant bonding. *Front. Psychol.* **2024**, *15*, 1402313. [CrossRef]
9. Kim, J.; Lee, J. Adult attachment styles across close relationships among Korean college students: A latent profile analysis. *J. Fam. Better Life* **2015**, *33*, 119–145.
10. Kennison, S.M.; Spooner, V.H. Childhood relationships with parents and attachment as predictors of resilience in young adults. *J. Fam. Stud.* **2023**, *29*, 15–27. [CrossRef]
11. Chin, B.N.; Kim, L.; Parsons, S.M.; Feeney, B.C. Attachment orientation and preferences for partners' emotional responses in stressful and positive situations. *Behav. Sci.* **2024**, *14*, 77. [CrossRef]
12. Hazan, C.; Shaver, P. Romantic love conceptualised as an attachment process. *J. Personal. Soc. Psychol.* **1987**, *52*, 511–524. [CrossRef]
13. Bartholomew, K.; Horowitz, L.M. Attachment styles among young adults: A test of a four-category model. *J. Personal. Soc. Psychol.* **1991**, *61*, 226. [CrossRef] [PubMed]
14. Kang, Y.R.; Kim, M.Y. An exploratory study on the lifestyle characteristics of the MZ generation—A focus on the 2010–2020 studies. *Korean Fash. Text. Res. J.* **2022**, *24*, 81–94. [CrossRef]
15. Lee, M.J.; Kim, G.H.; Lee, J.; Vo, N.H.; Lee, S.M. The effects of academic stress and academic failure tolerance on academic burnout among college students: Moderated mediation effects of interpersonal stress. *J. Korea Converg. Soc.* **2020**, *11*, 175–185.
16. Song, J.-Y. The effects of interpersonal relation and social support on college freshmen's adaptation to college life. *J. Korea Acad. Ind. Coop. Soc.* **2017**, *18*, 335–345.
17. Lee, H.-j. Beyond Marriage to Non–Dating: A Society without Romantic Relationships. Ajou University Newspaper and Broadcasting, Suwon, Republic of Korea. 2023. Available online: https://press.ajou.ac.kr/news/articleView.html?idxno=3349 (accessed on 15 December 2023).
18. Kim, N.; Lee, S.-j.; Seo, Y.-h.; Choi, J.-h.; Kim, S.-y.; Jeon, M.-y.; Lee, H.-e.; Lee, J.-y.; Kwon, J.-y. *Trend Korea 2019*; Future's Window Publications: Seoul, Republic of Korea, 2018; pp. 291–314.
19. Korean Statistical Information Service. Preliminary Results of Birth and Death Statistics for 2022. Available online: https://kostat.go.kr/board.es?mid=a20108100000&bid=11773&act=view&list_no=424347&tag=&nPage=1&ref_bid= (accessed on 15 December 2023).
20. Fromm, E. Love and its disintegration. *Pastor. Psychol.* **1956**, *7*, 37–44. [CrossRef]
21. Jarvis, J.A.; Corbett, A.W.; Thorpe, J.D.; Dufur, M.J. Too much of a good thing: Social capital and academic stress in South Korea. *Soc. Sci.* **2020**, *9*, 187. [CrossRef]
22. Hatfield, E.; Sprecher, S. Measuring passionate love in intimate relationships. *J. Adolesc.* **1986**, *9*, 383–410. [CrossRef]
23. May, R. *Man's Search for Himself*; Norton: New York, NY, USA, 1953.
24. Jang, M.K.; Lee, Y. A study of forms of expression in emblematic sign of love. *J. Korea Des. Forum* **2009**, *23*, 33–44. [CrossRef]
25. Lee, J.A. *The Colors of Love: An Exploration of the Ways of Loving*; New Press: Don Mills, ON, Canada, 1973.
26. Erikson, E.H. Inner and outer space: Reflections on womanhood. *Daedalus* **1964**, *93*, 582–606.
27. Fredrickson, B.L. What good are positive emotions? *Rev. Gen. Psych.* **1998**, *2*, 300–319. [CrossRef]
28. Levinson, B.M. Pets and personality development. *Psych. Rep.* **1978**, *42*, 1031–1038. [CrossRef]
29. Song, M.-J. A Study on Drama Therapy for Recognising Love. Master's Thesis, Department of Drama Therapy Graduate School of Culture and Arts Yong In University, Seoul, Republic of Korea, 2022.
30. Ram, J.J. A narrative research on 'definition of love' between male and female university students. *J. Fam. Relat.* **2014**, *19*, 125–142.
31. Oh, Y.M. A Study on the view of marriage and the types of love of College Students. *J. Holis. Edu.* **2019**, *23*, 165–186. [CrossRef]
32. Oh, S.O.; Park, T. Cultural study on university students' love repertoires and happiness. *Korean J. Soc. Theory* **2016**, *50*, 207–248.
33. Kim, Y.S.; Park, J.W. The difference of marital satisfaction and communication according to the type of love of middle-aged married person. *J. Korean Assoc. Psychother.* **2021**, *13*, 1–23.
34. Kim, Y.-G.; Park, M.-S. The research of college students' sexual culture in convergence ages (focused on the effect of the types of love to casual sex). *J. Digit. Converg.* **2016**, *14*, 295–301.
35. Sung, Y.S.; Im, S.H.; Kim, M.N.; Lee, J.Y. The color of love: Comparative study of passionate love, companionate love, and homosexual love in the ads. *Korean J. Adv.* **2007**, *18*, 83–110.
36. Choi, Y.S. The study about the ideal mate selection and components of love according to the university students' Enneagram personality types. *J. Enneagr. Stud.* **2010**, *7*, 121–156.
37. Choi, K.; Jun, J.-r. A study on the components of love as perceived by college students. *Korean Soc. Cult. Converg.* **2020**, *42*, 245–264. [CrossRef]
38. Hetsroni, A. Associations between television viewing and love styles: An interpretation using cultivation theory. *Psych. Rep.* **2012**, *110*, 35–50. [CrossRef]
39. Gabb, J.; Fink, J. Telling moments and everyday experience: Multiple methods research on couple relationships and personal lives. *Sociology* **2015**, *49*, 970–987. [CrossRef] [PubMed]
40. Kokab, S.; Ajmal, M.A. Perception of love in young adults. *Pakistan J. Soc. Clin. Psych.* **2012**, *9*, 4–48.
41. Dion, K.K.; Dion, K.L. Cultural perspectives on romantic love. *Person. Relat.* **1996**, *3*, 5–17. [CrossRef]

42. Sumter, S.R.; Valkenburg, P.M.; Peter, J. Perceptions of love across the lifespan: Differences in passion, intimacy, and commitment. *Int. J. Behav. Dev.* **2013**, *37*, 417–427. [CrossRef]
43. McKeown, B.; Thomas, D.B. *Q Methodology*; Sage Publications: New York, NY, USA, 2013; Volume 66.
44. Ramlo, S. Non-statistical, substantive generalisation: Lessons from Q methodology. *Int. J. Res. Meth. Edu.* **2024**, *47*, 65–78. [CrossRef]
45. Herrington, N.; Coogan, J. Q methodology: An overview. *Res. Teacher Edu.* **2011**, *1*, 24–28.
46. Kim, H.K. *Q Methodology*; Communication Books Publications: Seoul, Republic of Korea, 2008.
47. Lee, B.S. The fundamentals of Q methodology. *J. Res. Meth.* **2017**, *2*, 57–95. [CrossRef]
48. Stephenson, W. *The Study of Behavior: Q-technique and Its Methodology*; University of Chicago Press: Chicago, IL, USA, 1953.
49. Kil, B.-o.; Lee, S.-h.; Lee, S.-y.; Chung, H.-j. *Understanding and Application of Q Methodology*; Chungnam National University Press: Daejeon, Republic of Korea, 2020.
50. Lee, S.Y.; Kim, K.M. The perception of coaching questions for college students. *J. Korean Coach. Res.* **2019**, *12*, 47–65.
51. Kim, B. Understanding the Q methodology and its application to consumer research. *Asia Market. J.* **1999**, *1*, 7.
52. Hong, S.-R. Romantic attachment, self–esteem and love attitudes. *J. Fam. Better Life* **2007**, *25*, 169–182.
53. Yoo, K.-H. The study on the concept and development of love in adulthood. *Gend. Cult.* **2010**, *3*, 191–216.
54. Yu, Y.-H. A Study on the Love Styles and Sexual Attitudes of the University Students. Master's Thesis, Department of Child and Family Welfare Graduate School Ulsan University, Ulsan, Republic of Korea, 2016.
55. Kim, B.-H.; Cheong, M.-S. A study on the effects of gender differences between the importance of basic psychological needs and the components of love: Focusing on lovers. *J. Korea Contents Assoc.* **2021**, *21*, 529–540.
56. Yoonhee, S. An exploratory study on single adult males' attitudes toward love: A focus on sexism and gender role conflict. *J. Life-Span Stud.* **2022**, *12*, 41–56.
57. Lee, M.-j. Love Styles in Early Adulthood and Self–Esteem, Trust, and Relationship Satisfaction. Master's Thesis, Department of Home Management The Graduate School of Ewha Womans University, Seoul, Republic of Korea, 2000.
58. Bandinelli, C. Dating apps: Towards post-romantic love in digital societies. *Int. J. Cult. Pol.* **2022**, *28*, 905–919. [CrossRef]
59. Cassepp–Borges, V.; Gonzales, J.E.; Frazier, A.; Ferrer, E. Love and relationship satisfaction as a function of romantic relationship stages. *Trends Psych.* **2023**, 1–16. [CrossRef]
60. Ramlo, S. Theoretical significance in Q methodology: A qualitative approach to a mixed method. *Res. Sch.* **2015**, *22*, 73.
61. Kim, S.E. *Q Methodology and the Social Sciences*; CMPRESS: Seoul, Republic of Korea, 2016.
62. Hylton, P.; Kisby, B.; Goddard, P. Young people's citizen identities: A Q–methodological analysis of English youth perceptions of citizenship in Britain. *Societies* **2018**, *8*, 121. [CrossRef]
63. Kim, H.K. Q methodology and theory: Q sampling—Its nature, kind, and procedure. *J. Korean Soc. Sci. Stud. Sub.* **2007**, *14*, 19–39.
64. Kim, S.E. Theory and philosophy of the Q methodology. *Korean Soc. Pub. Admin.* **2010**, *20*, 1–25.
65. Baek, P. *Doing Q Methodological Research Theory, Method and Interpretation*; Communication Books: Seoul, Republic of Korea, 2008.
66. Kim, H.K. *Methodology, Philosophy of Science, Theory, Analysis and Application Q*; Communication Books: Seoul, Republic of Korea, 2008.
67. Meyers, S.A. Personality correlates of adult attachment style. *J. Soc. Psychol.* **1998**, *138*, 407–409. [CrossRef]
68. Kennedy, J.H. Romantic attachment style and ego identity, attributional style, and family of origin in first-year college students. *Coll. Stud. J.* **1999**, *33*, 171.
69. Marrero-Quevedo, R.J.; Blanco-Hernández, P.J.; Hernández-Cabrera, J.A. Adult attachment and psychological well-being: The mediating role of personality. *J. Adult Dev.* **2019**, *26*, 41–56. [CrossRef]
70. Frazier, P.A.; Esterly, E. Correlates of relationship beliefs: Gender, relationship experience and relationship satisfaction. *J. Soc. Pers. Relat.* **1990**, *7*, 331–352. [CrossRef]
71. Sternberg, R.J. A triangular theory of love. *Psych. Rev.* **1986**, *93*, 119–135. [CrossRef]
72. Sternberg, R.J. *The Triangle of Love: Intimacy, Passion, Commitment*; Basic Books: New York, NY, USA, 1988.
73. Madey, S.F.; Rodgers, L. The effect of attachment and Sternberg's triangular theory of love on relationship satisfaction. *Indiv. Diff. Res.* **2009**, *7*, 76–84.
74. Bierhoff, H.W.; Grau, I. *Romantische Beziehungen: Bindung, Liebe, Partnerschaft*; Huber: Göttingen, Germany, 1999.
75. De Munck, V.; Korotayev, A.; Khaltourina, D. A comparative study of the structure of love in the US and Russia: Finding a common core of characteristics and national and gender differences. *Ethn. Inter. J. Cult. Soc. Anthrop.* **2009**, *48*, 337–357.
76. Noh, E.J.; Park, J.Y.; Kim, Y.H. The relationship among adult attachment types, Love styles and dating of single people. *Hum. Ecol. Res.* **2006**, *44*, 31–42.
77. Levy, M.B.; Davis, K.E. Lovestyles and attachment styles compared: Their relations to each other and to various relationship characteristics. *J. Soc. Pers. Relat.* **1988**, *5*, 439–471. [CrossRef]
78. Lim, J.S. The relationship between attachment styles and love styles—With a focus on Korea, the US, and Germany. *Legis. Policies* **2008**, *2*, 185–207.
79. Cooley, C.H. The looking-glass self. The production of reality. *Essays Read. Soc. Interact.* **1902**, *6*, 126–128.
80. Yang, H.; Han, Y. The mediating effects of self-acceptance and personal growth on the effect of self-concept clarity on interpersonal competence for adults in their 20s and 30s. *Korean J. Hum. Eco.* **2022**, *31*, 707–715. [CrossRef]

81. Kim, Y.-J.; Sin, H.-C. The influence of meta-mood on interpersonal problems: The mediating effects of affect. *Korean J. Counsel.* **2013**, *14*, 839–856.
82. Chang, K.S. Social reproduction in an era of 'risk aversion': From familial fertility to women's fertility. *Fam. Cult.* **2011**, *23*, 1–23. [CrossRef]
83. Kim, E.; Kim, H. Institutional marriage value of the young generation in the mixture of Korean familism and individualism. *Kookmin Soc. Sci. Rev.* **2023**, *35*, 105–139. [CrossRef]
84. Lee, E. A qualitative research on the undergraduate students' romantic experience. *J. Hum. Soc. Sci.* **2020**, *21*, 679–691.
85. Lee, E.J. Research on Social Relationship Formation Through University Students' Dating Experiences. In Proceedings of the Journal of Family Relations Conference; 2017; pp. 61–70. Available online: https://www-riss-kr.sproxy.dongguk.edu/link?id=A104223635 (accessed on 15 June 2024).
86. Lloyd, S.A. Conflict in premarital relationships: Differential perceptions of males and females. *Fam. Relat.* **1987**, *36*, 290–294. [CrossRef]
87. Kang, J.W. The changes in discourse of romantic love in Korea. *Cult. Pol.* **2023**, *10*, 33–68.
88. Byoun, S.-J.; Choi, S.; Kim, H.-Y. Exploring the diverse family structures in South Korea: Experiences and perspectives of non-martial cohabitants. *Societies* **2021**, *11*, 90. [CrossRef]
89. Karandashev, V. Cultural diversity of romantic love experience. In *International Handbook of Love: Transcultural and Transdisciplinary Perspectives*; Springer International Publishing: Cham, Switzerland, 2021; pp. 59–79.

Disclaimer/Publisher's Note: The statements, opinions and data contained in all publications are solely those of the individual author(s) and contributor(s) and not of MDPI and/or the editor(s). MDPI and/or the editor(s) disclaim responsibility for any injury to people or property resulting from any ideas, methods, instructions or products referred to in the content.

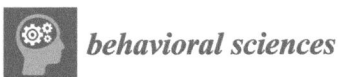

Article

What Is the Link of Closeness and Jealousy in Romantic Relationships?

Ana María Fernández [1,*], Maria Teresa Barbato [1], Pamela Barone [2], Belén Zavalla [1], Diana Rivera-Ottenberger [3] and Mónica Guzmán-González [4]

1. Laboratorio de Evolución y Relaciones Interpersonales, Universidad de Santiago de Chile, Santiago 9170022, Chile; maria.barbato@usach.cl (M.T.B.); belen.cordero@usach.cl (B.Z.)
2. Department of Psychology, Universitat de les Illes Balears, 07122 Palma, Spain; pamela.barone@uib.es
3. School of Psychology, Pontificia Universidad Católica de Chile, Santiago 7820436, Chile; dvrivera@uc.cl
4. School of Psychology, Universidad Católica del Norte, Antofagasta 1270709, Chile; moguzman@ucn.cl
* Correspondence: ana.fernandez@usach.cl

Abstract: From an evolutionary perspective, love and attachment foster closeness, while jealousy ensures exclusivity in romantic relationships. This study examined the links between jealousy and affective aspects of love, hypothesizing positive associations despite their apparent opposition. An online sample of 265 individuals in Chile and Spain completed measures of digital jealousy, closeness, love, felt loved, and attachment. Results revealed higher jealousy in Chile than in Spain. Across both countries, anxious attachment and closeness were significant predictors of jealousy, explaining nearly 30% of its variance. In Chile, feeling loved negatively predicted jealousy, suggesting that reassurance of the romantic bond may reduce jealousy in this cultural context. Notably, affective closeness—conceptualized as the inclusion of the self in the other—emerged as a novel predictor of jealousy, extending beyond the established role of anxious attachment. These findings underscore the nuanced interplay between cultural context, affective closeness, and attachment in shaping jealousy.

Keywords: close relationships; romantic bonds; emotions

1. Introduction

1.1. Love and Attachment

Love is a complex and multifaceted emotion that plays a crucial role in promoting enduring social bonds, especially within romantic relationships (Hatfield & Sprecher, 1986). From an evolutionary perspective, romantic love is a mechanism that encourages long-term commitment, facilitating caregiving and protection of offspring, both of which are essential for survival and reproductive success (Carter & Porges, 2013; Sorokowski et al., 2017). Love extends beyond romantic partnerships, influencing family and friendship dynamics, where consistent emotional closeness and actions that convey love are essential (Xia et al., 2023). In this context, the emotional connection one shares with others is crucial for feeling loved, not just within romantic relationships but across various forms of social bonds.

The theory of attachment supports this understanding by emphasizing that early relational experiences with caregivers shape mental models that influence adult relationships (Mikulincer & Shaver, 2017). These models underline how trust, emotional security, and mutual support within relationships foster emotional closeness, making such connections indispensable (Bowlby, 1982; Hazan & Shaver, 1987). Attachment bonds are fundamental not only in parent–child relationships but also in adult romantic relationships, reinforcing that emotional security and attachment are key to sustaining love over time (Eastwick, 2016; Ein-Dor, 2015). Yet, attachment theory is just one lens through which love can be understood. In addition, Fredrickson's (2013) theory of "positivity resonance" broadens the view of love, proposing it as a dynamic, momentary connection rooted in shared positive emotions, biobehavioral synchrony, and mutual care. This theory aligns with the idea that emotional closeness integrates a partner into one's sense of self, strengthening the bond (Aron et al., 1992). Secure attachment further reinforces positive emotional resonance, supporting the notion that love involves a complex interplay of emotional security and mutual care (Mikulincer & Shaver, 2017).

Despite the wide range of components that characterize love, the most commonly utilized framework for its measurement is Sternberg's Triangular Theory of Love. This theory portrays love in three dimensions: intimacy, passion, and commitment, which can be ranked to convey different types of love (Sternberg, 1986). Intimacy refers to feelings of closeness and emotional connection, passion relates to physical attraction and desire, and commitment involves the decision to maintain a relationship over time. Stenberg's model has significantly advanced the characterization of romantic relationships by providing a comprehensive structure to understand the dynamics of love cross-culturally (Cassepp-Borges et al., 2023; Kowal et al., 2024).

Moreover, the dimension of intimacy emphasizes that feelings of being loved are deeply rooted in mutual understanding and responsiveness between partners. This dimension can be measured through aspects of momentary connection, fostering deeper bonds and empathy within the relationship (Fredrickson, 2013; Gonzaga et al., 2006; Reis & Aron, 2008).

However, there is a complementary perspective on the nature of love, emphasizing the role of neuropsychological and emotional responses in shaping romantic experiences. For example, the concept of "feeling loved" highlights individual perceptions of love based on momentary emotional interactions, which may not always align with the structural components of intimacy, passion, and commitment (Ellis et al., 2022; Heshmati et al., 2017; Reis & Aron, 2008). The dynamics of love appear to be shaped not only by long-term relational structures but also by transient, emergent experiences of closeness and affection (Rykkje et al., 2015).

Recent research underscores the importance of measuring the subjective experience of "feeling loved" as a critical dimension in understanding relationships (Sasaki et al., 2023). This perspective enriches relational bonds by emphasizing the nuanced, reciprocal, and momentary aspects of love. Integrating this measurement with established theories deepens our understanding of how love operates across various relational contexts.

On the other hand, several studies have revealed that the way romantic love is experienced and expressed varies significantly across cultures and is shaped by societal norms and traditions (Karandashev, 2015). In Western cultures, love is often expressed explicitly through verbal affirmations and grand gestures, while in Chinese and Filipino traditions, it is more commonly conveyed through implicit actions and subtle behaviors (Nadal, 2012). Emotional investment also shows cultural differences, with North Americans tending to express higher levels of affection and passion compared to the more reserved approaches typical in East Asia (Schmitt et al., 2009). Moreover, cultural attitudes toward love differ, as more individualistic societies, such as Spain compared to Chile (Insights, 2020) (https://www.hofstede-insights.com/), emphasize autonomy and passionate connections, whereas collectivistic cultures prioritize familial bonds and societal harmony (Dion & Dion, 2006).

Across the majority of these studies, the extensive use of instruments enhances the ability to assess phenomena effectively, yet it remains unclear what specific aspects or characteristics of love are being evaluated. For instance, some cross-cultural studies on love employ standardized tools such as emotional investment scales to assess levels of affection, passion, and compassion across cultures (Schmitt et al., 2009). Similarly, De Munck et al. (2011) examined dimensions like altruism and physical attraction using self-report measures, while Sprecher et al. (1994) explored cross-cultural differences in the intensity of love through direct surveys. Longitudinal studies, such as those by Ingersoll-Dayton et al. (1996), have analyzed the evolution of romantic relationships over time, capturing shifts from initial intimacy to later emotional development in various cultural contexts. These tools, combined with ethnographic approaches, provide valuable insights into how universal emotions like love are shaped by cultural norms, revealing both shared and unique elements across societies.

Love not only fosters emotional security, mutual care, and intimacy but also evokes a range of powerful emotions that differentiate and define human relationships, from infancy through adulthood (Bode, 2023; Kowal et al., 2024). Among them, jealousy stands out as a pivotal emotion, intricately tied to the dynamics of close relationships and deeply influencing how love is experienced and expressed (Sullivan, 2021).

1.2. Jealousy

Jealousy represents a pivotal emotion in close human relationships, primarily examined in children within the framework of attachment theory (Bowlby, 1982; Fernández et al., 2022; Hart, 2010), as well as in the contexts of friendships and sibling dynamics (Rodriguez et al., 2015; Mikulincer & Shaver, 2017). Although often characterized as a troublesome emotion (Rodriguez et al., 2015), jealousy also plays a complementary role to love, serving to preserve romantic bonds (Fernández et al., 2023). From an evolutionary perspective, jealousy functions as a defense mechanism aimed at safeguarding relationships from perceived threats (Chung & Harris, 2018), particularly infidelity or emotional disengagement (Buss, 2013; Schützwohl, 2008). Commonly regarded as a reaction to the fear of losing a partner's affection (Buunk, 1997), jealousy fulfills an adaptive function by protecting the emotional and reproductive resources essential for sustaining long-term relationships (Buss, 2018). In this regard, love and jealousy operate synergistically to stabilize romantic partnerships (Conroy-Beam et al., 2015; Fletcher, 2015).

Research on jealousy has concentrated on its evolutionary and functional aspects, while also exploring the cultural and sexual variations that influence its expression. Cultural dimensions, such as collectivism and individualism, have been shown to influence how jealousy is experienced. Zandbergen and Brown (2015) found that collectivist societies prioritize relational harmony, often perceiving jealousy in the context of maintaining group stability, whereas individualistic cultures emphasize personal autonomy, framing jealousy as a threat to individual relationships. These cultural differences have been measured using tools like the Horizontal and Vertical Individualism and Collectivism Scale (Singelis et al., 1995), which provides valuable insights into the broader social frameworks that modulate emotional responses to jealousy.

In the context of romantic relationships, jealousy has been identified as a crucial emotion for protecting mating bonds (Buunk et al., 2019; Fernandez, 2017). It has primarily been studied through hypothetical infidelity scenarios and retrospective accounts of distress related to actual infidelity (Buss et al., 1992; Buss, 2018; Schützwohl, 2008). For example, men tend to exhibit greater distress by sexual infidelity, aligning with evolutionary concerns about paternity certainty, while women report heightened emotional jealousy, often linked to perceived threats to emotional commitment (Buss et al., 1992; Buunk & Fernandez, 2020; Larsen et al., 2021). These patterns have been captured using tools like the modified Emotional and Sexual Jealousy Scale (Buss et al., 1992) and the Self-Report Jealousy Scale

(Bringle et al., 1979), which quantify reactions to emotional and sexual threats. Experimental methods, including recalling personal betrayal experiences, exposure to attractive rivals, dramatized depictions in media (e.g., Cheaters), and subliminal priming with infidelity-related cues, have further highlighted the nuanced ways in which jealousy is elicited and expressed (Kuhle, 2011; Massar & Buunk, 2010; Sabini & Green, 2004).

Jealousy poses a significant threat to intimate relationships, as it is often considered a maladaptive and pathological emotion rooted in insecurity and negative self-esteem (Chin et al., 2017; Buss & Abrams, 2017). Previous research has linked jealousy to traits like narcissism, psychopathy, Machiavellianism, and low self-worth (Costa et al., 2015; Massar et al., 2017; Seeman, 2016). Despite its association with psychological distress and interpersonal conflict, jealousy remains universally prevalent, even in cultural contexts where traditional explanations—such as male dominance, aggression, or female emotional vulnerability—fail to fully explain its persistence and intensity (Kruger et al., 2013; Scelza, 2014). This paradox highlights the complexity of jealousy as an emotional phenomenon.

Qualitative approaches have complemented these findings by uncovering deeper themes, such as infidelity, expectations of time and commitment, self-esteem, and the influence of social media (Zandbergen & Brown, 2015). Additionally, innovative methods like economic games, which manipulate resource allocation between romantic partners and rivals, have provided new ways to study jealousy by offering real-time insights into emotional responses (Barbato et al., 2024). The rise of social media has introduced another layer, amplifying relational threats and rivalries in the digital sphere, and making it an increasingly important area of study (Tandon et al., 2021; Tukachinsky Forster, 2022).

1.3. Relationship Between Love and Jealousy

Therefore, both love and jealousy play complementary roles in promoting and preserving pair bonds (Chung & Harris, 2018). Love fosters prosocial behaviors and mutual benefits between reproductive partners (Fletcher, 2015), while jealousy helps prevent the loss of these benefits in the face of potential interlopers (Buss, 2018; Harris, 2003). These emotions together support the maintenance of long-term commitments, contributing to the evolutionary success of pair bonding by ensuring the continuity of shared resources, care, and reproductive fitness (Conroy-Beam et al., 2015; Cosmides & Tooby, 2013).

The relationship between love and jealousy is influenced by various factors such as attachment style (Attridge, 2013; Bartholomew & Horowitz, 1991), given the convergence of both constructs in the development of close bonds (Fernández et al., 2023). Evidence suggests that high attachment anxiety is strongly associated with increased jealousy (Sullivan, 2021). More specifically, individuals with anxious attachment often experience heightened suspicion, insecurity about their partner's availability, and concerns about potential abandonment, all of which can trigger jealousy (Collins & Feeney, 2000; Deng et al., 2023; Güçlü et al., 2017; Montalvini et al., 2014; Ng & Hou, 2017). In contrast, attachment avoidance—a tendency toward emotional independence due to early neglect or a lack of sensitive care—leads to self-reliance and discomfort with affection, often resulting in reduced jealousy (Lafontaine et al., 2018; Montalvini et al., 2014).

Therefore, the present research aims to explore the interplay between jealousy, emotional closeness, and love across two distinct cultural contexts: Chile and Spain. Drawing on attachment theory and theories of romantic love, this study examines how jealousy relates to key relational variables that influence the stability and dynamics of romantic relationships. Specifically, it is hypothesized that jealousy will show positive associations with emotional closeness, love (including its dimensions of intimacy, passion, and commitment), and attachment anxiety, as these variables are intertwined in shaping individuals' emotional responses. By exploring these dynamics, this study seeks to shed light on the role jealousy plays within the broader context of love, and how attachment, emotional closeness, and cultural factors shape the experience and expression of jealousy in romantic relationships.

2. Materials and Methods

2.1. Participants

This study employed a cross-sectional design with a convenience sample of 265 romantically involved individuals who completed all measures online using the PsyToolkit platform (Stoet, 2010). Participants were recruited through advertisements on social networks, resulting in a sample composed predominantly of heterosexual individuals (74.3%), of whom 71.9% were women. Only 29.2% of participants reported having children.

The sample included participants from Chile (40%) and Spain (60%). In the Chilean subsample, 78% were women compared to 72% in the Spanish subsample. There was a significantly shorter relationship duration in months among participants from Chile ($M = 46.97$, $SD = 6.46$) compared to those from Spain ($M = 89.18$, $SD = 15.63$; $t_{231.255} = -2.494$, $p < 0.05$). No significant differences were found between the two countries in terms of age or sex across any of the assessed variables ($Fs < 1.43$, $ps > 0.05$).

2.2. Measures

Sociodemographic questions. Participants provided information about their age, sex, employment status, duration of their current relationship, and number of children.

Jealousy. The digital jealousy scale (DJS) was used to measure jealousy in digital contexts (Gubler et al., 2023). This 9-item scale covers cognitive, affective, and behavioral aspects of jealousy. Participants were instructed to think about their current relationship and indicate their level of agreement with each statement on a 6-point Likert scale (1 = strongly disagree; 6 = strongly agree). Example items include "it worries me when a new woman/man appears on my partner's friends list" or "I look over my partner's shoulder when I know they are texting with someone else".

The original scale was developed in both German and English. For the current study, the items were translated into Spanish from the English version by a bilingual team, and a back-translation process was employed to ensure accuracy. In the original study, the DJS showed high construct reliability (McDonald's $\omega = 0.89$ in the German sample and McDonald's $\omega = 0.90$ in the English sample). Cronbach's alpha for the adapted DJS was 0.90. Gubler et al. (2023) found that digital jealousy and romantic jealousy (measured by a scale that does not refer to the context of social media) showed a very strong positive correlation ($r = 0.86$).

Love. The short version of the Triangular Love Scale (TLS-15) was used to measure love (Kowal et al., 2024). Based on Sternberg's triangular theory of love, the scale evaluates three core components, intimacy, passion, and commitment, commonly measured in romantic relationships. The abbreviated version consists of 15 items rated on a 5-point Likert scale (1 = never; 5 = always). Example items of each subscale include "I have a warm relationship with my partner" (intimacy), "I find my partner to be very personally attractive" (passion), and "I view my commitment to my partner as a solid one" (commitment).

The Spanish version of the TLS-15 has been previously validated and adapted for both Latin American and Spanish populations, showing high reliability in both contexts. In the Latin American sample, the reliability scores were intimacy: $\alpha = 0.92$, $\omega = 0.94$; passion: $\alpha = 0.89$, $\omega = 0.91$; and commitment: $\alpha = 0.90$, $\omega = 0.93$. In the Spanish sample, the scores were intimacy: $\alpha = 0.91$, $\omega = 0.93$; passion: $\alpha = 0.88$, $\omega = 0.90$; and commitment: $\alpha = 0.90$, $\omega = 0.90$ (Kowal et al., 2024). For the present sample, the reliability scores for the TLS-15 were the following: intimacy: $\alpha = 0.86$; passion: $\alpha = 0.81$; and commitment: $\alpha = 0.83$.

Closeness. An adapted version of the inclusion of other in the self (IOS) scale (Aron et al., 1992), a valid measure of perceived closeness between individuals (Gächter et al., 2015), was used. This single-item scale employs visual representations of overlapping circles to illustrate varying degrees of identification with the partner and affective closeness. Participants are asked to select the pair of circles that best represents their relationship with their romantic partner.

Felt loved. The Felt-Loved scale was used to assess how loved participants felt about their partners (Sasaki et al., 2023). Participants rated the following three items on a 7-point Likert scale (1 = not at all; 7 = very much): "I feel cared for/loved by my partner"; "I feel accepted/valued by my partner"; and "I feel understood/validated by my partner." The original study averaged the items to create an overall measure of felt love (α = 0.94; Sasaki et al., 2023). Cronbach's alpha for the current sample was 0.84.

Attachment. The Revised Adult Attachment Scale (RAAS), Close Relationship version (Collins, 1996), was used to assess adult attachment styles. This 18-item scale measures emotional closeness or distance in relationships using a 5-point Likert scale (1 = not at all characteristic of me; 5 = very characteristic of me). It evaluates three dimensions of attachment: closeness, dependence, and attachment-related anxiety and avoidance. Example items of each subscale are "I find it relatively easy to get close to people" (close); "I find it difficult to allow myself to depend on others" (depend); and "I often worry that other people don't really love me" (attachment-related anxiety and avoidance)

The validated Spanish version of the scale was used (Fernández & Dufey, 2015). Only the dimensions of anxiety (Cronbach's alpha = 0.90) and avoidance (Cronbach's alpha = 0.81) are reported in the current study.

2.3. Procedure

Data collection occurred between April and July 2024 using an online platform, where participants completed the questionnaires mentioned above. Following APA ethical standards, informed consent was obtained from all participants before participation. The study was approved by the Institutional Ethics Committee of the first author's university, ensuring adherence to confidentiality and ethical guidelines throughout the research process.

2.4. Data Analysis

Descriptive statistics were calculated to summarize the characteristics of the sample. Mean differences across countries were examined using independent t-tests, and effect sizes were calculated using Cohen's d.

Pearson correlations were performed to explore associations among the affective variables. Additionally, stepwise multiple regression analyses were conducted to identify the best predictors of jealousy. Separate regressions were conducted for the overall sample and by country (Chile and Spain) to examine potential cultural differences in the predictors of jealousy. All analyses were performed using SPSS 25 and JAMOVI 2.4.5. with significance levels set at $p < 0.05$.

3. Results

All participants in the sample were in a committed relationship when they completed the scales. Additionally, they reported having had on average 2.21 romantic relationships (SD = 1.24), having an average of 0.56 children (SD = 0.99).

The normality of the data was assessed using the Shapiro–Wilk test. The results indicated that all variables, including jealousy (W = 0.165, p = 0.000), IOS (W = 0.165, p = 0.000), intimacy (W = 0.193, p = 0.000), passion (W = 0.207, p = 0.000), commitment (W = 0.113, p = 0.000), felt loved (W = 208, p = 0.000), and anxious attachment (W = 0.125,

$p = 0.000$), did not meet the normality criterion, while avoidant attachment ($W = 0.053$, $p = 0.079$) was normally distributed.

Descriptive statistics by country are presented in Table 1, with Chilean participants reporting significantly more jealousy than the Spanish ($t = 3.653, p < 0.001$, Cohen's $d = 0.47$).

Table 1. Descriptive statistics and effect sizes for the variables by country.

	Chile		Spain		d	p
	M	SD	M	SD		
Jealousy	2.48	1.27	1.98	0.91	0.47	0.001
Intimacy	22.27	3.03	21.80	2.84	0.16	0.208
Passion	19.87	4.17	19.00	3.90	0.22	0.090
Commitment	22.03	3.72	21.94	2.94	0.03	0.828
IOS	3.74	4.00	3.73	4.00	0.01	0.954
Felt Loved	6.24	1.04	6.10	0.95	0.15	0.253
Anxious Attachment	2.37	1.07	2.37	0.83	0.00	0.997
Avoidant Attachment	2.34	0.64	2.42	0.58	0.12	0.340

Note. n = 265. Values of 0.20, 0.50, and 0.80 for Cohen's d (d) are commonly considered to be indicative of small, medium, and large effects, respectively.

When inquiring about the only demographic variable that was different across countries, the correlation between time in the relationship and the affective variables yielded that, in the Chileans, this was directly correlated to age ($r = 0.61, p < 0.001$), and inversely associated with jealousy ($r = -0.31, p < 0.01$) and anxious ($r = -0.38, p < 0.01$) and avoidant attachment ($r = -0.23, p < 0.01$). In the Spanish participants, only age, again, was positively correlated with time in the relationship ($r = 0.41, p < 0.001$).

Correlational analyses in the whole sample among the affective variables showed that jealousy was significantly and directly associated with IOS and anxious and avoidant attachment and inversely correlated with the dimensions of intimacy and commitment from the Love Scale, as well as the Felt-Loved scale (See Table 2).

Table 2. Correlation between jealousy and the affective variables.

Variables	2	3	4	5	6	7	8
1. Jealousy	−0.127 *	0.076	−0.173 *	0.364 ***	−0.240 ***	0.430 ***	0.178 **
2. Intimacy		0.667 ***	0.708 ***	0.013	0.815 ***	−0.174 **	−0.175 **
3. Passion			0.587 ***	0.095	0.577 ***	0.019	−0.042
4. Commitment				0.036	0.677 ***	−0.194 **	−0.122
5. IOS					−0.054	−0.236 **	−0.169 **
6. Felt loved						0.243 **	0.071
7. Anxious Att.							0.445 ***
8. Avoidant Att.							-----

Note. The table presents Pearson correlation coefficients (r) between jealousy and the affective variables: love (including the dimensions intimacy, passion, and commitment), closeness (assessed using IOS), felt loved, and attachment (anxious attachment and avoidant attachment). * $p < 0.05$, ** $p < 0.01$, and *** $p < 0.001$.

A stepwise regression predicting jealousy from the affective variables yielded anxious attachment, IOS, and felt loved as the best predictors of jealousy ($R^2 = 0.28, F_{3, 254} = 33.264$. $p < 001$). Jealousy was positively predicted by anxious attachment ($\beta = 0.325. t = 5.772, p < 0.001$) and IOS ($\beta = 0.279, t = 5.082, p < 0.001$) and negatively predicted by felt loved ($\beta = -0.176, t = -2.910, p < 0.001$).

As can be seen in Figure 1, two additional stepwise regressions were run predicting jealousy by country. In Chile, 41.9% of the variance in jealousy ($F_{3, 89} = 20.650, p < 001$) was positively explained by IOS ($\beta = 0.395. t = 4.433, p < 0.001$) and anxious attachment

($\beta = 0.218$, $t = 2.364$, $p < 0.05$) and negatively predicted by felt loved ($\beta = -0.251$, $t = -2.827$, $p < 0.05$). In Spain, 21.9% of the variance in jealousy ($F_{2, 165} = 23.157$, $p < 0.001$) was predicted by anxious attachment ($\beta = 0.400$, $t = 5.749$, $p < 0.001$) and IOS ($\beta = 0.188$, $t = 2.705$, $p < 0.01$).

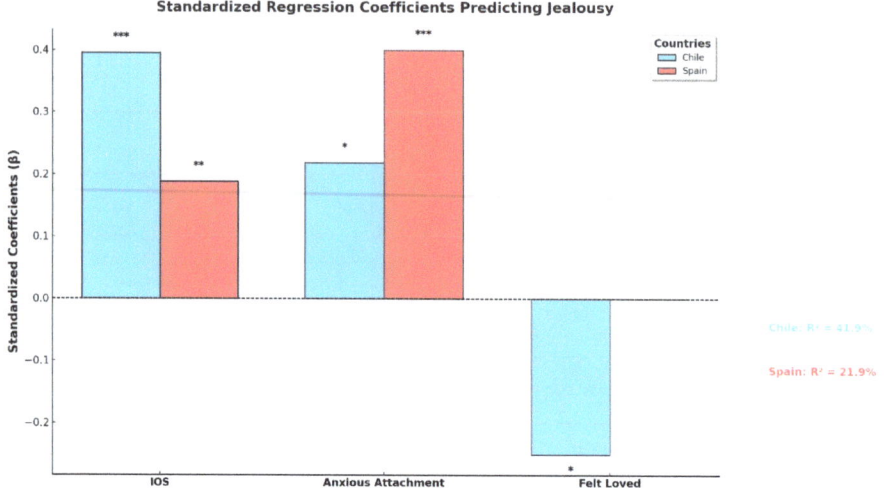

Figure 1. Predictors of jealousy by country. Note: * $p < 0.05$, ** $p < 0.01$, and *** $p < 0.001$.

4. Discussion

This study posits that love and jealousy are emotions that help protect a significant romantic relationship, rather than being reverse affective variables, as might commonly be expected. Therefore, jealousy was predicted to be associated with relationship closeness and insecure attachment, a hypothesis that was supported by our results from two Spanish-speaking samples, one from South America and the other from Europe.

The results reveal distinct patterns in how demographic and affective variables interact across the two countries. For Chilean participants, relationship duration correlates significantly with a broader range of variables, including age, jealousy, and attachment styles. This suggests a more complex interplay between relationship duration and emotional dynamics in Chile. Longer relationships may foster lower attachment insecurity and jealousy, which aligns with the classical literature that links jealousy to insecure attachment (Rodriguez et al., 2015). Additionally, shorter relationship duration may signal lower commitment. In contrast, among Spanish participants, relationship duration was found to correlate exclusively with age. This possibly reflects a distinct cultural approach to relationship dynamics, where the passage of time exerts less influence on affective experiences. Furthermore, the absence of a significant association between relationship duration and jealousy in the Spanish sample may be explained by a more individualistic orientation in the Spanish sample than in the Chilean group. It could also be linked to a higher prevalence of avoidant attachment styles in more individualistic societies (Sakman & Sümer, 2024). Supporting this interpretation, Deng et al. (2023) reported that individuals with avoidant tendencies tend to experience less pervasive jealousy in Russia.

Jealousy is consistently associated with anxious attachment and the perception of the inclusion of other in the self (IOS) across both samples, highlighting the universal role of attachment insecurity and relational closeness in this affection. However, the perception of being loved (felt loved) emerged as a protective factor against jealousy, particularly in the Chilean sample. This outcome suggests that feelings of relational security may mitigate jealousy more strongly in Chile, reflecting cultural nuances in emotional regulation or relational expectations (Collins & Feeney, 2000), which could be related to the shorter relationship duration of this group compared to the Spanish. For example, Sasaki et al. (2023) found that feeling loved fosters emotional security and mutual appreciation within a couple, serving as a protective factor for relationship stability. This variable may act as a buffer against negative emotions, reducing their potential to disrupt relational harmony. By reinforcing positive affect and strengthening emotional bonds, feeling loved helps couples navigate challenges more effectively, reducing conflict escalation, enhancing resilience, and mitigating romantic jealousy. Alternatively, the shorter relationship duration observed in the Chilean sample could be associated with an enhanced sensibility to jealousy, as limited romantic stability is known to increase jealousy (Chursina, 2023).

The variance in jealousy explained by the regression models differs notably between countries, with the Chilean data explaining nearly twice the variance observed in Spain. This disparity underscores the potentially greater emotional complexity or cultural significance of jealousy in Chilean relationships. The stronger role of feeling loved among Chilean participants highlights the protective influence of emotional validation and perceived affection, which seems less critical in the Spanish sample (see Watkins et al., 2019).

The findings suggest that jealousy, rather than being merely an indicator of insecurity or distrust, may reflect the emotional intensity characteristic of close relationships. In the Chilean sample, the perception of feeling loved served as a significant protective factor, stressing the role of relational security in mitigating jealousy. Greater emotional closeness appears to moderate jealousy, as reciprocal connections within relationships enable individuals to manage these emotions more effectively (Attridge, 2013; Sasaki et al., 2023).

The difference in the impact of feeling loved between Chile and Spain may stem from the varying emphasis on emotional connection within these cultural contexts. Individualistic societies often prioritize autonomy and passionate connections, while collectivist cultures place greater value on family ties and social harmony (Nadal, 2012). These cultural differences extend to responses to jealousy, particularly in situations involving sexual infidelity, where factors such as commitment expectations and the influence of social media play significant roles (Zandbergen & Brown, 2015). In Chile, shorter average relationship durations may reflect distinct relational expectations shaped by cultural or generational factors. For instance, younger generations or individuals from collectivist cultures may approach relationship maintenance behaviors with heightened sensitivity to emotional security and perceived trustworthiness. Previous research suggests that relational expectations evolve with cultural norms and age groups, influencing thresholds for acceptable behavior on social media (Tandon et al., 2021). These evolving norms could explain why shorter relationships in Chile exhibit greater sensitivity to feeling loved, compared to the longer and potentially more stable relationships observed in Spain.

The findings point to the importance of considering cultural context when examining jealousy and its predictors. In Chile, jealousy seems deeply intertwined with affective security and emotional closeness, whereas, in Spain, attachment anxiety and perceived relational closeness (IOS) play dominant roles, with a weaker association with feeling loved. These distinctions may reflect cultural differences in attachment processes, relational priorities, or societal norms surrounding romantic relationships. For example, Sakman and Sümer (2024) found that there is an association between attachment anxiety and interdependence—the more individuals view themselves in relation to others, the more attachment anxiety they experience—which may underlie greater feelings of jealousy in the Chilean context since there is higher relational closeness and possibly interdependence.

While this study illuminates key predictors of jealousy, the cross-sectional nature, small sample size, and convenience sampling limit causal interpretations. Additionally, jealousy was measured using a digital jealousy scale, which may not fully capture the broader context of jealousy in romantic relationships. Another limitation of this study was that the distribution of sexes within the sample was not balanced, which could influence the generalizability of the findings. Furthermore, as most participants were in heterosexual relationships, we were unable to analyze potential differences in affective variables based on relationship type, like in polyamorous or fluid relationships.

Future research should explore longitudinal designs to track changes in affective variables over time and examine how cultural factors shape emotional regulation in relationships. Additionally, investigating other cultural contexts would further elucidate the universality or variability of these dynamics. It is also important to use more comprehensive measures of jealousy that extend beyond digital contexts, capturing a wider array of jealousy experiences. Moreover, forthcoming studies should aim for more balanced samples across sexes as well as more diverse samples that include various relationship types, allowing for meaningful comparisons across these groups. Power analyses to justify sample sizes and ensure robust and generalizable findings should also be incorporated. Finally, the non-pathological and subtle nature of normal relationship jealousy that was studied should not be confused with other kinds of destructive relationship affects and behaviors within romantic relationships (i.e., Rodriguez et al., 2015), which were not the focus of the research.

5. Conclusions

This study reaffirms the idea that love and jealousy may be evolved protective factors of romantic relationships. It stresses the complex, culturally nuanced nature of jealousy in romantic relationships. The findings emphasize the interplay of attachment, relational closeness, and feeling loved, highlighting the need to consider both individual and cultural factors in understanding emotional experiences within romantic partnerships.

Author Contributions: Conceptualization, A.M.F., M.T.B., D.R.-O., M.G.-G. and P.B.; methodology, A.M.F. and P.B.; software, B.Z.; writing—original draft preparation, A.M.F. and M.T.B.; writing—review and editing, A.M.F., B.Z., M.T.B., P.B., M.G.-G. and D.R.-O. visualization, B.Z. All authors have read and agreed to the published version of the manuscript.

Funding: This research was funded by Project "AYUDANTE Dicyt_032456FT", Vicerrectoría de Investigación, Innovación y Creación, Universidad de Santiago de Chile, and the Fondecyt Project #1181114 of the Government of Chile.

Institutional Review Board Statement: The study was conducted in accordance with the Declaration of Helsinki and approved by the ETHICS COMMITTEE of UNIVERSIDAD DE SANTIAGO DE CHILE (protocol code 443, 21 June 2018).

Informed Consent Statement: Informed consent was obtained from all subjects involved in the study.

Data Availability Statement: Data analyzed during this study are not publicly available due to confidentiality agreements with participants but are available from the corresponding author upon reasonable request.

Conflicts of Interest: The authors declare no conflicts of interest.

References

Aron, A., Aron, E. N., & Smollan, D. (1992). Inclusion of other in the Self Scale and the structure of interpersonal closeness. *Journal of Personality and Social Psychology*, 63(4), 596–612. [CrossRef]

Attridge, M. (2013). Jealousy and relationship closeness: Exploring the good (reactive) and bad (suspicious) sides of romantic jealousy. *SAGE Open*, 3(1), 2158244013476054. [CrossRef]

Barbato, M. T., Fernández, A. M., Rodriguez-Sickert, C., Muñoz, J. A., Polo, P., & Buss, D. (2024). Jealousy as predicted by allocation and reception of resources in an economic game. *Evolutionary Psychology*, 22(4), 14747049241289232. [CrossRef] [PubMed]

Bartholomew, K., & Horowitz, L. M. (1991). Attachment styles among young adults: A test of a four-category model. *Journal of Personality and Social Psychology*, *61*(2), 226. [CrossRef] [PubMed]

Bode, A. (2023). Romantic love evolved by co-opting mother-infant bonding. *Frontiers in Psychology*, *14*, 1176067. [CrossRef] [PubMed]

Bowlby, J. (1982). *Attachment and loss*. (Attachment (2nd ed.), Vol. 1). Basic Books.

Bringle, R. G., Roach, S., Andler, C., & Evenbeck, S. E. (1979). Measuring the intensity of jealous reactions. *Journal of Supplemental Abstract Service*, *9*, 23–24.

Buss, D. M. (2013). Sexual jealousy. *Psihologijske Teme*, *22*(2), 155–182.

Buss, D. M. (2018). Sexual and emotional infidelity: Evolved gender differences in jealousy prove robust and replicable. *Perspectives on Psychological Science*, *13*(2), 155–160. [CrossRef] [PubMed]

Buss, D. M., & Abrams, M. (2017). Jealousy, infidelity, and the difficulty of diagnosing pathology: A CBT approach to coping with sexual betrayal and the green-eyed monster. *Journal of Rational-Emotive & Cognitive-Behavior Therapy*, *35*, 150–172. [CrossRef]

Buss, D. M., Larsen, R. J., Westen, D., & Semmelroth, J. (1992). Sex differences in jealousy: Evolution, physiology, and psychology. *Psychological Science*, *3*(4), 251–256. [CrossRef]

Buunk, B. P. (1997). Personality, birth order and attachment styles as related to various types of jealousy. *Personality and Individual Differences*, *23*(6), 997–1006. [CrossRef]

Buunk, A. P., & Fernandez, A. M. (2020). Don't cheat like I did: Possessive jealousy and infidelity in close relationships. *Interpersona*, *14*(2), 211–216. [CrossRef]

Buunk, A. P., Massar, K., Dijkstra, P., & Fernández, A. M. (2019). Intersexual and intrasexual competition and their relation to jealousy. In *The Oxford handbook on evolutionary psychology and behavioral endocrinology* (pp. 125–236). Oxford University Press. [CrossRef]

Carter, C. S., & Porges, S. W. (2013). The biochemistry of love. An oxytocin hypothesis. *EMBO Reports*, *14*(1), 12–16. [CrossRef] [PubMed]

Cassepp-Borges, V., Gonzales, J. E., Frazier, A., & Ferrer, E. (2023). Love and relationship satisfaction as a function of romantic relationship stages. *Trends in Psychology*, 1–16. [CrossRef]

Chin, K., Atkinson, B. E., Raheb, H., Harris, E., & Vernon, P. A. (2017). The dark side of romantic jealousy. *Personality and Individual Differences*, *115*, 23–29. [CrossRef]

Chung, M., & Harris, C. R. (2018). Jealousy as a specific emotion: The dynamic functional model. *Emotion Review*, *10*(4), 272–287. [CrossRef]

Chursina, A. V. (2023). The impact of romantic attachment styles on jealousy in young adults. *Psychology in Russia*, *16*(3), 222–232. [CrossRef]

Collins, N. L. (1996). Working models of attachment: Implications for explanation, emotion, and behavior. *Journal of Personality and Social Psychology*, *71*(4), 810–832. [CrossRef] [PubMed]

Collins, N. L., & Feeney, B. C. (2000). A safe haven: An attachment theory perspective on support seeking and caregiving in intimate relationships. *Journal of Personality and Social Psychology*, *78*(6), 1053. [CrossRef]

Conroy-Beam, D., Goetz, C. D., & Buss, D. M. (2015). Why do humans form long-term mateships? An evolutionary game-theoretic model. In J. Olson, & M. Zanna (Eds.), *Advances in experimental social psychology* (pp. 1–39). Academic Press. [CrossRef]

Cosmides, L., & Tooby, J. (2013). Evolutionary psychology: New perspectives on cognition and motivation. *Annual Review of Psychology*, *64*(1), 201–229. [CrossRef] [PubMed]

Costa, A. L., Sophia, E. C., Sanches, C., Tavares, H., & Zilberman, M. L. (2015). Pathological jealousy: Romantic relationship characteristics, emotional and personality aspects, and social adjustment. *Journal of Affective Disorders*, *174*, 38–44. [CrossRef] [PubMed]

De Munck, V. C., Korotayev, A., de Munck, J., & Khaltourina, D. (2011). Cross-cultural analysis of models of romantic love among US residents, Russians, and Lithuanians. *Cross-Cultural Research*, *45*(2), 128–154. [CrossRef]

Deng, M., Tadesse, E., Khalid, S., Zhang, W., Song, J., & Gao, C. (2023). The influence of insecure attachment on undergraduates' jealousy: The mediating effect of self-differentiation. *Frontiers in Psychology*, *14*, 1153866. [CrossRef]

Dion, K. K., & Dion, K. L. (2006). Individualism, collectivism, and the psychology of love. In R. J. Sternberg, & K. Weis (Eds.), *The new psychology of love* (pp. 298–312). Yale University Press.

Eastwick, P. W. (2016). The emerging integration of close relationships research and evolutionary psychology. *Current Directions in Psychological Science*, *25*(3), 183–190. [CrossRef]

Ein-Dor, T. (2015). Attachment dispositions and human defensive behavior. *Personality and Individual Differences*, *81*, 112–116. [CrossRef]

Ellis, O., Heshmati, S., & Oravecz, Z. (2022). What makes early adults feel loved? Cultural consensus of felt love experiences in early adulthood. *Applied Developmental Science*, *28*(2), 166–177. [CrossRef]

Fernandez, A. M. (2017). Sexual jealousy among women. In T. Shackelford, & V. Weekes-Shackelford (Eds.), *Encyclopedia of Evolutionary Psychological Science* (pp. 1–8). Springer International Publishing. [CrossRef]

Fernández, A. M., Acevedo, Y., Baeza, C. G., Dufey, M., & Puga, I. (2022). Jealousy protest to a social rival compared to a nonsocial rival in Chilean infants 10–20 months' old. *Infancy*, *27*(5), 997–1003. [CrossRef]

Fernández, A. M., Barbato, M. T., Cordero, B., & Acevedo, Y. (2023). What's love got to do with jealousy? *Frontiers in Psychology*, *14*, 1249556. [CrossRef]

Fernández, A. M., & Dufey, M. (2015). Adaptação da escala dimensional revisada de apego adulto de Collins para o contexto chileno. *Psicologia: Reflexão e Crítica*, *28*, 242–252. [CrossRef]

Fletcher, G. J. (2015). Accuracy and bias of judgments in romantic relationships. *Current Directions in Psychological Science*, *24*(4), 292–297. [CrossRef]

Fredrickson, B. L. (2013). Positive emotions broaden and build. *Advances in Experimental Social Psychology*, *47*(1), 1–53. [CrossRef]

Gächter, S., Starmer, C., & Tufano, F. (2015). Measuring the closeness of relationships: A comprehensive evaluation of the 'inclusion of the other in the self' scale. *PLoS ONE*, *10*(6), e0129478. [CrossRef] [PubMed]

Gonzaga, G. C., Turner, R. A., Keltner, D., Campos, B., & Altemus, M. (2006). Romantic love and sexual desire in close relationships. *Emotion*, *6*(2), 163–179. [CrossRef] [PubMed]

Gubler, D. A., Schlegel, K., Richter, M., Kapanci, T., & Troche, S. J. (2023). The green-eyed monster in social media—Development and validation of a digital jealousy scale. *Psychological Test Adaptation and Development*, *4*(1), 13–27. [CrossRef]

Güçlü, O., Şenormancı, Ö., Şenormancı, G., & Köktürk, F. (2017). Gender differences in romantic jealousy and attachment styles. *Psychiatry and Clinical Psychopharmacology*, *27*(4), 359–365. [CrossRef]

Harris, C. R. (2003). Factors associated with jealousy over real and imagined infidelity: An examination of the social-cognitive and evolutionary psychology perspectives. *Psychology of Women Quarterly*, *27*(4), 319–329. [CrossRef]

Hart, S. L. (2010). The ontogenesis of jealousy in the first year of life: A theory of jealousy as a biologically-based dimension of temperament. In S. L. Hart, & M. Legerstee (Eds.), *Handbook of jealousy: Theory, research, and multidisciplinary approaches* (pp. 57–82). Wiley Blackwell.

Hatfield, E., & Sprecher, S. (1986). Measuring passionate love in intimate relationships. *Journal of Adolescence*, *9*(4), 383–410. [CrossRef]

Hazan, C., & Shaver, P. (1987). Romantic love conceptualized as an attachment process. *Journal of Personality and Social Psychology*, *52*(3), 511–524. [CrossRef]

Heshmati, S., Oravecz, Z., Pressman, S., Batchelder, W. H., Muth, C., & Vandekerckhove, J. (2017). What does it mean to feel loved: Cultural consensus and individual differences in felt love. *Journal of Social and Personal Relationships*, *36*(1), 214–243. [CrossRef]

Ingersoll-Dayton, B., Campbell, R., Kurokawa, Y., & Saito, M. (1996). Separateness and togetherness: Interdependence over the life course in Japanese and American marriages. *Journal of Social and Personal Relationships*, *13*(3), 385–398. [CrossRef]

Insights, H. (2020). *National culture*. Available online: https://www.hofstede-insights.com/ (accessed on 22 December 2024).

Karandashev, V. (2015). A Cultural Perspective on Romantic Love. *Online Readings in Psychology and Culture*, *5*(4), 2. [CrossRef]

Kowal, M., Sorokowski, P., Dinić, B. M., Pisanski, K., Gjoneska, B., Frederick, D. A., Pfuhl, G., Milfont, T. L., Bode, A., Aguilar, L., García, F. E., Roberts, S. C., Abad-Villaverde, B., Kavčič, T., Miroshnik, K. G., Ndukaihe, I. L. G., Šafárová, K., Valentova, J. V., Aavik, T., . . . Sternberg, R. J. (2024). Validation of the short version (TLS-15) of the Triangular Love Scale (TLS-45) across 37 languages. *Archives of Sexual Behavior*, *53*(2), 839–857. [CrossRef]

Kruger, D. J., Fisher, M. L., Edelstein, R. S., Chopik, W. J., Fitzgerald, C. J., & Strout, S. L. (2013). Was that cheating? Perceptions vary by sex, attachment anxiety, and behavior. *Evolutionary Psychology*, *11*, 159–171. [CrossRef] [PubMed]

Kuhle, B. (2011). Did you have sex with him? Do you love her? An in vivo test of sex differences in jealous interrogations. *Personality and Individual Differences*, *51*(8), 1044–1047. [CrossRef]

Lafontaine, M. F., Guzmán-González, M., Péloquin, K., & Levesque, C. (2018). I am not in your shoes: Low perspective taking mediating the relation among attachment insecurities and physical intimate partner violence in Chilean university students. *Journal of Interpersonal Violence*, *33*(22), 3439–3458. [CrossRef]

Larsen, P. H. H., Bendixen, M., Grøntvedt, T. V., Kessler, A. M., & Kennair, L. E. O. (2021). Investigating the emergence of sex differences in jealousy responses in a large community sample from an evolutionary perspective. *Scientific Reports*, *11*(1), 6485. [CrossRef]

Massar, K., & Buunk, A. P. (2010). Judging a book by its cover: Jealousy after subliminal priming with attractive and unattractive faces. *Personality and Individual Differences*, *49*(6), 634–638. [CrossRef]

Massar, K., Winters, C. L., Lenz, S., & Jonason, P. K. (2017). Green-eyed snakes: The associations between psychopathy, jealousy, and jealousy induction. *Personality and Individual Differences*, *115*, 164–168. [CrossRef]

Mikulincer, M., & Shaver, P. R. (2017). Adult Attachment and compassion. In E. M. Seppälä, E. Simon-Thomas, S. L. Brown, M. C. Worline, C. D. Cameron, & J. R. Doty (Eds.), *Oxford handbooks online* (pp. 79–90). Oxford University Press. [CrossRef]

Montalvini, P. R., Lucero, M., & López, G. B. (2014). Estilos de apego y su relación con el patrón alimenticio de restricción-sobrealimentación en sujetos dietantes crónicos. *Revista Chilena de Neuropsicología*, *9*(1–2), 8–11.

Nadal, K. L. (2012). Mahal: Expressing love in Filipino and Filipino American families. In M. A. Paludi (Ed.), *The psychology of love. Volume 3: Meaning and culture* (pp. 23–26). Praeger.

Ng, S. M., & Hou, W. K. (2017). Contentment duration mediates the associations between anxious attachment style and psychological distress. *Frontiers in Psychology*, *8*, 258. [CrossRef]

Reis, H. T., & Aron, A. (2008). Love: What is it, why does it matter, and how does it operate? *Perspectives on Psychological Science*, 3(1), 80–86. [CrossRef]

Rodriguez, L. M., DiBello, A. M., Øverup, C. S., & Neighbors, C. (2015). The price of distrust: Trust, anxious attachment, jealousy, and partner abuse. *Partner Abuse*, 6(3), 298–319. [CrossRef] [PubMed]

Rykkje, L., Eriksson, K., & Råholm, M.-B. (2015). Love in connectedness: A theoretical study. *SAGE Open*, 5(1), 2158244015571186. [CrossRef]

Sabini, J., & Green, M. C. (2004). Emotional responses to sexual and emotional infidelity: Constants and differences across genders, samples, and methods. *Personality and Social Psychology Bulletin*, 30(11), 1375–1388. [CrossRef] [PubMed]

Sakman, E., & Sümer, N. (2024). Cultural correlates of adult attachment dimensions: Comparing the US and Turkey. *Cross-Cultural Research*, 58(2–3), 208–237. [CrossRef]

Sasaki, E., Overall, N. C., Reis, H. T., Righetti, F., Chang, V. T., Low, R. S. T., Henderson, A. M. E., McRae, C. S., Cross, E. J., Jayamaha, S. D., Maniaci, M. R., & Reid, C. J. (2023). Feeling loved as a strong link in relationship interactions: Partners who feel loved may buffer destructive behavior by actors who feel unloved. *Journal of Personality and Social Psychology*, 125(2), 367–396. [CrossRef]

Scelza, B. A. (2014). Jealousy in a small-scale, natural fertility population: The roles of paternity, investment and love in jealous response. *Evolution and Human Behavior*, 35, 103–108. [CrossRef]

Schmitt, D. P., Youn, G., Bond, B., Brooks, S., Frye, H., Johnson, S., Klesman, J., Peplinski, C., Sampias, J., Sherrill, M., & Stoka, C. (2009). When will I feel love? The effects of culture, personality, and gender on the psychological tendency to love. *Journal of Research in Personality*, 43(5), 830–846. [CrossRef]

Schützwohl, A. (2008). The intentional object of romantic jealousy. *Evolution and Human Behavior*, 29(2), 92–99. [CrossRef]

Seeman, M. V. (2016). Pathological jealousy. An interactive condition. *Psychiatry*, 79(4), 379–388. [CrossRef] [PubMed]

Singelis, T. M., Triandis, H. C., Bhawuk, D. P., & Gelfand, M. J. (1995). Horizontal and vertical dimensions of individualism and collectivism: A theoretical and measurement refinement. *Cross-Cultural Research*, 29(3), 240–275. [CrossRef]

Sorokowski, P., Sorokowska, A., Butovskaya, M., Karwowski, M., Groyecka, A., Wojciszke, B., & Pawłowski, B. (2017). Love influences reproductive success in humans. *Frontiers in Psychology*, 8, 1922. [CrossRef] [PubMed]

Sprecher, S., Sullivan, Q., & Hatfield, E. (1994). Mate selection preferences: Gender differences examined in a national sample. *Journal of Personality and Social Psychology*, 66(6), 1074–1080. [CrossRef]

Sternberg, R. J. (1986). A triangular theory of love. *Psychological Review*, 93(2), 119–135. [CrossRef]

Stoet, G. (2010). PsyToolkit: A software package for programming psychological experiments using Linux. *Behavior Research Methods*, 42, 1096–1104. [CrossRef]

Sullivan, K. T. (2021). Attachment style and jealousy in the digital age: Do attitudes about online communication matter? *Frontiers in Psychology*, 12, 678542. [CrossRef]

Tandon, A., Dhir, A., & Mäntymäki, M. (2021). Jealousy due to social media? A systematic literature review and framework of social media-induced jealousy. *Internet Research*, 31(5), 1541–1582. [CrossRef]

Tukachinsky Forster, R. (2022). The green side of parasocial romantic relationships: An exploratory investigation of parasocial jealousy. *Psychology of Popular Media*, 12(3), 279–293. [CrossRef]

Watkins, C. D., Leongómez, J. D., Bovet, J., Żelaźniewicz, A., Korbmacher, M., Varella, M. A. C., Fernandez, A. M., Wagstaff, B., & Bolgan, S. (2019). National income inequality predicts cultural variation in mouth to mouth kissing. *Scientific Reports*, 9, 6698. [CrossRef] [PubMed]

Xia, M., Chen, Y., & Dunne, S. (2023). What makes people feel loved? An exploratory study on core elements of love across family, romantic, and friend relationships. *Family Process*, 63(3), 1304–1318. [CrossRef]

Zandbergen, D. L., & Brown, S. G. (2015). Culture and gender differences in romantic jealousy. *Personality and Individual Differences*, 72, 122–127. [CrossRef]

Disclaimer/Publisher's Note: The statements, opinions and data contained in all publications are solely those of the individual author(s) and contributor(s) and not of MDPI and/or the editor(s). MDPI and/or the editor(s) disclaim responsibility for any injury to people or property resulting from any ideas, methods, instructions or products referred to in the content.

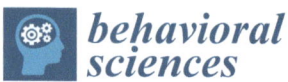

Article

Loneliness and Relationship Well-Being: Investigating the Mediating Roles of Relationship Awareness and Distraction among Romantic Partners

Thomas B. Sease [1,*], Emily K. Sandoz [2], Leo Yoke [3], Julie A. Swets [4] and Cathy R. Cox [1]

1. Institute of Behavioral Research, Texas Christian University, Fort Worth, TX 76129, USA; c.cox@tcu.edu
2. Psychology Department, University of Louisiana at Lafayette, Lafayette, LA 70504, USA; emily.sandoz@louisiana.edu
3. San Fransico Center for Compassion Focused Therapies, San Francisco, CA 94102, USA; leo.yoke@sfcompassion.com
4. Eastern Washington University at Bellevue College, Bellevue, WA 98007, USA; jswets@ewu.edu
* Correspondence: thomas.b.sease@tcu.edu

Abstract: Loneliness arises when there is a discrepancy between one's desired and actual social connection with others. Studies examining the effects of loneliness in romantic relationships show that people who are lonely are less satisfied and committed to their romantic relationships. The present study explored the association between loneliness and romantic relationship well-being. Using a cross-sectional design, loneliness was correlated with relationship commitment, trust, and conflict. Relationship awareness, but not relationship distraction, statistically mediated the association between loneliness, relationship conflict, and relationship trust. The indirect effect of loneliness on relationship well-being was only present in people reporting low and medium levels of psychological inflexibility. Implications are discussed for acceptance- and mindfulness-based interventions for persons in romantic relationships.

Keywords: loneliness; social connection; romantic relationship; trust; conflict; well-being

1. Introduction

Loneliness arises when there is a discrepancy between one's desired and actual social connection with others [1,2]. Research has shown that loneliness is a universally experienced affective state [3–5], with nearly 11% of all people reporting feelings of loneliness at any one time [6,7]. Loneliness differs from concepts like solitude in that people who are lonely generally crave the social connection they are lacking [8]. Failure to respond effectively to feelings of loneliness and reconnect with others can have deleterious effects, having been correlated with decreased physical and psychological well-being [9–11].

1.1. Loneliness

As a non-scientific term, the word "loneliness" is commonly used in situations that emphasize a person's physical proximity with other people. For example, someone who spends a considerable amount of time alone may be referred to as a "loner" and thought of as a "lonely person". This colloquial usage of the word contrasts the scientific literature, which instead uses the term loneliness to describe the experience of being psychologically isolated. This point is perhaps best exemplified by scientific definitions describing loneliness as the absence of meaningful social relationships [1,2,12,13]. Empirical studies have identified reliable precursors of loneliness, such as social anxiety, rejection sensitivity, and social rejection [14–16]. These data showing that loneliness can be precipitated in experimental settings suggest that loneliness is likely context-dependent rather than context-independent [17,18]. For example, people commonly report feeling lonely following the loss of a loved one or the dissolution of a close relationship.

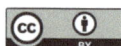

Citation: Sease, T.B.; Sandoz, E.K.; Yoke, L.; Swets, J.A.; Cox, C.R. Loneliness and Relationship Well-Being: Investigating the Mediating Roles of Relationship Awareness and Distraction among Romantic Partners. *Behav. Sci.* **2024**, *14*, 439. https://doi.org/10.3390/bs14060439

Academic Editors: Mehmet Mehmetoglu, Bianca P. Acevedo and Adam Bode

Received: 1 March 2024
Revised: 8 May 2024
Accepted: 15 May 2024
Published: 24 May 2024

Copyright: © 2024 by the authors. Licensee MDPI, Basel, Switzerland. This article is an open access article distributed under the terms and conditions of the Creative Commons Attribution (CC BY) license (https://creativecommons.org/licenses/by/4.0/).

Extant literature also suggests that loneliness is associated with patterns of behavior across various levels of analysis [19–22]. For example, people who are lonely show more cardiovascular activation, a risk factor for chronic heart disease, than people who are not lonely [23]. Feelings of loneliness are a robust predictor of psychopathology [24–26] and have been positively correlated with social avoidance and withdrawal in young adults [27]. Collectively, interpreting these findings suggest loneliness is a response class of behaviors precipitated in situations where we lack social connection.

1.2. Loneliness in Romantic Relationships

Several theorists have noted humans' fundamental need to belong and their desire for meaningful social relationships [28–31] Romantic relationships have specifically been identified as having a unique effect on health; for example, married persons report feeling more supported, having less stress, and experiencing greater well-being as compared to their single counterparts [32,33]. Similar results have also been shown among relationship partners prior to marriage [34]. According to Myers [35], the associative link between relationship status and well-being is not merely explained by relationship status alone, but that the quality of the partnership matters. For instance, higher relationship quality (e.g., satisfaction, commitment, trust) is associated with increased levels of happiness, life satisfaction, positive affect, and self-esteem [34,36,37]. Conversely, lower relationship quality (e.g., higher conflict, less trust, more relationship anxiety) is related to increased levels of anxiety, depression, aggression, and substance abuse, as well as poorer immune and endocrine functioning [38–42].

There exist a handful of studies that have examined the association between loneliness and relationship well-being. These studies have mostly investigated partner satisfaction and commitment as a predictor of loneliness [43–46]. Certainly, these associations can be interpreted bidirectionally as people who are lonely find their relationships less satisfying. This alternative interpretation of the data may be especially relevant for people experiencing chronic feelings of loneliness. Said differently, the interpersonal consequences of loneliness may be especially salient for people with "trait-based loneliness"—that is, loneliness that is present for a person in general across many different contexts. An 8-year longitudinal study including heterosexual dyads in a romantic relationship showed that loneliness prospectively predicted one's own relationship dissatisfaction and their partner's relationship dissatisfaction [47]. As such, a potential next step to better understanding the association between loneliness and romantic relationship well-being is to identify mechanisms participating in this relationship, so that clinical interventions can be tailored to redress the negative interpersonal outcomes connected to loneliness.

1.3. Potential Mechanisms: Relationship Awareness and Distraction

Mindfulness is one concept that could be involved in the relationship between loneliness and relationship well-being [48]. That is, mindfulness has been shown to confer several interpersonal benefits [49–51] and may therefore impact how loneliness affects people in romantic relationships. The term mindfulness has been broadly defined as a behavioral process including (1) an acute awareness of thoughts and feelings as being separate from reality, (2) the ability to remain present with intrusive thoughts without avoidance, (3) a predisposition towards accepting negative internal experiences, and (4) letting go of aversive thoughts without becoming preoccupied with their content [52]. In practice, mindfulness is a purported mechanism of change among many third-wave psychotherapies, yielding moderate to large effect sizes in youth [53], older adults [54], people with depression and anxiety [55], disordered eating [56], and psychosis [57]. Mindfulness-based interventions foster therapeutic change by deemphasizing the content of subtle events and building skills in areas related to emotion regulation, psychological flexibility, and compassion.

Additionally, relationship awareness, or the tendency to remain in the present moment and actively engaged with one's romantic partnership [58–60], and relationship distraction, or being continually out of touch or neglectful of one's romantic relationship [61], could be mindfulness-based processes mediating the association between loneliness and romantic relationship well-being. Longitudinal evidence has shown relationship awareness and distraction are differentially associated with positive (e.g., satisfaction, dedication, affection) and negative (e.g., relationship anxiety, conflict, insensitivity) relationship outcomes [61]. Conceptually, loneliness may decrease peoples' sensitivity to cues of social reinforcement and increase their sensitivity to cues of social punishment. Indeed, people who are lonely are less likely to detect commitment cues (i.e., receiving words of affirmation from a close friend or romantic partner) when compared to their non-lonely counterparts [62] and show an increased sensitivity to romantic relationship threat [63]. Taken together, the current study investigated relationship awareness and relationship distraction as potential mediators of the relationship between loneliness and romantic relationship well-being.

Another variable that could impact the associative link between loneliness, relationship awareness, relationship distraction, and romantic relationship well-being is psychological inflexibility. Psychological inflexibility has been conceptualized as the "rigid dominance of psychological reactions over chosen values and contingencies in guiding action" [64]. Being more psychologically inflexible, as compared to more psychologically flexible, has deleterious effects, such as increased anxiety and depression [65]. Psychological inflexibility also negatively impacts romantic relationship well-being. In a recent meta-analysis, psychological inflexibility was correlated with lower relationship satisfaction, lower sexual satisfaction, higher conflict, and more physical aggression [66]. Thus, someone that is more psychologically flexible may be able to overcome the negative consequences associated with loneliness in romantic relationships. In other words, psychological inflexibility may moderate the anticipated indirect effect of loneliness on decreased romantic relationship well-being through relationship awareness and relationship distraction.

1.4. Current Study

Studies focusing on loneliness in the context of romantic relationships have demonstrated that loneliness can be precipitated by feelings of relationship dissatisfaction [43–46]. However, one question that remains is how loneliness may lead someone to experience interpersonal difficulties in close relationships. Uncovering manipulable processes supporting the association between loneliness and romantic relationship well-being could afford therapists additional clinical targets with the potential to improve client outcomes.

The purpose of this study was to identify a pathway through which loneliness contributes to decreased relationship well-being among people in a romantic relationship. The authors hypothesized that loneliness would be negatively associated with relationship awareness and positively associated with relationship distraction. It was also expected that relationship awareness and relationship distraction would simultaneously mediate the association between loneliness and relationship well-being. Finally, a first stage moderated mediation model investigated psychological inflexibility as a moderator of the indirect effect loneliness had on relationship well-being. Although the moderated-mediation model was deemed exploratory in nature, we expected the indirect effect of loneliness on romantic relationship outcomes to only be significant at high levels of psychological flexibility. In other words, we did not expect loneliness to decrease relationship well-being for people reporting low levels of psychological inflexibility.

2. Method

2.1. Participants

Two hundred and twenty people showed an initial interest in the study by starting the survey and 210 people completed more than 75% of the study survey. After removing data from participants who (1) missed an attention check item, (2) did not provide consent for us to use their data, and (3) reported that they were not currently in a romantic relationship, the final sample consisted of 201 people ranging in age from 19–72 ($M = 37.53$, $SD = 11.70$). As illustrated in Table 1, most of the people in this study were women ($n = 138$, 68.7%), White ($n = 165$, 82.0%), heterosexual ($n = 170$, 84.6%), and married ($n = 112$, 55.7%).

Table 1. Descriptive Statistics.

Characteristic	n (%)
Gender Identity	
Woman	138 (68.7%)
Man	60 (30.0%)
Non-Binary or Transgender	3 (0.03%)
Race	
White	165 (82.1%)
BIPOC	36 (17.9%)
Sexual Orientation	
Heterosexual	170 (84.6%)
Gay or Lesbian	5 (2.5%)
Bisexual	21 (10.4%)
Another Sexuality	5 (2.5%)
Relationship Status	
Married	112 (55.6%)
Engaged	13 (6.5%)
Domestic Partnership	14 (7.0%)
Committed Relationship	57 (28.4%)
Casually dating someone	5 (2.5%)

Note. BIPOC = Black, Indigenous, or People of Color.

2.2. Procedure

Two hundred and ten people were recruited from Cloud Research [67], an online platform that provides academic researchers with high quality data by prescreening workers on Amazon's Mechanical Turk (MTurk). Inclusion criteria required respondents to be (1) at least 18 years old, (2) fluent in the English language, (3) live in the United States, and (4) be in a romantic relationship. Study participation was restricted to people who have completed between 0–500 surveys on MTurk with an approval rating greater than or equal to 0.95. All respondents were compensated $1 for participating in this study.

The study survey was created in Qualtrics with a hyperlink posted online through Cloud Research. Respondents were presented with a vague title (i.e., "Research Study for People in a Romantic Relationship") and a description of the study that included its purpose and inclusion criteria. People who were interested in the study could click on the survey link, which connected participants to the informed consent page. Participants who provide informed consent could proceed with the remainder of the survey, which was composed of counterbalanced instruments of loneliness, attentive awareness, relationship distraction, relationship trust, relationship conflict, relationship commitment, and demographic questions. Four attention checks presented on a Likert scale (e.g., "Select *Strongly Disagree* for this item") were randomly incorporated throughout the survey. One open-ended question requiring participants to type "I am not a robot" in a text blank was also included. People who missed any of the five attention checks were excluded from data analysis. Similarly, participants who provided information during the study that would make them ineligible for the project (e.g., not being in a romantic relationship) were removed from the dataset. Missing attention checks and providing information that would make someone ineligible for the study did not affect participants' right to compensation. This study was pre-registered prior to the start of data collection and all materials associated with this study are available at https://osf.io/u4sc8/?view_only=9215b02fccd04bf0ad5a9794ef034e3e (accessed on 17 July 2022). Data collection for this project was completed in August 2022, and this study was approved by the first author's Institutional Review Board prior to data collection.

2.3. Measures

2.3.1. Demographics

A brief demographics form was administered at the end of the study to capture respondents' age, gender identity, sexuality, and race. This form also included questions asking about participants' romantic relationships (e.g., length, dating vs. married, etc.).

2.3.2. Relationship Conflict

The 6-item Relationship Conflict Scale [68] was presented on a 7-point Likert scale (1 = *Strongly Disagree*, 7 = *Strongly Agree*) to measure the amount of conflict in respondents' romantic relationships. Sample items include: "There is a lot of conflict in my relationship," "My partner and I have a lot of conflicts", and "My partner and I are always in agreement on major issues" (reversed). The Relationship Conflict Scale has been tested among people in romantic relationships, showing good internal reliability ($\alpha = 0.83$) and validity [68]. Scores for relationship conflict were calculated by taking the mean of all items, with higher scores indicating more conflict.

2.3.3. Relationship Commitment

Relationship commitment was assessed using the commitment scale on the Investment Model Scale [69]. This instrument was presented on a 9-point Likert scale (0 = *Do not Agree at All*, 8 = *Agree Completely*) and measured relationship commitment using items such as, "I am committed to maintaining my relationship with my partner," "I am oriented toward the long-term future of my relationship," and "It is likely I will date someone other than my partner in the next year" (reversed). The relationship commitment subscale has shown strong psychometric properties in past research [69] and was scored by taking the mean of all items.

2.3.4. Relationship Trust

Relationship trust was measured using the 17-item Trust in Close Relationships Scale [70]. Items for this scale were presented on a 7-point Likert scale (-3 = *Strongly Disagree*, 3 = *Strongly Agree*) and instructed respondents to answer each question as it pertains to their romantic partner. Sample items include: "My partner has proven to be trustworthy, and I am willing to let him/her engage in activities which other partners find too threatening," "I have found my partner is usually dependable," and "My partner is very unpredictable. I never know how he/she is going to act from one day to the next" (reversed). Items that used gendered language, such as "Even when my partner makes excuses which sound rather unlikely, I am confident that he/she is telling the truth". were changed to use they/them pronouns to describe their partner. The Trust in Close Relationships Scale has demonstrated an acceptable internal reliability score ($\alpha = 0.70$) and validity [70]. Scores for relationship trust were computed by taking the mean of all items.

2.3.5. Loneliness

Loneliness was assessed using the well-established UCLA Loneliness scale [71,72]. This 20-item instrument was presented on a 4-point Likert scale (0 = *I never feel this way*, 3 = *I often feel this way*) and asked respondents to rate how often they experience feelings of social isolation. Example items include: "I am unable to reach out and communicate with those around me", "I find myself waiting for people to call or write", and "My interests and ideas are not shared by those around me". Studies evaluating the psychometric properties of the UCLA Loneliness Scale have revealed this instrument is both reliable and valid [73,74]. For people in romantic relationships, the UCLA Loneliness Scale has shown an internal reliability score of 0.93 [75]. Loneliness scores were computed by taking the mean of all items, with higher scores indicating more loneliness.

2.3.6. Relationship Awareness and Distraction

Relationship awareness and distraction were measured using the newly developed Attentive Awareness in Relationships Scale [61]. The AAIRS is a 16-item instrument presented on a 7-point Likert scale (1 = *Strongly Disagree*, 7 = *Strongly Agree*). Respondents are instructed to answer each item as it pertains to respondents' sensitivity to the needs of their romantic relationship. Sample items include: "I was in touch with the ebb and flow of feelings in my romantic relationship" and "I was distracted and did not pay much attention to my romantic relationship" for relationship awareness and distraction, respectively. The AAIRS is an item response theory optimized instrument, demonstrating acceptable internal consistency (α = 0.87 for relationship awareness; α = 0.93 for relationship distraction), convergent, divergent, and predictive validity [61]. Relationship awareness and relationship distraction scores were calculated by taking the mean of all items within their respective scale.

2.3.7. Psychological Inflexibility

Psychological inflexibility was measured using the Multidimensional Psychological Flexibility Inventory [75]. This study used the shortened 12-item psychological inflexibility scale that is presented on a 7-point Likert scale (1 = *Strongly Disagree*, 7 = *Strongly Agree*). Sample items include: "When I had a bad memory, I tried to distract myself to make it go away", "I thought some of my emotions were bad or inappropriate and I shouldn't feel them", and "I criticized myself for having irrational or inappropriate emotions". The MPFI is an item response theory optimized instrument that has shown acceptable internal reliability (α = 0.88–0.92), convergent, content, and divergent validity [75]. The MPFI was scored by taking the mean of all items, with higher scores meaning more psychological inflexibility.

2.3.8. Analytic Plan

Using R Studio [76], descriptive statistics and regression diagnostics were examined for all variables of interest. Pearson's product-moment correlation investigated the associations among loneliness, relationship awareness, distraction, and measures of relationship well-being. To test the study's main hypothesis, three parallel mediation models were fitted to the data with loneliness predicting each indicator of relationship well-being through the proposed mediators (i.e., mindful awareness, mindful distraction). The indirect effect of loneliness on relationship well-being was estimated by simultaneously taking the product of the a_1 and a_2 path and the b_1 and b_2 path [77]. These effects included 5000 bootstrap reiterations with a 95% confidence interval [78]. A Monte Carlo power analysis [79] including 20,000 replications suggested that between 270 and 277 people were required to observe a significant indirect effect through each mediator—assuming a large effect size (r = 0.60) between the mediators and a moderate effect size (r = 0.40) among all other variables. With a final sample of 201, the power analysis revealed that this study was underpowered.

Next, a pre-registered exploratory analysis tested whether psychological inflexibility moderated the association between loneliness and mindful awareness using hierarchical multiple linear regression. Simple slope analysis [80] was used to decompose the 2-way interaction between loneliness and mindful awareness at low (1 *SD* below the mean), medium (at the mean), and high (1 *SD* above the mean) levels of psychological inflexibility. Non-significant predictors were removed from the mediation model and then combined with the moderation results in a first-stage moderated mediation model. A critical value of 0.05 determined statistical significance and the data for this study were not analyzed until all participant responses were collected.

3. Results

Descriptive statistics and internal reliability scores for all measures are displayed in Table 2. Correlation analyses showed that all measures were significantly associated in a theoretically consistent direction.

Table 2. Descriptive Statistics and Bivariate Correlations.

Scale	Mean (SD)	1	2	3	4	5	6	7
1. Loneliness	0.98 (0.72)	0.96						
2. Inflexibility	3.02 (1.03)	0.59	0.93					
3. Awareness	4.73 (0.91)	−0.30	−0.28	0.93				
4. Distraction	2.11 (0.84)	0.35	0.35	−0.76	0.90			
5. Trust	5.44 (1.23)	−0.45	−0.47	0.52	−0.47	0.94		
6. Conflict	2.63 (1.47)	0.41	0.44	−0.43	0.42	−0.82	0.92	
7. Commitment	8.25 (1.52)	−0.25	−0.31	0.38	−0.40	0.56	−0.46	0.87

Note. All correlations were statistically significant at a critical p value of 0.05. Internal reliability scores (α) are displayed on the diagonal.

To test the authors' main hypothesis, three parallel mediation models investigated whether relationship awareness and relationship distraction simultaneously mediated the association between loneliness and measures of relationship well-being (see Figure 1). Loneliness was significantly associated with relationship commitment ($b = -0.43$, $SE = 0.12$, $t = 3.59$, $p < 0.001$), trust ($b = -0.76$, $SE = 0.11$, $t = 7.04$, $p < 0.001$), and conflict ($b = 0.84$, $SE = 0.13$, $t = 6.42$, $p < 0.001$). More importantly, loneliness was negatively associated with relationship awareness ($b = -0.37$, $SE = 0.09$, $t = 4.43$, $p < 0.001$; a_1 path) and positively associated with relationship distraction ($b = 0.40$, $SE = 0.08$, $t = 5.25$, $p < 0.001$; a_2 path). While controlling for other variables in the model, relationship awareness was associated with relationship trust ($b = 0.50$, $SE = 0.12$, $t = 4.16$, $p < 0.001$; b_1 path) whereas the association between relationship distraction and relationship trust did not reach statistical significance ($b = -0.12$, $SE = 0.13$, $t = 0.95$, $p = 0.343$; b_2 path). The indirect effect of loneliness on relationship trust through relationship awareness was significant, 95% C.I. [−0.32, −0.08], suggesting relationship awareness statistically mediated the relationship between loneliness and relationship trust.

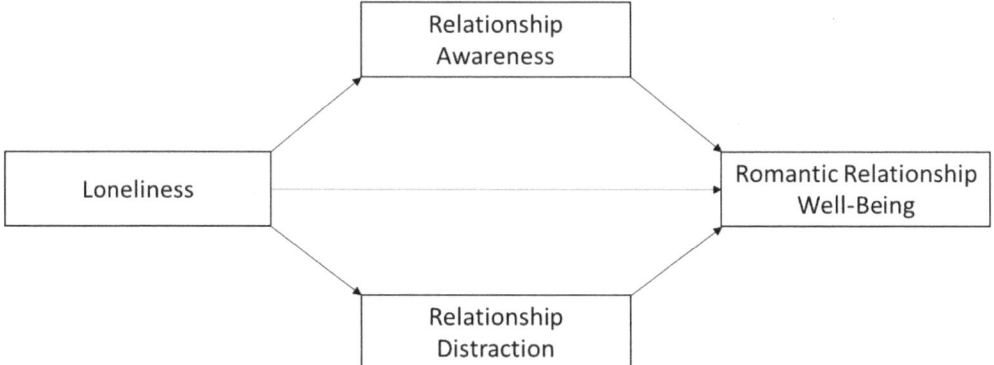

Figure 1. Theorized Path Model.

Similar results were observed when relationship conflict was entered into the regression model as the dependent variable. When holding other variables in the model constant, relationship awareness was negatively associated with relationship conflict ($b = -0.41$, $SE = 0.15$, $t = 2.71$, $p < 0.001$; b_1 path) and relationship distraction not significantly related to relationship conflict ($b = 0.21$, $SE = 0.17$, $t = 1.28$, $p = 0.201$; b_2 path). The indirect effect including 5000 bootstrap reiterations and a 95% confidence interval for relationship awareness was significant, 95% C.I. [0.04, 0.31]. In contrast, when relationship commitment was examined as the outcome variable, relationship distraction was correlated with relationship commitment ($b = -0.33$, $SE = 0.15$, $t = 2.20$, $p = 0.029$; b_1 path) but not relationship awareness ($b = 0.25$, $SE = 0.14$, $t = 1.82$, $p = 0.07$; b_2 path). The indirect effect, however, was non-significant for both relationship distraction, 95% C.I. [−0.31,0.01] and awareness, 95% C.I. [−0.23,0.03], meaning there was no mediational effect.

As an exploratory analysis, a hierarchical multiple linear regression tested whether psychological inflexibility moderated the association between loneliness and relationship awareness (see Table 3). At Step 1, the main effects of loneliness (centered) and psychological inflexibility (centered) were entered into the regression model as predictors of relationship awareness. Then, the interaction between loneliness and psychological inflexibility was entered into the model as a predictor variable, while controlling for their main effects. Results showed that the interaction between loneliness and psychological inflexibility was significant when predicting relationship awareness ($b = 0.21$, $SE = 0.07$, $t = 2.82$, $p = 0.005$). Simple slope analysis showed that there was a negative association between loneliness and relationship awareness at low ($b = -0.54$, $SE = 0.14$, $t = 3.79$, $p < 0.001$) and medium ($b = -0.33$, $SE = 0.11$, $t = 3.12$, $p < 0.001$) levels of psychological inflexibility (see Figure 2). In contrast, the association between loneliness and relationship awareness was non-significant at high levels of psychological inflexibility ($b = -0.11$, $SE = 0.11$, $t = 1.00$, $p = 0.320$).

Table 3. Moderation Analysis.

	B	B	SE	t	Sig.	R^2
Step 1						10.6%
Loneliness	−0.26	−0.21	0.10	2.50	<0.001	
Inflexibility	−0.14	−0.16	0.07	1.89	0.060	
Step 2						14.0%
Loneliness	−0.33	−0.26	0.11	3.12	<0.001	
Inflexibility	−0.14	−0.16	0.07	2.02	0.045	
Interaction	0.21	0.17	0.07	2.82	0.005	

Note. Interaction = Loneliness × Psychological Inflexibility.

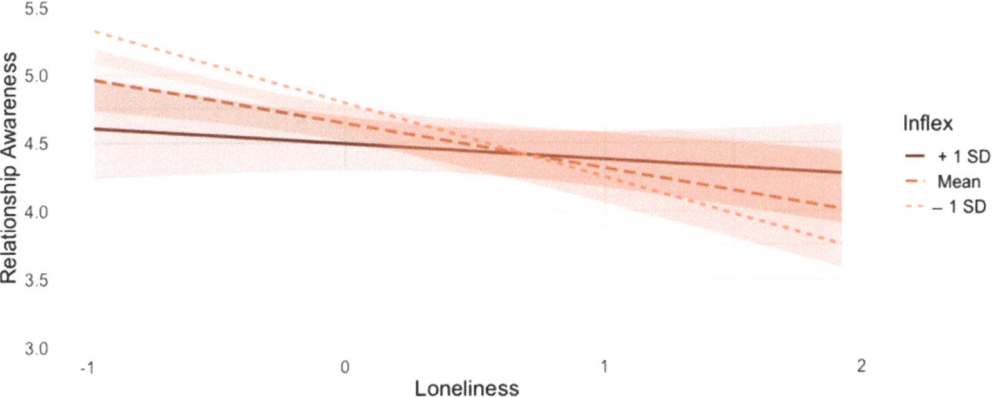

Figure 2. Two-way Interaction between Loneliness and Psychological Inflexibility; Note. Inflex = Psychological Inflexibility.

In extension of the results above, a first stage moderated mediation model examined psychological inflexibility as a moderator of the mediational effect relationship awareness had on the relationship between loneliness and measures of relationship well-being (see Figures 3 and 4). Results showed that the indirect effect of loneliness on relationship trust through relationship awareness was significant at low, 95% C.I. [−0.50, −0.15], and medium, 95% C.I. [−0.32, −0.07], levels of psychological inflexibility. Conversely, at high levels of psychological inflexibility, the indirect effect was non-significant, 95% C.I. [−0.20, 0.08]. Likewise, the mediational effect of relationship awareness on the relation between loneliness and relationship conflict was only present at low, 95% C.I. [0.13, 0.50], and medium levels, 95% C.I. [0.06, 0.32], of psychological inflexibly, but not high, 95% C.I. [−0.08, 0.20].

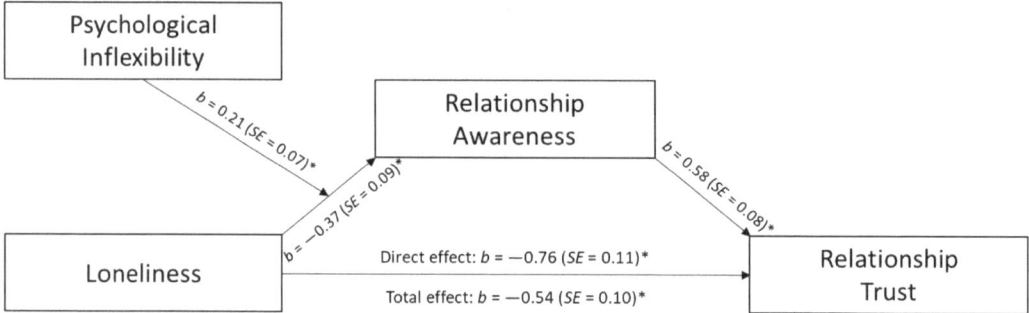

Figure 3. Predicting Relationship Trust; Note. * $p < 0.01$.

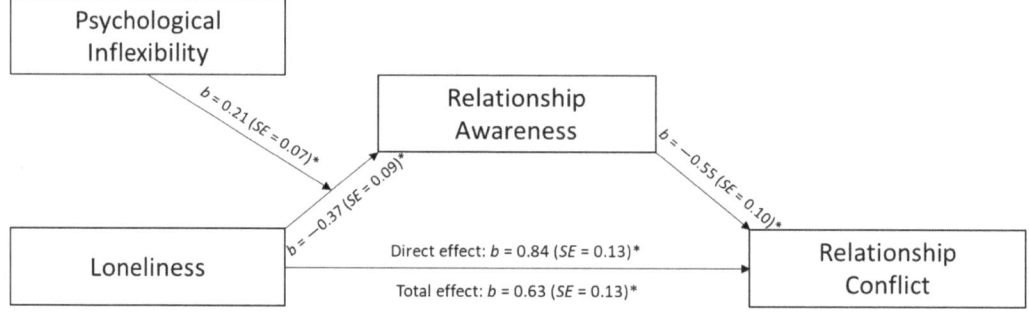

Figure 4. Predicting Relationship Conflict. Note. * $p < 0.01$.

4. Discussion

Loneliness is an affective state ubiquitous to the human condition that contributes to poor physical and psychological health [9–11]. In this study, we investigated whether relationship awareness and relationship distraction—two processes of mindfulness relevant in romantic relationships—statistically mediated the association between loneliness and measures of romantic relationship well-being. We found that relationship awareness, but not relationship distraction, had a mediational effect on the relationship between loneliness and relationship conflict as well as the relationship between loneliness and relationship trust. More specifically, people who reported feeling lonely were more likely to report less awareness in their romantic relationships. This decreased attentiveness in persons' romantic relationships was correlated with more self-reported conflict and less trust of their partner.

Further, we tested whether psychological inflexibility moderated these mediational results. A significant two-way interaction between loneliness and psychological inflexibility was observed; loneliness was only correlated with less relationship awareness at low and medium levels of psychological inflexibility. Upon further investigation, the association between psychological inflexibility and relationship awareness was significant, even while controlling for the effects of loneliness. It thus appears that, in the current study, the effect of loneliness on relationship awareness did not matter if the person was also reporting high levels of psychological inflexibility. These results converge with extant literature showing the negative effects psychological inflexibility has on romantic relationships [see 66 for a full review], and suggests that the practical implications derived from the mediational effect observed in this study may be most relevant for people with low levels of psychological inflexibility.

These results have direct implications for mindful- and acceptance-based interventions, such as Acceptance and Commitment Therapy [81]. Loneliness is a common psychological concern for people presenting with depression, anxiety disorders, schizophrenia, and suicidal ideation [15,25,26], and is associated with less positive treatment outcomes [82]. Thus, the information gathered from this study can be used to identify and target processes in psychotherapy that contribute to poor psychosocial functioning in several clinical populations. For clients in romantic relationships, this study identified a manipulable process (i.e., relationship awareness) that statistically mediated the relationship between loneliness and measures of romantic relationship well-being. Therapists working with romantic partners may aim to increase clients' attentiveness to their partner to bolster positive relationship outcomes. Indeed, interventions using mindfulness as the purported mechanism of change have shown preliminary effectiveness in improving relationship acceptance and satisfaction [83–85], suggesting techniques focusing on mindful awareness may show similar benefits.

Limitations and Future Directions

This study used a cross-sectional design to investigate the role that relationship awareness and distraction had on the association between loneliness and relationship well-being. This eliminates the possibility of inferring causation from the proposed mediation model, and thus, a temporal relationship among these variables cannot be established. Succeeding studies will need to replicate this project's findings longitudinally to conclude the directionality of these associations. It may also be useful to explore other mediators that may be involved in explaining the relationships between loneliness and interpersonal outcomes in romantic relationships. In other words, the meditation models in this study only explained 36.5% and 27.8% of the observed variance in relationship trust and conflict, respectively. Thus, forthcoming work could focus on other behavioral characteristics associated with loneliness that may contribute negative interpersonal outcomes.

Second, given this study's relatively small sample size, our design was unpowered, and it would be useful to replicate these findings using a larger, more representative sample. People in couples' therapy could be recruited and asked to complete assessments before every session to test whether fluctuations in loneliness affect relationship instability in the manner proposed here. Ideally, these investigations would include responses from both partners to assess how one partner's feelings of loneliness affect their partner's behavior in a manner that could be detrimental for the relationship. For example, Actor Partner Interdependence Modeling [86] allows researchers to statistically control for the dependence between romantic partners and create models that can be used to determine how one partner's behavior affects their own and their partner's behavior.

Finally, how relationship well-being was operationalized is perhaps the largest limitation of this study. Relationship well-being was conceptualized as romantic relationships low in commitment, low in trust, and high in conflict. Although these variables have been repeatedly correlated with poor relationship outcomes among romantic partners [87–90], there are several variables that could have been justifiably included as a proxy for relationship well-being (e.g., relationship satisfaction, infidelity, affection). Along with these measures being self-report assessments, future work in the area would benefit from using behavioral assessments of relationship instability, including the number of conflicts per week, infidelity, or relationship dissolution [91]. This would provide more tangible empirical evidence demonstrating that decreased relationship awareness in response to loneliness is determinantal for people in romantic relationships.

5. Conclusions

This project investigated the roles relationship awareness and relationship distraction played on the association between loneliness and romantic relationship well-being. The results showed that loneliness was associated with less self-reported relationship awareness, which in turn was associated with more relationship conflict and less relationship trust. Psychological inflexibility was also found to moderate the association between loneliness and relationship awareness. Specifically, the indirect effect of loneliness on relationship outcomes through relationship awareness was only present at low- to medium-levels of psychological inflexibility. These data provide insight into how loneliness may contribute to worsened interpersonal outcomes in romantic relationships. As such, this study provides useful information that can be incorporated into the curriculum of clinical programs designed to redress feelings of isolation for people in romantic relationships.

Author Contributions: Conceptualization, T.B.S.; Methodology, T.B.S., J.A.S. and C.R.C.; Writing—original draft, T.B.S., E.K.S., L.Y. and C.R.C.; Writing—review & editing, T.B.S., E.K.S., L.Y. and C.R.C.; Funding acquisition, C.R.C. All authors have read and agreed to the published version of the manuscript.

Funding: Publication fees for this article were provided by TCU Library's Open Access fund.

Institutional Review Board Statement: The study was approved by the Institutional Review Board (or Ethics Committee) of Texas Christian University (protocol code IRB#2022-102; 7 November 2022).

Informed Consent Statement: Informed consent and consent for data use was obtained from all participants involved in the study.

Data Availability Statement: Data will be made available upon request by the corresponding author.

Conflicts of Interest: The authors declare no conflict of interest.

References

1. Francis, G.M. Loneliness: Measuring the abstract. *Int. J. Nurs. Stud.* **1976**, *13*, 153–160. [CrossRef]
2. Younger, J.B. The alienation of the sufferer. *Adv. Nurs. Sci.* **1995**, *17*, 53–72. [CrossRef]
3. Lasgaard, M. Reliability and validity of the Danish version of the UCLA Loneliness Scale. *Personal. Individ. Differ.* **2007**, *42*, 1359–1366. [CrossRef]
4. Wilson, D.; Cutts, J.; Lees, I.; Mapungwana, S.; Maunganidze, L. Psychometric properties of the revised UCLA Loneliness Scale and two short-form measures of loneliness in Zimbabwe. *J. Personal. Assess.* **1992**, *59*, 72–81. [CrossRef]
5. Wu, C.H.; Yao, G. Psychometric analysis of the short-form UCLA Loneliness Scale (ULS-8) in Taiwanese undergraduate students. *Personal. Individ. Differ.* **2008**, *44*, 1762–1771. [CrossRef]
6. Beutel, M.E.; Klein, E.M.; Brähler, E.; Reiner, I.; Jünger, C.; Michal, M.; Wiltink, J.; Wild, P.S.; Münzel, T.; Lackner, K.J.; et al. Loneliness in the general population: Prevalence, determinants and relations to mental health. *BMC Psychiatry* **2017**, *17*, 97. [CrossRef]
7. Surkalim, D.L.; Luo, M.; Eres, R.; Gebel, K.; van Buskirk, J.; Bauman, A.; Ding, D. The prevalence of loneliness across 113 countries: Systematic review and meta-analysis. *BMJ* **2022**, *376*, e067068. [CrossRef] [PubMed]
8. Copel, L.C. A conceptual model. *J. Psychosoc. Nurs. Ment. Health Serv.* **1988**, *26*, 14–19. [CrossRef] [PubMed]
9. Mushtaq, R.; Shoib, S.; Shah, T.; Mushtaq, S. Relationship between loneliness, psychiatric disorders and physical health? A review on the psychological aspects of loneliness. *J. Clin. Diagn. Res.* **2014**, *8*, WE01. [CrossRef]
10. Park, C.; Majeed, A.; Gill, H.; Tamura, J.; Ho, R.C.; Mansur, R.B.; Narsi, F.; Lee, Y.; Rosenblat, J.D.; Wong, E.; et al. The effect of loneliness on distinct health outcomes: A comprehensive review and meta-analysis. *Psychiatry Res.* **2020**, *294*, 113514. [CrossRef]
11. Richard, A.; Rohrmann, S.; Vandeleur, C.L.; Schmid, M.; Barth, J.; Eichholzer, M. Loneliness is adversely associated with physical and mental health and lifestyle factors: Results from a Swiss national survey. *PLoS ONE* **2017**, *12*, e0181442. [CrossRef] [PubMed]
12. Portnoff, G. Loneliness: Lost in the landscape of meaning. *J. Psychol.* **1988**, *122*, 545–555. [CrossRef]
13. Ryan, M.C.; Patterson, J. Loneliness in the elderly. *J. Gerontol. Nurs.* **1987**, *13*, 6–9. [CrossRef] [PubMed]
14. Gao, S.; Assink, M.; Cipriani, A.; Lin, K. Associations between rejection sensitivity and mental health outcomes: A meta-analytic review. *Clin. Psychol. Rev.* **2017**, *57*, 59–74. [CrossRef] [PubMed]

15. Lim, M.H.; Rodebaugh, T.L.; Zyphur, M.J.; Gleeson, J.F. Loneliness over time: The crucial role of social anxiety. *J. Abnorm. Psychol.* **2016**, *125*, 620. [CrossRef] [PubMed]
16. Xiao, B.; Bullock, A.; Liu, J.; Coplan, R. Unsociability, peer rejection, and loneliness in Chinese early adolescents: Testing a cross-lagged model. *J. Early Adolesc.* **2021**, *41*, 865–885. [CrossRef]
17. Matthews, T.; Danese, A.; Wertz, J.; Odgers, C.L.; Ambler, A.; Moffitt, T.E.; Arseneault, L. Social isolation, loneliness and depression in young adulthood: A behavioral genetic analysis. *Soc. Psychiatry Psychiatr. Epidemiol.* **2016**, *51*, 339–348. [CrossRef] [PubMed]
18. Spithoven, A.W.M.; Cacioppo, S.; Goossens, L.; Cacioppo, J.T. Genetic contributions to loneliness and their relevance to the evolutionary theory of loneliness. *Perspect. Psychol. Sci.* **2019**, *14*, 376–396. [CrossRef] [PubMed]
19. Brown, E.G.; Gallagher, S.; Creaven, A.M. Loneliness and acute stress reactivity: A systematic review of psychophysiological studies. *Psychophysiology* **2018**, *55*, e13031. [CrossRef] [PubMed]
20. Cacioppo, S.; Capitanio, J.P.; Cacioppo, J.T. Toward a neurology of loneliness. *Psychol. Bull.* **2014**, *140*, 1464. [CrossRef]
21. Hawkley, L.C.; Cacioppo, J.T. Loneliness and pathways to disease. *Brain Behav. Immun.* **2003**, *17*, 98–105. [CrossRef] [PubMed]
22. Hawkley, L.C.; Cacioppo, J.T. Loneliness matters: A theoretical and empirical review of consequences and mechanisms. *Ann. Behav. Med.* **2010**, *40*, 218–227. [CrossRef]
23. Cacioppo, J.T.; Hawkley, L.C.; Crawford, L.E.; Ernst, J.M.; Burleson, M.H.; Kowalewski, R.B.; Malarkey, W.B.; Van Cauter, E.; Berntson, G.G. Loneliness and health: Potential mechanisms. *Psychosom. Med.* **2002**, *64*, 407–417. [CrossRef] [PubMed]
24. Chau, A.K.; Zhu, C.; So, S.H.W. Loneliness and the psychosis continuum: A meta-analysis on positive psychotic experiences and a meta-analysis on negative psychotic experiences. *Int. Rev. Psychiatry* **2019**, *31*, 471–490. [CrossRef] [PubMed]
25. Erzen, E.; Çikrikci, Ö. The effect of loneliness on depression: A meta-analysis. *Int. J. Soc. Psychiatry* **2018**, *64*, 427–435. [CrossRef] [PubMed]
26. McClelland, H.; Evans, J.J.; Nowland, R.; Ferguson, E.; O'Connor, R.C. Loneliness as a predictor of suicidal ideation and behavioral: A systematic review and meta-analysis of prospective studies. *J. Affect. Disord.* **2020**, *274*, 880–896. [CrossRef] [PubMed]
27. Watson, J.; Nesdale, D. Rejection sensitivity, social withdrawal, and loneliness in young adults. *J. Appl. Soc. Psychol.* **2012**, *42*, 1984–2005. [CrossRef]
28. Baumeister, R.F.; Leary, M.R. The need to belong: Desire for interpersonal attachments as a fundamental human motivation. *Psychol. Bull.* **1995**, *117*, 497–529. [CrossRef] [PubMed]
29. Bowlby, J. *Attachment and Loss: Attachment*; Basic Books: New York, NY, USA, 1969; Volume I.
30. Deci, E.L.; Ryan, R.M. The what and why of goal pursuits: Human needs and the self-determination of behavior. *Psychol. Inq.* **2000**, *11*, 227–268. [CrossRef]
31. Maslow, A. *Deficiency motivation growth motivation In Nebraska Symposium on Values*; Jones, M., Ed.; University of Nebraska Press: Lincoln, NE, USA, 1955; Volume 1, pp. 1–30.
32. Diener, E.; Gohm, C.L.; Suh, E.; Oishi, S. Similarity of the relations between marital status and subjective well-being across cultures. *J. Cross-Cult. Psychol.* **2000**, *31*, 419–436. [CrossRef]
33. Walen, H.R.; Lachman, M.E. Social support and strain from partner, family, and friends: Costs and benefits for men and women in adulthood. *J. Soc. Pers. Relatsh.* **2000**, *17*, 5–30. [CrossRef]
34. Dush, C.M.K.; Amato, P.R. Consequences of relationship status and quality for subjective well-being. *J. Soc. Pers. Relatsh.* **2005**, *22*, 607–627. [CrossRef]
35. Myers, D. The funds, friends, and faith of happy people. *Am. Psychol.* **2000**, *55*, 56–67. [CrossRef] [PubMed]
36. Dyrdal, G.M.; Røysamb, E.; Nes, R.B.; Vittersø, J. Can a happy relationship predict a happy life? A population-based study of maternal well-being during the life transition of pregnancy, infancy, and toddlerhood. *J. Happiness Stud.* **2011**, *12*, 947–962. [CrossRef] [PubMed]
37. Love, A.B.; Holder, M.D. Can romantic relationship quality mediate the relation between psychopathy and subjective well-being? *J. Happiness Stud.* **2015**, *17*, 2407–2429. [CrossRef]
38. Hawkins, D.N.; Booth, A. Unhappily ever after: Effects of long-term, low-quality marriages on well-being. *Soc. Forces* **2005**, *84*, 451–471. [CrossRef]
39. Horwitz, A.V.; White, H.R.; Howell-White, S. Becoming married and mental health: A longitudinal study of a cohort of young adults. *J. Marriage Fam.* **1996**, *58*, 895–907. [CrossRef]
40. Kiecolt-Glaser, J.K.; Newton, T.L. Marriage and health: His and hers. *Psychol. Bull.* **2001**, *127*, 472–503. [CrossRef] [PubMed]
41. Sampson, R.J.; Laub, J.H.; Wimer, C. Does marriage reduce crime? A counterfactual approach to within-individual causal effects. *Criminology* **2006**, *44*, 465–508. [CrossRef]
42. Umberson, D.; Williams, K.; Powers, D.A.; Liu, H.; Needham, B. You make me sick: Marital quality and health over the life course. *J. Health Soc. Behav.* **2006**, *47*, 1–16. [CrossRef]
43. Burke, T.J.; Segrin, C. Bonded or stuck? Effects of personal and constraint commitment on loneliness and stress. *Personal. Individ. Differ.* **2014**, *64*, 101–106. [CrossRef]
44. Givertz, M.; Woszidlo, A.; Segrin, C.; Knutson, K. Direct and indirect effects of attachment orientation on relationship quality and loneliness in married couples. *J. Soc. Pers. Relatsh.* **2013**, *30*, 1096–1120. [CrossRef]

45. Pereira, M.G.; Taysi, E.; Fincham, F.D.; Machado, J.C. Communication, relationship satisfaction, attachment and physical/psychological symptoms: The mediating role of loneliness. *Online Braz. J. Nurs.* **2015**, *14*, 1–25.
46. Pereira, M.G.; Taysi, E.; Orcan, F.; Fincham, F. Attachment, infidelity, and loneliness in college students involved in a romantic relationship: The role of relationship satisfaction, morbidity, and prayer for partner. *Contemp. Fam. Ther.* **2014**, *36*, 333–350. [CrossRef]
47. Mund, M.; Johnson, M.D. Lonely me, lonely you: Loneliness and the longitudinal course of relationship satisfaction. *J. Happiness Stud.* **2021**, *22*, 575–597. [CrossRef]
48. Quinn-Nilas, C. Self-reported trait mindfulness and couples' relationship satisfaction: A meta-analysis. *Mindfulness* **2020**, *11*, 835–848. [CrossRef]
49. Anand, L.; Sadowski, I.; Per, M.; Khoury, B. Mindful parenting: A meta-analytic review of intrapersonal and interpersonal parental outcomes. *Curr. Psychol.* **2023**, *42*, 8367–8383. [CrossRef]
50. Donald, J.N.; Sahdra, B.K.; Van Zanden, B.; Duineveld, J.J.; Atkins, P.W.; Marshall, S.L.; Ciarrochi, J. Does your mindfulness benefit others? A systematic review and meta-analysis of the link between mindfulness and prosocial behaviour. *Br. J. Psychol.* **2019**, *110*, 101–125. [CrossRef] [PubMed]
51. Malin, Y. Others in mind: A systematic review and meta-analysis of the relationship between mindfulness and prosociality. *Mindfulness* **2023**, *14*, 1582–1605. [CrossRef]
52. Chadwick, P.; Hember, M.; Symes, J.; Peters, E.; Kuipers, E.; Dagnan, D. Responding mindfully to unpleasant thoughts and images: Reliability and validity of the Southampton Mindfulness Questionnaire (SMQ). *Br. J. Clin. Psychol.* **2008**, *47*, 451–455. [CrossRef]
53. Zack, S.; Saekow, J.; Kelly, M.; Radke, A. Mindfulness based interventions for youth. *J. Ration. Emotive Cogn. Behav. Ther.* **2014**, *32*, 44–56. [CrossRef]
54. Kishita, N.; Takei, Y.; Stewart, I. A meta-analysis of third wave mindfulness-based cognitive behavioral therapies for older people. *Int. J. Geriatr. Psychiatry* **2017**, *32*, 1352–1361. [CrossRef] [PubMed]
55. Hoffmann, S.G.; Gómez, A.F. Mindfulness-based interventions for anxiety and depression. *Psychiatry Clin.* **2017**, *40*, 739–749. [CrossRef] [PubMed]
56. Linardon, J.; Gleeson, J.; Yap, K.; Murphy, K.; Brennan, L. Meta-analysis of the effects of third-wave behavioral interventions on disordered eating and body image concerns: Implications for eating disorder prevention. *Cogn. Behav. Ther.* **2019**, *48*, 15–38. [CrossRef] [PubMed]
57. Louise, S.; Fitzpatrick, M.; Strauss, C.; Rossell, S.L.; Thomas, N. Mindfulness- and acceptance-based interventions for psychosis: Our current understanding and a meta-analysis. *Schizophr. Res.* **2018**, *192*, 57–63. [CrossRef] [PubMed]
58. Acitelli, L.K. Gender differences in relationship awareness and marital satisfaction among young married couples. *Personal. Soc. Psychol. Bull.* **1992**, *18*, 102–110. [CrossRef]
59. Kimmes, J.G.; Jaurequi, M.E.; May, R.W.; Srivastava, S.; Fincham, F.D. Mindfulness in the context of romantic relationships: Initial development and validation of the Relationship Mindfulness Measure. *J. Marital. Fam. Ther.* **2018**, *44*, 575–589. [CrossRef] [PubMed]
60. Snell, W.E., Jr. The Relationship Awareness Scale: Measuring Relational Consciousness, Relational-Monitoring, and Relational Anxiety. In Proceedings of the Fourth Annual International Conference on Personal Relationships, Vancouver, BC, Canada, July 1988.
61. Daks, J.S.; Rogge, R.D.; Fincham, F.D. Distinguishing the correlates of being mindfully vs. mindlessly coupled: Development and validation of the Attentive Awareness in Relationships Scale (AAIRS). *Mindfulness* **2021**, *12*, 1361–1376. [CrossRef]
62. Yamaguchi, M.; Smith, A.; Ohtsubo, Y. Loneliness predicts insensitivity to partner commitment. *Personal. Individ. Differ.* **2017**, *105*, 200–207. [CrossRef]
63. Nowland, R.; Talbot, R.; Qualter, P. Influence of loneliness and rejection sensitivity on threat sensitivity in romantic relationships in young and middle-aged adults. *Personal. Individ. Differ.* **2018**, *131*, 185–190. [CrossRef]
64. Bond, F.W.; Hayes, S.C.; Baer, R.A.; Carpenter, K.M.; Guenole, N.; Orcutt, H.K.; Waltz, T.; Zettle, R.D. Preliminary psychometric properties of the Acceptance and Action Questionnaire–II: A revised measure of psychological inflexibility and experiential avoidance. *Behav. Ther.* **2011**, *42*, 676–688. [CrossRef] [PubMed]
65. Yao, X.; Xu, X.; Chan, K.L.; Chen, S.; Assink, M.; Gao, S. Associations between psychological inflexibility and mental health problems during the COVID-19 pandemic: A three-level meta-analytic review. *J. Affect. Disord.* **2023**, *320*, 148–160. [CrossRef]
66. Daks, J.S.; Rogge, R.D. Examining the correlates of psychological flexibility in romantic relationship and family dynamics: A meta-analysis. *J. Context. Behav. Sci.* **2020**, *18*, 214–238. [CrossRef]
67. Litman, L.; Robinson, J.; Abberbock, T. TurkPrime.com: A versatile crowdsourcing data acquisition platform for the behavioral sciences. *Behav. Res. Methods* **2017**, *49*, 433–442. [CrossRef]
68. Gordon, A.M.; Chen, S. Do you get where I'm coming from?: Perceived understanding buffers against the negative impact of conflict on relationship satisfaction. *J. Personal. Soc. Psychol.* **2016**, *110*, 239. [CrossRef] [PubMed]
69. Rusbult, C.E.; Martz, J.M.; Agnew, C.R. The investment model scale: Measuring commitment level, satisfaction level, quality of alternatives, and investment size. *Pers. Relatsh.* **1998**, *5*, 357–387. [CrossRef]
70. Rempel, J.K.; Holmes, J.G.; Zanna, M.P. Trust in close relationships. *J. Personal. Soc. Psychol.* **1985**, *49*, 95. [CrossRef]

71. Russell, D.; Peplau, L.A.; Cutrona, C.E. The revised UCLA Loneliness Scale: Concurrent and discriminant validity evidence. *J. Personal. Soc. Psychol.* **1980**, *39*, 472. [CrossRef] [PubMed]
72. Russell, D.W. UCLA Loneliness Scale (Version 3): Reliability, validity, and factor structure. *J. Personal. Assess.* **1996**, *66*, 20–40. [CrossRef]
73. Alsubheen, S.A.; Oliveira, A.; Habash, R.; Goldstein, R.; Brooks, D. Systematic review of psychometric properties and cross-cultural adaptation of the University of California and Los Angeles loneliness scale in adults. *Curr. Psychol.* **2021**, *42*, 11819–11833. [CrossRef]
74. Cole, A.; Bond, C.; Qualter, P.; Maes, M. A systematic review of the development and psychometric properties of loneliness measures for children and adolescents. *Int. J. Environ. Res. Public Health* **2021**, *18*, 3285. [CrossRef] [PubMed]
75. Rolffs, J.L.; Rogge, R.D.; Wilson, K.G. Disentangling components of flexibility via the hexaflex model: Development and validation of the Multidimensional Psychological Flexibility Inventory (MPFI). *Assessment* **2018**, *25*, 458–482. [CrossRef]
76. RStudio Team. *RStudio: Integrated Development Environment for R. RStudio*; PBC: Boston, MA, USA, 2022. Available online: http://www.rstudio.com/ (accessed on 1 January 2024).
77. Preacher, K.J.; Hayes, A.F. SPSS and SAS procedures for estimating indirect effects in simple mediation models. *Behav. Res. Methods Instrum. Comput.* **2004**, *36*, 717–731. [CrossRef] [PubMed]
78. Shrout, P.E.; Bolger, N. Mediation in experimental and nonexperimental studies: New procedures and recommendations. *Psychol. Methods* **2002**, *7*, 422. [CrossRef]
79. Schoemann, A.M.; Boulton, A.J.; Short, S.D. Determining power and sample size for simple and complex mediation models. *Soc. Psychol. Personal. Sci.* **2017**, *8*, 379–386. [CrossRef]
80. Rosnow, R.L.; Rosenthal, R. Definition and interpretation of interaction effects. *Psychol. Bull.* **1989**, *105*, 143–146. [CrossRef]
81. Hayes, S.C.; Strosahl, K.D.; Bunting, K.; Twohig, M.; Wilson, K.G. What is acceptance and commitment therapy? In *A Practical Guide to Acceptance and Commitment Therapy*; Springer: Boston, MA, USA, 2004; pp. 3–29.
82. Wang, J.; Mann, F.; Lloyd-Evans, B.; Ma, R.; Johnson, S. Associations between loneliness and perceived social support and outcomes of mental health problems: A systematic review. *BMC Psychiatry* **2018**, *18*, 1–16. [CrossRef] [PubMed]
83. Kappen, G.; Karremans, J.C.; Burk, W.J. Effects of a short online mindfulness intervention on relationship satisfaction and partner acceptance: The moderating role of trait mindfulness. *Mindfulness* **2019**, *10*, 2186–2199. [CrossRef]
84. Khaddouma, A.; Coop Gordon, K.; Strand, E.B. Mindful mates: A pilot study of the relational effects of mindfulness-based stress reduction on participants and their partners. *Fam. Process* **2017**, *56*, 636–651. [CrossRef]
85. Vajda, D.; Kiss, E.C. Effects of a mindfulness-based intervention on psychological distress and romantic relationships: Results of a pilot study. *J. Community Med. Public Health Care* **2016**, *3*, 1–6. [CrossRef]
86. Cook, W.L.; Kenny, D.A. The actor–partner interdependence model: A model of bidirectional effects in developmental studies. *Int. J. Behav. Dev.* **2005**, *29*, 101–109. [CrossRef]
87. Anderson, T.L.; Emmers-Sommer, T.M. Predictors of relationship satisfaction in online romantic relationships. *Commun. Stud.* **2006**, *57*, 153–172. [CrossRef]
88. Cramer, D. Emotional support, conflict, depression, and relationship satisfaction in a romantic partner. *J. Psychol.* **2004**, *138*, 532–542. [CrossRef] [PubMed]
89. Impett, E.A.; Beals, K.P.; Peplau, L.A. Testing the investment model of relationship commitment and stability in a longitudinal study of married couples. *Curr. Psychol.* **2001**, *20*, 312–326. [CrossRef]
90. Rhoades, G.K.; Stanley, S.M.; Markman, H.J. Should I stay or should I go? Predicting dating relationship stability from four aspects of commitment. *J. Fam. Psychol.* **2010**, *24*, 543. [CrossRef]
91. Gottman, J.M. *What Predicts Divorce: The Relationship between Marital Processes and Marital Outcomes*; Lawrence Erlbaum Associates, Inc.: Mahwah, NJ, USA, 1994.

Disclaimer/Publisher's Note: The statements, opinions and data contained in all publications are solely those of the individual author(s) and contributor(s) and not of MDPI and/or the editor(s). MDPI and/or the editor(s) disclaim responsibility for any injury to people or property resulting from any ideas, methods, instructions or products referred to in the content.

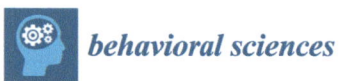

Article

Psychometric Validation of the Dating Violence Questionnaire (DVQ-R) in Ecuadorians

Miriam Jacqueline Muñoz-Aucapiña [1], Rosa Elvira Muñoz-Aucapiña [1], Inmaculada García-García [2], María Adelaida Álvarez-Serrano [3,*], Ana María Antolí-Jover [3] and Encarnación Martínez-García [2,4,5]

[1] Department of Nursing, Faculty of Health Sciences, University Católica Santiago de Guayaquil, Guayaquil 090615, Ecuador; miriam.munoz@cu.ucsg.edu.ec (M.J.M.-A.); rosa.munoz@cu.ucsg.edu.ec (R.E.M.-A.)
[2] Department of Nursing, Faculty of Health Sciences, University of Granada, 18016 Granada, Spain; igarcia@ugr.es (I.G.-G.); emartinez@ugr.es (E.M.-G.)
[3] Department of Nursing, Faculty of Health Sciences, University of Granada, 51001 Ceuta, Spain; antolijover@ugr.es
[4] Virgen de las Nieves University Hospital, 18014 Granada, Spain
[5] Instituto de Investigación Biosanitaria ibs.GRANADA, Granada, Spain
* Correspondence: adealvarez@ugr.es

Academic Editors: Heng Choon Oliver Chan, Bianca P. Acevedo and Adam Bode

Received: 6 September 2024
Revised: 5 December 2024
Accepted: 7 January 2025
Published: 15 January 2025
Corrected: 3 April 2025

Citation: Muñoz-Aucapiña, M. J., Muñoz-Aucapiña, R. E., García-García, I., Álvarez-Serrano, M. A., Antolí-Jover, A. M., & Martínez-García, E. (2025). Psychometric Validation of the Dating Violence Questionnaire (DVQ-R) in Ecuadorians. *Behavioral Sciences*, *15*(1), 68. https://doi.org/10.3390/bs15010068

Copyright: © 2025 by the authors. Licensee MDPI, Basel, Switzerland. This article is an open access article distributed under the terms and conditions of the Creative Commons Attribution (CC BY) license (https://creativecommons.org/licenses/by/4.0/).

Abstract: Gender-based violence among young people is a pressing global problem, causing injury and disability to women and posing physical, mental, sexual, and reproductive health risks. This study aimed to psychometrically validate the Dating Violence Questionnaire—Revised (DVQ-R) in a sample of 340 Ecuadorian university students. The study included 340 male and female students from two universities in Ecuador. The reliability and validity of the questionnaire were rigorously assessed by exploratory and confirmatory factor analyses, which revealed a four-factor model as the most parsimonious solution (RMSEA = 0.012). The factors were labelled as follows: 'emotional neglect and contempt', 'physical violence and aggression', 'coercion and control', and 'emotional manipulation and testing'. The validated scale yielded a Cronbach's alpha (α) of 0.839, with individual alpha values of 0.872, 0.764, 0.849, and 0.729 for each dimension. Convergent validity was established, as the mean variance extracted per factor exceeded 0.4. Divergent validity was confirmed, as the variance retained by each factor was greater than the variance shared between them (mean variance extracted per factor > ϕ^2). These results indicate that the DVQ-R is a valid and reliable instrument to assess dating violence among Spanish-speaking young adults, which supports future research and prevention programmes.

Keywords: dating violence; nursing students; gender violence; validation study

1. Introduction

Dating violence among young people is now reported in many countries (Gebrie et al., 2022; Oyarzún et al., 2021; World Health Organizatión, 2021). Its definition encompasses any type of physical violence, sexual violence, stalking, or psychological aggression (including coercive acts) by a current or former partner, both in adolescence and adulthood (Miller & McCaw, 2019).

Globally, dating violence has received increasing attention due to its high prevalence. In the United States, for example, according to a report by the Centers for Disease Control and Prevention (CDC), approximately 10% of college students report having experienced physical violence in their dating relationships, while 11% have experienced sexual violence in these relationships (Wiklund et al., 2010).

In Europe, statistics also reveal a high prevalence of dating violence. According to data from the European Union Agency for Fundamental Rights (FRA), 33% of young women have experienced some form of physical or sexual violence in their youth. This problem is recurrently observed in the university environment (Neilson et al., 2023), where according to studies carried out in 2015 by the American Association of Universities on 27 university campuses, more than 20% of university students report having been victims of sexual aggression (Association of American Universities, 2015). In Spain, the first research on violence against women in the university context revealed that 62% of students knew of or had experienced situations of this type within these institutions (Valls et al., 2016). In addition, cultural contexts seem to have a strong influence on students' perceptions of IPV. In this context, studies suggest that university students in North America, predominantly in the United States, have less favourable attitudes towards IPV than their counterparts in Asia, South America, or Europe (Buquet Corleto, 2011; Zark & Satyen, 2022). On the other hand, An et al. (2023), in their study of Hispanic/Latino and non-Hispanic white students across seven universities, found that Hispanic/Latino students had higher rates of intimate partner violence victimisation and perpetration than their white counterparts. In a similar vein, an acceptance of violence in these populations, influenced by social norms, was found in Quito, Ecuador (Medina Maldonado et al., 2022).

Consequently, several studies have found that dating violence is a common experience among young adults, with prevalence differing across countries and contexts (Coulter et al., 2017). The existence of gender inequalities, patriarchal stereotypes, and socio-cultural norms that perpetuate violence play a key role in its persistence.

In Latin America, where strong gender disparities and very traditional behaviours prevail, dating violence is a serious problem (Red de Desarrollo Social de América Latina y el Caribe, 2017). In university environments, young people explore their dating relationships more freely (Kaukinen, 2014), and while some adopt communication skills to express their feelings, others adopt risky behaviours and various methods of physical, sexual, and psychological coercion to validate their love and affection in their dating relationships. It is significantly more common for women than men to be the victim in these situations (Bhochhibhoya et al., 2021).

In Ecuador, the situation is no different. The National Survey on Family Relations and Gender Violence published in 2019 indicates that six out of ten women between 15 and 45 years of age have suffered some type of violence at least once in their lives. The most frequent is psychological violence (1/2), followed by physical (2/5), patrimonial (4/10), and sexual (1/4). Of these women, 45.0% were between 15 and 17 years old (INEC, 2019).

However, there are no specific official data that provide a detailed analysis of the prevalence of dating violence among young people, which has limited the implementation of specific programmes to address and prevent this problem.

Considering that dating relationships in young people constitute a key aspect for the shaping of future interaction patterns in couple relationships (Gómez et al., 2014; Wiklund et al., 2010), their quantification represents a priority to identify the problem and promote measures aimed at the prevention and eradication of violence (Galdo Castiñeiras et al., 2023). To this end, different instruments have been developed, including self-administered questionnaires such as Aggression in Dating Situations (AADS), the Acceptance of Violence Questionnaire (AVQ), the Conflict Tactics Scale (CTS), the Conflict in Adolescent Dating Relationships Inventory (CADRI), and the Justification of Verbal/Coercive Tactics Scale (JVCT) (Yanez Peñúñuri et al., 2019). However, the Dating Violence Questionnaire (DVQ-R) is especially recommended for young people aged 15–26 years, due to its greater structural stability (Rodríguez Díaz et al., 2017). This instrument was created in Spain by authors such as (Rodríguez Franco et al., 2010), with a first version of 42 items, and has been widely used in research contexts to better understand the prevalence and characteristics of dating violence. It was later revised and modified, resulting in the DVQ-R version with 20 items. This modification, made to improve the reliability and validity of the scale, sought to simplify certain items and adapt them to reduce both cultural and interpretation biases that were observed in different contexts (Alfaro Urquiola, 2020). The revised version used in this study offers a more robust measurement and has been validated and used in different university settings in countries such as Spain, Mexico, Colombia, Peru, Argentina, and Bolivia, but so far it has not been validated in men and women in the Ecuadorian context (Alfaro Urquiola, 2020; Martínez Gómez et al., 2021; Rodríguez Díaz et al., 2017).

For all these reasons, universities have become ideal environments for exploring multiple aspects related to IPV in young people. The aim of this study was to carry out the psychometric validation of the Dating Violence Questionnaire (DVQ-R) in an Ecuadorian university population.

2. Materials and Methods

2.1. Design

In order to adapt and evaluate the psychometric properties of the DVQ-R, a cross-sectional study was conducted. The questionnaire was administered to young men and women from two Ecuadorian universities: the private Universidad Católica Santiago de Guayaquil and the public Universidad de Guayaquil. Data collection took place during the months of June to September of the academic year 2021/2022.

2.2. Sample, Participants, and Measures

The accessible population of the study was nursing students of various academic levels, corresponding to a total of 1657 students enrolled in the period 2021/2022.

Although in the process of validating a questionnaire, there is no single criterion for establishing the sample size, one of the most considered guidelines suggests having between 5 and 10 participants per item (The R Foundation, n.d.). Therefore, following this criterion, in the specific case of the DVQ-R composed of 20 items, a minimum total sample size of between 100 and 200 participants is suggested.

2.3. Instrument

The questionnaire was divided into two blocks. The first collected information on socio-demographic variables: year of birth; sex (male, female); university (Universidad Católica de Santiago de Guayaquil, Universidad Estatal de Guayaquil); relationship status (No, Yes); relationship duration (1–3 months, 3–6 months, 1–3 years, >3 years). The second block was based on the Dating Violence Questionnaire—Revised (DVQ-R) (Rodríguez Díaz et al., 2017), which was later validated for samples of Ecuadorian women aged 18 to 30 by Cherrez Santos et al. (2022). This study remains the ideal reference for exclusively female samples in this age group and population. This instrument is a simplified version of the Dating Violence Questionnaire (DVQ) (Rodríguez Franco et al., 2010). It is aimed at adolescents involved in dating relationships, or who have been in a relationship in the last six months, with a minimum duration of one month. It includes 20 items and uses a Likert-type scale with five response options (0 = Never to 4 = Always). It can be administered individually or in a group, lasting approximately five to ten minutes. This questionnaire assesses five dimensions of dating violence, which are shown below:
1. Coercive violence: explicit behaviours aimed at pressuring the partner to force his or her will or behaviour, represented by items 1, 9, 25, and 38.

2. Sexual violence: sexist or sexual behaviours, such as unwanted play on the part of the partner or feeling forced to perform acts and touching, represented by items 2, 10, 26, and 39.
3. Physical violence: includes hitting, shoving, direct injury, or indirect injury through damage to objects with emotional significance for the victim, represented by items 5, 13, 20, and 21.
4. Detachment violence: behaviours related to an attitude of indifference and discourtesy towards the partner and his or her feelings, represented by items 6, 14, 30, and 32.
5. Humiliation violence: behaviours of personal criticism directed against the partner's self-esteem and personal pride, neglect, and denial of support, as well as behaviours aimed at lowering the esteem of the person, represented by items 15, 23, 40, and 41.

2.4. Validation of the Instrument

The content validity, internal consistency, construct validity, convergent validity, and discriminative validity of the DVQ-R were evaluated for the Ecuadorian youth population. In the adaptation process, a group of experts made up of nursing professionals with experience in both clinical and teaching settings, and who were familiar with the work of the DVQ-R, considered the discrepancies found by other authors and issued their opinion regarding the coherence, relevance, and thematic clarity of the instrument (Amar & Laughon, 2020). In addition, content validity was assessed by a group of 10 students with socio-demographic characteristics similar to those of the final sample.

Construct validity was assessed by exploratory factor analysis (EFA) and confirmatory factor analysis (CFA) in two stages. Exploratory factor analysis (EFA) was conducted to identify the dimensions of the questionnaire, followed by confirmatory factor analysis (CFA) to validate the factor structure, using the total sample.

EFA was performed using the principal component analysis (PCA) method with oblimin rotation. Each factor of the questionnaire was modelled as a variable and the number of factors was determined for eigenvalues greater than 1. To estimate the reliability of the questionnaire, the internal consistency of each factor was measured by calculating Cronbach's alpha coefficient. Convergent validity was also calculated to estimate the average variance extracted (AVE). An AVE greater than 0.4 indicates that the measurement questions can better reflect the characteristics of each variable in the model (Owens et al., 2024). The discriminative reliability of the scale was tested using the correlation matrix between the factors.

To determine the overall fit of the proposed model, a CFA with the WLSMV (weighted least squares mean and variance adjusted) estimator was performed on the covariance matrix. In addition, a parallel CFA with the 5-dimensional structure described by Rodríguez Franco et al. (2010) was performed to compare the results. The WLSMV estimator was used to estimate the goodness-of-fit parameters, using additional indices to the C and additive fit indices (Knaul et al., 2020) mentioned by Bentler PM and Lévy Mangin (Cerdán Torregrosa et al., 2023; Dion et al., 2023; Romero Méndez et al., 2021).

2.5. Data Analysis

Descriptive analyses and AFE were performed using IBM-SPSS version 25 for MAC. On the other hand, CFA and figure analyses were performed with R version 4.4.1 (14 June 2024) in the R statistical environment using specific packages (The R Foundation, n.d.).

2.6. Ethical Considerations

The study was approved by the Ethics Committee of Hospital Clínica Kennedy HCK-CEISH-20-0031, Guayas province (Ecuador). All participants received a written information sheet and signed an informed consent form. In addition, the author of the original scale was contacted to request permission for the adaptation and validation of the questionnaire.

3. Results

3.1. Description of the Study Sample

The sample was used in its entirety for both exploratory factor analysis (EFA) and confirmatory factor analysis (CFA), which allowed us to explore and thoroughly validate the dimensions of the questionnaire. This approach ensures an adequate representation of the population studied, whose socio-demographic and relational characteristics are shown in Table 1.

Table 1. Socio-demographic and time-related variables of relationships in the study population (n = 340).

	Total n = 340	
	M	D.S
Age	25	4.716
	n	%
Sex		
Female	269	79.1
Male	71	20.9
University		
UCSG	208	61.2
UG	132	38.8
Couple		
No	194	57.1
Yes	146	42.9
Time relationship		
<1 month	3	0.9
1–12 months	20	5.9
1–3 ages	43	12.6
>3 ages	80	23.5

3.2. Content Validity

An expert team of nurses with clinical and teaching experience who were familiar with the work of the DVQ-R confirmed that all proposed items were clearly worded, relevant, and consistent with the construct being measured, i.e., different forms of intimate partner violence victimization. To further enhance the validity of the instrument, content validity was also assessed by a group of 10 students whose socio-demographic characteristics closely matched those of the final sample. The feedback from this group helped ensure that the questions were understandable and relevant to the target population, reflecting their experiences and perceptions of dating violence. For those items where potential confusion was detected, additional explanations were included in parentheses to ensure greater clarity and facilitate respondents' understanding.

3.3. Construct, Convergent, and Discriminant Validity

3.3.1. Exploratory Factor Analysis (EFA)

In order to explore the best factor structure, an exploratory factor analysis (EFA) was conducted. The KMO test value was 0.895 and Bartlett's test of sphericity was significant ($p = 0.001$). During this first analysis, the existence of four factors was demonstrated; although item 4 showed a communality lower than 0.5 (0.366), it was decided to keep it due to its valuable contribution to the construct.

In the final solution, eigenvalues greater than 1 showed the existence of four factors. This solution converged in five iterations and explained 59.73%. The items had factor loadings above 0.50 within their factor and communalities above 0.50 (Table 2). The factor loadings of all items were above the 0.50 threshold (0.537 to 0.811), and the average variance extracted (AVE) was above 0.4.

Table 2. Exploratory factor analysis (EFA) results.

	Communalities	Factor 1	Factor 2	Factor 3	Factor 4
Item 1	0.560				0.741
Item 2	0.694			0.811	
Item 5	0.587		0.755		
Item 6	0.366	0.602			
Item 9	0.545				0.65
Item 10	0.667			0.719	
Item 13	0.619		0.646		
Item 14	0.629	0.613			
Item 15	0.648		0.797		
Item 20	0.594		0.763		
Item 21	0.581	0.712			
Item 23	0.581				0.739
Item 25	0.796			0.900	
Item 26	0.607	0.736			
Item 30	0.523	0.650			
Item 32	0.509				0.537
Item 38	0.643			0.771	
Item 39	0.556	0.687			
Item 40	0.626	0.719			
Item 41	0.615	0.758			
AVE		0.48	0.47	0.60	0.40

The Dating Violence Questionnaire presents four factors in the context of Ecuadorian culture with 20 items. The four factors identified were qualitatively labelled by the research team as follows: Factor 1 includes eight items related to the 'Emotional Neglect and Contempt Dimension': items 6, 14, 21, 26, 30, 39, 40, and 41. Factor 2 contains four items related to the 'Physical Violence and Aggression Dimension': items 5, 13, 15, and 20. Factor 3 contains four items related to the 'Coercion and Control Dimension': Items 2, 10, 25, and 38. Finally, Factor 4 contains four items related to the 'Manipulation and Emotional Testing Dimension': Items 1, 9, 23, and 32.

3.3.2. Convergent and Discriminant Validity

Convergent validity was established, as the mean variance extracted per factor exceeded 0.4, with values of 0.48, 0.47, 0.60, and 0.40, respectively.

Discriminant validity between factors was confirmed when the variance retained by each factor was greater than the variance shared between them (AVE > ϕ^2). The results demonstrated validity among the four factors, as detailed in Table 3.

Table 3. Internal discriminant validity of the scale.

Factor No. 1	Factor No. 2	AVE1	AVE2	φ	φ²	
F1	F2	0.48	0.47	0.33	0.11	SÍ
F1	F3	0.48	0.60	0.51	0.26	SÍ
F1	F4	0.48	0.40	0.48	0.23	SÍ
F2	F3	0.47	0.60	0.23	0.05	SÍ
F2	F4	0.47	0.40	0.29	0.09	SÍ
F3	F4	0.60	0.40	0.35	0.12	SÍ

F1: Emotional Neglect and Contempt Dimension; F2: Coercion and Control Dimension; F3: Physical Violence and Aggression Dimension; F4: Manipulation and Emotional Testing Dimension; AVE1: Average Variance Extracted factor No. 1; AVE2: Average Variance Extracted factor No. 2; φ: interfactorial correlation; φ²: variance.

3.3.3. Internal Consistency

The internal consistency analysis is shown in Table 4. Cronbach's alpha coefficient (α) was 0.839 for the total scale, and all factors scored above 0.7.

Table 4. Alfa coefficient (α) for the four factors of DVQ-R.

Factor	Number of Items	α
F1. Emotional Neglect and Contempt Dimension	8	0.872
F2. Physical Violence and Aggression Dimension	4	0.764
F3. Coercion and Control Dimension	4	0.849
F4. Manipulation and Emotional Testing Dimension	4	0.729
Total scale	20	0.839

3.3.4. Confirmatory Factor Analysis (CFA)

A CFA was then carried out to test the exploratory factor structure of the four-factor model. The results were compared with the five-factor model developed by Rodríguez Franco et al. (2010).

For the estimation of the goodness-of-fit parameters, the WLSMV estimator was used; the fit indices are presented in Table 5. Figure 1 shows the model with the normalized scores. The chi-square (χ^2) values are statistically significant in both models; however, the four-factor measurement model presents a better fit, indicating that the items correctly reflected the latent constructs (Table 5). In particular, the RMSEA value of 0.012 indicates an excellent fit, well below the 0.05 threshold. In addition, the CFI and TLI values of 0.999 reflect a superior fit, exceeding the recommended threshold of 0.90. The GFI and AGFI values also support this conclusion, with values of 0.993 and 0.989, respectively.

Table 5. Expected fit indices for a structural equation model and indices obtained for the confirmatory factor analysis (CFA).

Adjustment Index	Expected	Original Model	4-Factor Model
χ^2	>0.05	0.001	0.001
CMIN/DF	<5	3.849	1.052
GFI	0.90–1	0.976	0.993
AGFI	0.90–1	0.961	0.989
RMR	≈0.5	0.097	0.048
RMSEA	<0.05	0.092	0.012
CFI	0.90–1	0.971	0.999
NFI	0.90–1	0.962	0.989
TLI	0.90–1	0.966	0.999

Abbreviations: χ^2: chi-square; CMIN/DF: discrepancy between chi-square and degrees of freedom; GFI: goodness-of-fit index; AGFI: weighted fit index; RMR: root mean square residual index; RMSEA: root mean square error of approximation; CFI: comparative fit index; NFI: normalized fit index; NNFI or TLI: non-normalized fit index.

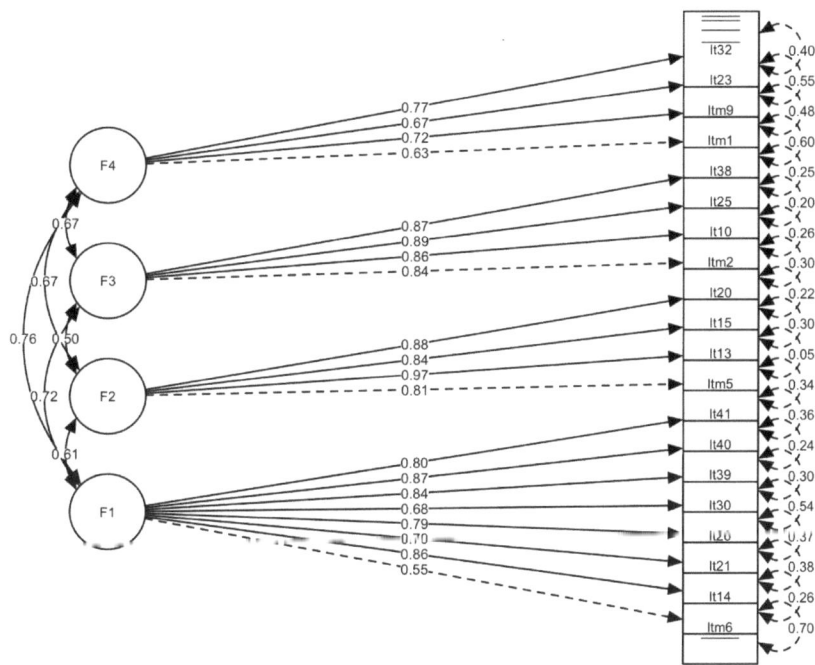

Figure 1. Confirmatory factor analysis of the four-factor model. Confirmatory factor analysis of the four-factor model, with standardised weights and measurement errors for each of the items included in the DVQ-R scale.

3.4. Item Analysis

Table 6 shows a summary of the scores obtained for each factor of the questionnaire, providing a concise overview of the different types of violence experienced by the sample. In particular, Factor 4, 'manipulation and emotional testing', stands out with a mean of 2.03 (S.D. = 0.788). Next, Factor 1, 'emotional neglect and contempt', has a mean of 1.91 (S.D. = 0.806). Factor 3, 'coercion and control', has a mean score of 1.51 with a standard deviation of 0.403. Finally, Factor 2, 'physical violence and aggression', has the lowest score, with a mean of 1.23 (standard deviation of 0.235).

Table 6. Descriptive statistics of the DVQ-R.

	Mean	SD
Factor 1. Emotional Neglect and Contempt Dimension	1.91	0.806
Factor 2. Physical Violence and Aggression Dimension	1.23	0.235
Factor 3. Coercion and Control Dimension	1.51	0.403
Factor 4. Manipulation and Emotional Testing Dimension	2.03	0.788

4. Discussion

To make progress in the fight for gender equality and the eradication of gender-based violence, it is crucial to address the existence of this problem (Amar & Laughon, 2020; Knaul et al., 2020; Owens et al., 2024; Verbeek et al., 2023). Moreover, authors such as Cerdan et al. and other researchers show that violence is currently occurring at increasingly earlier stages (Cerdán Torregrosa et al., 2023; Dion et al., 2023; Romero Méndez et al., 2021), which requires adequate identification and quantification. This study has attempted to evaluate the reliability, validity, and internal consistency of the Dating Violence Questionnaire—

Revised (DVQ-R), adapted to the specific culture and context of Ecuador in a university population of men and women (Appendix A). It is therefore the first in this setting, thus joining those carried out in this line in other countries (Alfaro Urquiola, 2020; Martínez Gómez et al., 2021; Rodríguez Díaz et al., 2017). Furthermore, the results suggest that the questionnaire could be useful for research in other socio-cultural contexts in Latin America, given the similarity of cultural and social patterns in the region.

Compared to previous psychometric validation studies, substantial discrepancies have been observed in both the structure of the questionnaire and the characteristics of the sample. The original model of the DVQ-R postulated five dimensions, including sexual violence, whereas in our study, sexual violence did not emerge as an independent dimension, as Romero et al. have previously documented in Mexico (Anitha & Lewis, 2018). In fact, the prevalence of psychological dating violence shows higher incidence rates compared to physical and sexual violence. However, prevalence studies in high-income countries, such as the United States, Canada, the United Kingdom, and Australia, report levels of IPV that are mainly sexual (Terrazas Carrillo et al., 2024). Furthermore, the absence of sexual violence as a separate dimension might indicate that, in our sample, experiences of sexual violence are more closely related to other forms of maltreatment. This result underscores the interconnectedness of different types of violence in Ecuadorian university dating and highlights the importance of prevention strategies that address these interrelated complexities.

Also, a fusion of elements related to coercion and control was observed in the new dimension 'coercion and control', suggesting that experiences of violence may manifest differently in university contexts. This reinforces the importance of adapting measurement tools to the specific characteristics of the population studied (Campbell et al., 2021; Łukaszek, 2022; Mulumeoderhwa & Harris, 2015). The identification of the dimension 'coercion and control' as an independent factor highlights the uniqueness of these aspects among youth populations. The structural difference found here underlines the need to specifically address power and control dynamics in prevention interventions and policies, recognizing their importance in young adult relationships (De Sousa et al., 2023; Swan et al., 2021; Wong et al., 2023).

Furthermore, these discrepancies could be related to differences in the samples studied. Although young adults share some psychosocial traits with adolescents, they face different emotional and decision-making challenges, which may affect how they perceive and report dating violence (Łukaszek, 2022; Swan et al., 2021). This justifies the need to adapt and validate tools such as the DVQ-R for university populations, ensuring that they capture the specific dynamics of this age group.

Additionally, the separation of 'manipulation and emotional testing' as a distinct dimension reflects the complexity of emotional interactions in dating (Cherrez Santos et al., 2022). This suggests the need to address manipulation tactics and emotional testing separately when addressing dating violence.

To ensure the robustness of the revised structure of the DVQ-R, both internal consistency and construct validity were assessed. Internal consistency, as measured by Cronbach's alpha, demonstrated high reliability for all four factors, ranging from 0.729 to 0.872. This strong consistency reflects the findings of other studies, reaffirming the reliability of the scale. Convergent validity was established, with an average variance extracted (AVE) greater than 0.4 for all factors, confirming that the items of each factor adequately capture the intended constructs. Discriminant validity was also achieved, as the variance retained by each factor was greater than the variance shared between factors (AVE > ϕ^2). These results confirm that the four dimensions represent distinct and independent aspects of dating violence.

The revised four-factor structure was further supported by the model fit indices, which showed significant improvements compared to the original model. Specifically, the discrepancy between chi-square and degrees of freedom (CMIN/DF) improved from 3.849 in the original model to 1.052 in the revised model, while the root mean square error of approximation (RMSEA) decreased from 0.092 to 0.012, indicating an overall better fit. Other indices, such as the goodness-of-fit index (GFI) and the comparative fit index (CFI), also showed improvements, reaching near-perfect values in the revised model (GFI = 0.993, CFI = 0.999), confirming that the updated structure better represents the underlying data for this population.

Finally, the inclusion of both men and women in this study, as opposed to only women, as in Cherrez Santos et al. (2022), was intended to diversify the experiences captured in the DVQ-R. Our results are consistent with those documented by Sanmartín-Andújar et al. (2023), in which the largest differences between men and women were observed in the items of the control domain. This is consistent with multiple studies suggesting that relationship dynamics vary significantly between sexes. These differences in gender dynamics suggest that interventions and prevention strategies should be tailored to address the unique experiences of men and women, especially in terms of power and control (Vives Cases et al., 2021).

In addition, this study represents a first effort to validate the DVQ-R in the Ecuadorian context, a significant contribution given the paucity of research on dating violence in this population. The validation of this instrument allows for a more accurate assessment of the prevalence of dating violence in university students, which is essential for developing effective prevention policies and intervention programmes in Ecuador (Cherrez Santos et al., 2022). The high internal consistency and construct validity demonstrated in this research further support the applicability of the scale in this context, laying the groundwork for future studies in the region.

Limitations

This study has certain limitations that should be highlighted. Although the sample size was sufficient to achieve the objectives set and therefore the internal validity of the study can be considered adequate, the fact that it focused only on a population of university students limits its external validity. To overcome this limitation, this design would need to be replicated with more diverse samples of Ecuadorian youth from different educational contexts. Furthermore, although measures were taken to guarantee the maximum anonymity of the people participating in the study and that the nature of their participation was voluntary, the introduction of social desirability bias in the responses to the questionnaire cannot be ruled out. It should also be borne in mind that cultural differences within the university population and the particularities of the academic environment may have played a significant role in shaping the factor structure. Therefore, the importance of considering cultural diversity, even within the same country, and the need to adapt measurement tools to specific contexts, such as the university environment, should be emphasized. Despite these limitations, we believe that the study offers valuable insights into dating violence in the university context in Ecuador. The incorporation of the opinions of the group of experts brought rigour and coherence to the process of cultural adaptation and validation, helping to maintain a close link between the meaning of the items and the constructs to be explored. Finally, the method followed allowed us to design a questionnaire with solid psychometric properties that we hope will prove useful in the future.

5. Conclusions

The adaptation of the Dating Violence Questionnaire (DVQ-R) to this sample of Ecuadorian university students highlighted significant differences with respect to the original, both in the structure of the questionnaire and in the characteristics of the sample. The new emerging dimensions, the inclusion of people of both sexes, and the influence of the cultural and university context, as well as the specific attention given to the age variable, offer valuable perspectives for future research. Additionally, these results suggest that the adapted questionnaire could be useful for research in other sociocultural contexts in Latin America, given the similarities in cultural and social patterns across the region. These findings underscore the importance of tailoring measurement tools to the specific dynamics of different populations, which will be essential for developing effective prevention strategies and interventions aimed at addressing IPV in university settings.

Author Contributions: M.J.M.-A.: Conceptualization, Investigation, Methodology, Supervision, Writing—original draft. R.E.M.-A.: Investigation, Supervision, Writing—review and editing. I.G.-G.: Methodology, Supervision, Writing—review and editing. M.A.Á.-S.: Data curation, Formal analysis, Methodology, Investigation, Writing—original draft. A.M.A.-J.: Conceptualization, Writing—review and editing. E.M.-G.: Conceptualization, Supervision, Writing—review and editing. All authors have read and agreed to the published version of the manuscript.

Funding: This research was funded by the Universidad Catolica de Santiago de Guayaquil, grant number 0030-2022. The funder had no role in the study design; in the collection, analysis, or interpretation of the data; writing the manuscript; or the decision to submit the paper for publication.

Institutional Review Board Statement: The study was conducted in accordance with the Declaration of Helsinki and approved by the Ethics Committee of the Hospital Clinica Kennedy HCK-CEISH-20-0031, Guayas province (Ecuador), approval date: 14 January 2022.

Informed Consent Statement: Due informed consent was obtained from all participants involved in the study.

Data Availability Statement: Data are contained within the article.

Conflicts of Interest: The authors declare no conflicts of interest.

Appendix A. Dating Violence Questionnaire (DVQ-R)

1. He/she tests your love, setting traps to check if you cheat on him/her if you love him/her or if you are faithful to him/her.
2. You feel obliged (0) to have sex in order not to give explanations.
5. He/she has hit you (5).
6. He/she is good at studying, but he/she is late for appointments, doesn't keep his/her promises and is irresponsible.
9. Talks to you about love affairs that he/she imagines you have.
10. Insists on touching you in ways that you don't like and don't want.
13. Has hit, pushed, shoved, or pulled you.
14. Does not recognize any responsibility for the relationship or for what happens to both of you.
15. Criticizes you, underestimates your character and/or humiliates your self-esteem.
20. Has thrown blunt objects at you.
21. Hurt you with an object.
23. Ridiculed the way you express yourself.
25. Stopped you from leaving.
26. You feel forced to perform certain sexual acts.
30. Ignores your feelings.

32. Stops talking to you or disappears for several days without explanation as a way of showing his/her anger.
38. Invades your space (listens to loud music when you are studying, interrupts you when you are alone, etc.), invades your privacy (reads your messages, listens to your phone conversations, etc.).
39. Forces you to undress when you don't want to.
40. Has ridiculed or insulted your beliefs, religion, or social class.
41. Ridicules or insults you for the ideas you hold.

Titles for each factor:

Factor 1: Emotional Neglect and Contempt

- Items: 6, 14, 21, 26, 30, 39, 40 and 41.
- Description: This factor appears to be related to behaviours involving emotional disregard and neglect in the relationship, including ridiculing beliefs and lack of acknowledgement towards each other's feelings.

Factor 2: Physical Violence and Aggression

- Items: 5, 13, 15, and 20.
- Description: This factor appears to be related to behaviours of physical violence and aggression, including hitting, pushing, and shoving, and humiliation towards the partner.

Factor 3: Coercion and Control

- Items: 2, 10, 25, and 38.
- Description: This factor encompasses controlling and coercive behaviours, including unwanted sexual pressures and invasion of the partner's privacy and personal space.

Factor 4: Manipulation and Emotional Testing

- Items: 1, 9, 23, and 32.
- Description: This factor involves manipulative behaviours and emotional testing, such as setting traps to assess fidelity and manipulating each other's emotions through tactics such as prolonged silence.

References

Alfaro Urquiola, A. L. (2020). Validación del cuestionario de violencia en el noviazgo (CUVINO-R) en una muestra de jóvenes paceños. *Ajayu*, *18*(1), 102–120. Available online: http://www.scielo.org.bo/scielo.php?script=sci_arttext&pid=S2077-21612020000100005 (accessed on 30 October 2024).

Amar, A., & Laughon, K. (2020). Gender violence prevention in middle school male athletics programs. *JAMA Pediatrics*, *174*(3), 233–234. [CrossRef]

An, S., Choi, G. Y., Yun, S. H., Joon Choi, Y., Son, E., Cho, H., Gharbi, V. C., & Hong, S. (2023). Intimate partner violence among hispanic/latinx and white college students. *Violence and Victims*, *38*(4), 513–535. [CrossRef] [PubMed]

Anitha, S., & Lewis, R. (2018). *Gender based violence in university communities: Policy, prevention and educational initiatives* (1.a ed.). Bristol University Press. [CrossRef]

Association of American Universities. (2015). *AAU climate survey on sexual assault and sexual misconduct*. Available online: https://www.aau.edu/key-issues/aau-climate-survey-sexual-assault-and-sexual-misconduct-2015 (accessed on 11 November 2024).

Bhochhibhoya, S., Maness, S. B., Cheney, M., & Larson, D. (2021). risk factors for sexual violence among college students in dating relationships: An ecological approach. *Journal of Interpersonal Violence*, *36*(15–16), 7722–7746. [CrossRef]

Buquet Corleto, A. (2011). Transversalización de la perspectiva de género en la educación superior. Problemas conceptuales y prácticos. *Perfiles Educativos*, *XXXIII*, 211–225.

Campbell, J. C., Sabri, B., Budhathoki, C., Kaufman, M. R., Alhusen, J., & Decker, M. R. (2021). Unwanted Sexual Acts Among University Students: Correlates of Victimization and Perpetration. *Journal of Interpersonal Violence*, *36*(1–2), NP504–NP526. [CrossRef] [PubMed]

Cerdán Torregrosa, A., Nardini, K., & Vives Cases, C. (2023). «I reject it, but that's what normally happens»: Grey zones of gender-based violence and gender roles in young people. *Journal of Interpersonal Violence*, *38*(11–12), 7656–7677. [CrossRef]

Cherrez Santos, A. V., Alulema-Sanchez, S., & Juarros Basterretxea, J. (2022). Propiedades psicométricas del dating violence questionnaire—R en mujeres de Ecuador. *R.E.M.A. Revista Electrónica de Metodología Aplicada*, 24(1), 1–12. [CrossRef]

Coulter, R. W. S., Mair, C., Miller, E., Blosnich, J. R., Matthews, D. D., & McCauley, H. L. (2017). Prevalence of past-year sexual assault victimization among undergraduate students: Exploring differences by and intersections of gender identity, sexual identity, and race/ethnicity. *Prevention Science: The Official Journal of the Society for Prevention Research*, 18(6), 726–736. [CrossRef]

De Sousa, D., Paradis, A., Fernet, M., Couture, S., & Fortin, A. (2023). «I felt imprisoned»: A qualitative exploration of controlling behaviors in adolescent and emerging adult dating relationships. *Journal of Adolescence*, 95(5), 907–921. [CrossRef]

Dion, J., Hébert, M., Sadikaj, G., Girouard, A., Godbout, N., Martin-Storey, A., Blais, M., & Bergeron, S. (2023). Dating violence trajectories in adolescence: How do they relate to sexual outcomes in Canada? *Archives of Sexual Behavior*, 52(7), 2749–2765. [CrossRef] [PubMed]

Galdo Castiñeiras, J. A., Hernández Morante, J. J., & Morales Moreno, I. (2023). Educational intervention to decrease justification of adolescent dating violence: A comparative quasi-experimental study. *Healthcare*, 11(8), 1156. [CrossRef]

Gebrie, S., Wasihun, Y., Abegaz, Z., & Kebede, N. (2022). Gender-based violence and associated factors among private college female students in Dessie City, Ethiopia: Mixed method study. *BMC Women's Health*, 22(1), 513. [CrossRef]

Gómez, M. P., Delgado, A. O., & Gómez, Á. H. (2014). Violencia en relaciones de pareja de jóvenes y adolescentes. *Revista Latinoamericana de Psicología*, 46(3), 148–159. [CrossRef]

INEC. (2019). *Encuesta nacional sobre relaciones familiares y violencia de género contra las mujeres (ENVIGMU)*. INEC. Available online: https://www.ecuadorencifras.gob.ec/documentos/web-inec/Estadisticas_Sociales/Violencia_de_genero_2019/Boletin_Tecnico_ENVIGMU.pdf (accessed on 30 July 2024).

Kaukinen, C. (2014). Dating violence among college students: The risk and protective factors. *Trauma, Violence & Abuse*, 15(4), 283–296. [CrossRef]

Knaul, F. M., Bustreo, F., & Horton, R. (2020). Countering the pandemic of gender-based violence and maltreatment of young people: The Lancet Commission. *The Lancet*, 395(10218), 98–99. [CrossRef]

Łukaszek, M. (2022). Patterns of university students' risky sexual experiences and their characteristics. *International Journal of Environmental Research and Public Health*, 19(21), 14239. [CrossRef] [PubMed]

Martínez Gómez, J. A., Bolívar Suárez, Y., Yanez Peñuñuri, L. Y., & Gaviria Gómez, A. M. (2021). Validación del cuestionario de violencia entre novios (DVQ-R) para víctimas en jóvenes adultos colombianos y mexicanos. *RELIEVE—Revista Electrónica de Investigación y Evaluación Educativa*, 27(2). [CrossRef]

Medina Maldonado, V., del Mar Pastor Bravo, M., Vargas, E., Francisco, J., & Ruiz, I. J. (2022). Adolescent dating violence: Results of a mixed study in Quito, Ecuador. *Journal of Interpersonal Violence*, 37(17–18), NP15205–NP15230. [CrossRef]

Miller, E., & McCaw, B. (2019). Intimate partner violence. *New England Journal of Medicine*, 380(9), 850–857. [CrossRef]

Mulumeoderhwa, M., & Harris, G. (2015). Forced sex, rape and sexual exploitation: Attitudes and experiences of high school students in South Kivu, Democratic Republic of Congo. *Culture, Health & Sexuality*, 17(3), 284–295. [CrossRef]

Neilson, E. C., Gulati, N. K., Stappenbeck, C. A., George, W. H., & Davis, K. C. (2023). Emotion regulation and intimate partner violence perpetration in undergraduate samples: A review of the literature. *Trauma, Violence & Abuse*, 24(2), 576–596. [CrossRef]

Owens, J., Aboul Enein, B. H., Bernstein, J., Dodge, E., & J Kelly, P. (2024). Reducing violence against women and girls in the Arab League: A systematic review of preventive interventions. *Trauma, Violence & Abuse*, 25, 2219–2233. [CrossRef]

Oyarzún, J., Pereda, N., & Guilera, G. (2021). The prevalence and severity of teen dating violence victimization in community and at-risk adolescents in Spain. *New Directions for Child and Adolescent Development*, 2021(178), 39–58. [CrossRef]

Red de Desarrollo Social de América Latina y el Caribe. (2017). *Violencia en las relaciones de noviazgo entre adolescentes en Brasil y Honduras: Resumen ejecutivo*. Available online: https://dds.cepal.org/redesoc/portal/publicaciones/ficha/?id=4650 (accessed on 30 October 2024).

Rodríguez Díaz, F. J., Herrero, J., Rodríguez Franco, L., Bringas Molleda, C., Paíno Quesada, S. G., & Pérez, B. (2017). Validation of dating violence questionnarie-R (DVQ-R). *International Journal of Clinical and Health Psychology*, 17(1), 77–84. [CrossRef]

Rodríguez Franco, L., López Cepero Borrego, J., Rodríguez Díaz, F. J., Bringas Molleda, C., Antuña Bellerín, M. de los Á., & Estrada Pineda, C. (2010). Validation of the dating violence questionnaire, DVQ (cuestionario de violencia entre novios CUVINO) among Spanish-speaking youth: Analysis of results in Spain, Mexico and Argentina. *Anuario de Psicología Clínica y de La Salud*, 6, 43–50.

Romero Méndez, C. A., Rojas Solís, J. L., & Greathouse Amador, L. M. (2021). Co-ocurrencia de distintos tipos de violencia interpersonal en adolescentes mexicanos. *Pedagogia Social Revista Interuniversitaria*, 38, 137–150. [CrossRef]

Sanmartín-Andújar, M., Vila Fariñas, A., Pérez Ríos, M., Rey Brandariz, J., Candal Pedreira, C., Martín-Gisbert, L., Rial-Vázquez, J., Ruano Ravina, A., & Varela Lema, L. (2023). Perception of dating violence among adolescents. Transversal study. *Revista Española de salud pública*, 97, e202306056. [PubMed]

Swan, L. E. T., Mennicke, A., & Kim, Y. (2021). Reproductive coercion and interpersonal violence victimization experiences among college students. *Journal of Interpersonal Violence*, 36(23–24), 11281–11303. [CrossRef]

Terrazas Carrillo, E., Sabina, C., Vásquez, D. A., & Garcia, E. (2024). Cultural Correlates of dating violence in a combined gender group of Latino college students. *Journal of Interpersonal Violence*, *39*(3–4), 785–810. [CrossRef]
The R Foundation. (n.d.). *R: El proyecto R para el cálculo estadístico*. Available online: https://www.r-project.org/ (accessed on 30 October 2024).
Valls, R., Puigvert, L., Melgar, P., & Garcia Yeste, C. (2016). Breaking the silence at Spanish universities: Findings from the first study of violence against women on campuses in Spain. *Violence Against Women*, *22*(13), 1519–1539. [CrossRef]
Verbeek, M., Weeland, J., Luijk, M., & van de Bongardt, D. (2023). Sexual and dating violence prevention programs for male youth: A systematic review of program characteristics, intended psychosexual outcomes, and effectiveness. *Archives of Sexual Behavior*, *52*(7), 2899–2935. [CrossRef]
Vives Cases, C., Pérez Martínez, V., Davó Blanes, M., Sánchez SanSegundo, M., Gil González, D., Abiétar, D. G., Sánchez Martínez, F., Forcadell Díez, L., Pérez, G., & Sanz Barbero, B. (2021). Dating violence and associated factors among male and female adolescents in Spain. *PLoS ONE*, *16*(11), e0258994. [CrossRef]
Wiklund, M., Bengs, C., Malmgren Olsson, E.-B., & Ohman, A. (2010). Young women facing multiple and intersecting stressors of modernity, gender orders and youth. *Social Science & Medicine*, *71*(9), 1567–1575. [CrossRef]
Wong, J. S., Bouchard, J., & Lee, C. (2023). The effectiveness of college dating violence prevention programs: A meta-analysis. *Trauma, Violence & Abuse*, *24*(2), 684–701. [CrossRef]
World Health Organización. (2021). *Devastatingly pervasive: 1 in 3 women globally experience violence*. Available online: https://www.who.int/news/item/09-03-2021-devastatingly-pervasive-1-in-3-women-globally-experience-violence (accessed on 10 July 2024).
Yanez Peñúñuri, L. Y., Hidalgo Rasmussen, C. A., & Chávez Flores, Y. V. (2019). Revisión sistemática de instrumentos de violencia en el noviazgo en Iberoamérica y evaluación de sus propiedades de medida. *Ciência & Saúde Coletiva*, *24*, 2249–2262. [CrossRef]
Zark, L., & Satyen, L. (2022). Cross-cultural differences in student attitudes toward intimate partner violence: A systematic review. *Trauma, Violence & Abuse*, *23*(3), 1007–1022. [CrossRef]

Disclaimer/Publisher's Note: The statements, opinions and data contained in all publications are solely those of the individual author(s) and contributor(s) and not of MDPI and/or the editor(s). MDPI and/or the editor(s) disclaim responsibility for any injury to people or property resulting from any ideas, methods, instructions or products referred to in the content.

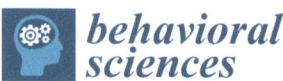 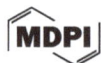

Review

Refuting Six Misconceptions about Romantic Love

Sandra J. E. Langeslag

Department of Psychological Sciences, University of Missouri—St. Louis, St. Louis, MO 63121, USA; langeslags@umsl.edu

Abstract: Scientific research on romantic love has been relatively sparse but is becoming more prevalent, as it should. Unfortunately, several misconceptions about romantic love are becoming entrenched in the popular media and/or the scientific community, which hampers progress. Therefore, I refute six misconceptions about romantic love in this article. I explain why (1) romantic love is not necessarily dyadic, social, or interpersonal, (2) love is not an emotion, (3) romantic love does not just have positive effects, (4) romantic love is not uncontrollable, (5) there is no dedicated love brain region, neurotransmitter, or hormone, and (6) pharmacological manipulation of romantic love is not near. To increase progress in our scientific understanding of romantic love, I recommend that we study the intrapersonal aspects of romantic love including the intensity of love, that we focus our research questions and designs using a component process model of romantic love, and that we distinguish hypotheses and suggestions from empirical findings when citing previous work.

Keywords: love; close relationships; misconceptions; myths; emotions; brain; neuroscience

Citation: Langeslag, S.J.E. Refuting Six Misconceptions about Romantic Love. *Behav. Sci.* **2024**, *14*, 383. https://doi.org/10.3390/bs14050383

Academic Editors: Bianca P. Acevedo and Adam Bode

Received: 7 March 2024
Revised: 15 April 2024
Accepted: 30 April 2024
Published: 2 May 2024

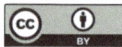

Copyright: © 2024 by the author. Licensee MDPI, Basel, Switzerland. This article is an open access article distributed under the terms and conditions of the Creative Commons Attribution (CC BY) license (https://creativecommons.org/licenses/by/4.0/).

1. Introduction

There is a growing interest in the science of romantic love, as evident from the increased number of publications on this topic, the organization of scientific conferences devoted to research on love, and the publication of special journal issues like this one. This growing interest is exciting and warranted for two reasons. First, love pertains to virtually everyone. For example, more than 80% of adolescents in a study in the US reported to have been involved in at least one romantic relationship by the age of 18 [1] and love has been observed in almost all cultures that have been studied [2]. Second, when people fall in love, it greatly impacts their lives. People are sometimes even willing to change their friends, job, country, or religion to be with their beloved [3]. It is important that we conduct thorough scientific research on romantic love and that we disseminate the results broadly. Unfortunately, there are several misconceptions about romantic love that are permeating popular media, the scientific community, or both. Some of these misconceptions stem from lay people's and scientists' assumptions about romantic love. Other misconceptions stem from hypotheses or interpretations put forth in scientific articles being cited in other articles as empirical evidence. Collectively, these misconceptions are hampering the progress of the scientific understanding of romantic love. In this article, I refute six of those misconceptions and provide recommendations for research.

The misconceptions refuted in this article concern romantic love, which is love for a significant other (as opposed to love for family members or friends, for example) and can be experienced regardless of whether someone is in a romantic relationship with the beloved. Scientists have proposed several taxonomies of love, each with various numbers and different types of love, e.g., [4–7]. Because the word "love" does not have a plural form, I use the term "love feelings" to refer to a collection of different love types (note that the term "feeling" does not necessarily refer to an emotion [8]). In my work, I have distinguished between the following types of romantic love: infatuation (or passionate love), attachment (or companionate love), and sexual desire (cf. [5]). Infatuation is the overwhelming, amorous feeling for one individual that is typically most intense during the early stage of love (i.e., when individuals are not (yet) in a relationship with their beloved or are in a new relationship). Attachment, on the other hand, is the comforting feeling of emotional bonding with another individual that takes some time to develop, often in the context of a romantic relationship [5,6,9]. Sexual desire is the craving for sexual gratification [5]. Even though some of the arguments below may depend on certain definitions or taxonomies of love, those arguments are never the sole argument used to refute a misconception. Therefore, the overall refutation of each misconception does not hinge on specific definitions or taxonomies of love.

2. Romantic Love Is Not Necessarily Dyadic, Social, or Interpersonal

The first misconception is that romantic love is dyadic, social, or interpersonal, and that it only exists within romantic relationships. For example, one anonymous reviewer of one of my manuscripts commented that "It's odd that ~1/6 of the sample who were purportedly "in love" were not in a relationship with the target of their love." While romantic love has obvious interpersonal aspects (i.e., people are in love with another person and romantic relationships involve more than one person by definition), romantic love is not *necessarily* dyadic, social, or interpersonal, and can be experienced outside of the context of a romantic relationship.

In contrast to what the reviewer seemed to think, it does not take two to love. For example, people may develop love feelings for someone before they become involved in a romantic relationship with that person [9], or may still experience love feelings after a romantic relationship has ended [10]. People may experience love feelings that are not reciprocated and may love someone they have never been and will never be in a romantic relationship with. People can even experience love feelings for someone they have never interacted with. For example, people can experience love at first sight [11] and some people develop one-sided, parasocial attachment to celebrities [12]. Interestingly, people even report experiencing parasocial attachment to fictional characters in movies, TV shows, video games, and books [13,14]. Finally, people may experience sexual arousal in the absence of (thoughts of) another individual, such as during masturbation, which suggests that sexual desire, which has been considered a type of love by some researchers [5], may not require a target at all.

So, romantic love is not necessarily dyadic, social, or interpersonal, and does not only exist within romantic relationships. Therefore, we need to broaden our approach and study the intrapersonal aspects of romantic love as well. This does not require the study of dyads who are in a relationship with each other, but can be achieved by studying individuals who are experiencing love feelings, regardless of their relationship status. This also means that besides fitting into the realm of social psychology/neuroscience, research on romantic love fits into the realm of affective and cognitive (neuro)science.

Due to the social emphasis of previous research on romantic love, researchers have often focused on relationship satisfaction rather than intrapersonal love feelings. It is important to note, though, that romantic love is not the same as relationship satisfaction. People can be satisfied with a relationship if it fulfils some need (e.g., money, housekeeping, sex, protection, child care, status, personal growth), rather than experiencing love for their partner [15]. And, in abusive relationships, conversely, it is possible that the victim is in love with their abuser while being unsatisfied with the relationship. In a sample of married individuals, the correlation between relationship satisfaction and attachment level was high but nowhere near perfect (.68), and the correlation between relationship satisfaction and infatuation level was only .18 [16]. And, in a meta-analysis of 25 questionnaire studies, the correlations between relationship satisfaction and the intensity of different types of love (i.e., infatuation, attachment, eros, and mania) ranged between $-.02$ and .56 [17]. These findings confirm that even though relationship satisfaction and intensity of love feelings may be related, they are distinct concepts.

Because romantic love is distinct from relationship satisfaction, relationship satisfaction—while interesting in its own right—should not be used as a proxy for love intensity in research. Relationship satisfaction can be assessed using items such as "How happy/satisfied are you in your relationship with___?" or using questionnaires such as the Couples Satisfaction Index (CSI-32) [18] or the Revised Dyadic Adjustment Scale (RDAS) [19]. Intensity of love feelings, on the other hand, can be assessed using items such as "How in love with/infatuated with/attached to___are you?" or questionnaires such as Infatuation and Attachment Scales [9].

3. Love Is Not an Emotion

The second misconception is that love is an emotion (similar to fear, anger, sadness, surprise, disgust, and joy, for example). Lay people typically consider love to be an emotion [20,21] and so do some scientists [22,23]. Although it depends on how emotions are defined, there are several reasons to assume that love is not an emotion.

As mentioned above, although scientists do not agree on how many and which types of love exist, they do agree that there are multiple types of love [4–7]. There being multiple types of love is one reason to assume that love *as a whole* is not an emotion [24]. There are also reasons to assume that the different types of love themselves are not emotions either. First, love elicits various emotions depending on the situation. When infatuation is requited, for example, it may elicit the emotion joy [25], yet it may elicit the emotion sadness when it is unrequited [26]. Note that this is different from how emotions can elicit meta-emotions, which are emotions about one's own emotions [27]. An example of a meta-emotion is when someone is anxious about an upcoming presentation and then feels shame about being anxious. The emotions elicited as a result of love, in contrast, are not *about* being in love. For example, someone who is in love may feel jealous when their beloved attends to others, but they are not jealous about being in love. Second, it has been shown that distraction after a romantic breakup decreased negative affect but not the intensity of love, and that negative reappraisal of an ex-partner decreased love intensity yet increased negative affect [10,28]. These observed dissociations indicate that love regulation and emotion regulation are conceptually distinct. That is, love regulation targets love feelings (such as infatuation and attachment), whereas emotion regulation targets emotions (such as fear, anger, sadness, surprise, disgust, and joy) [10]. Third, another reason why love feelings are not emotions is that love feelings can be very long lasting, whereas emotions are usually shorter lasting. Research has shown that emotions typically last for a half hour up to several days. The longest lasting emotion was sadness, with a median duration until a first return to baseline of 48 h (i.e., 2 days) and a median duration until permanent return to baseline of 120 h (i.e., 5 days) [29]. In contrast, it is not uncommon for infatuation to last for weeks or months and for attachment to last for years or decades [9,30].

Rather than an emotion, scientists have categorized love as an attitude [31], a script [32], or a motivation or drive (similar to craving, hunger, and thirst) [24,33–35]. Although refuting the misconception that love is an emotion may just seem a quibble about semantics, it does suggest that we should not assume that any knowledge we have about emotions generalizes to romantic love.

4. Romantic Love Does Not Just Have Positive Effects

The third misconception is that romantic love has mainly positive effects, which has contributed to the relative paucity of scientific interest in romantic love (e.g., in terms of the number of publications, journals, scientific societies, and grant mechanisms). Of course, love has a plethora of positive effects on people and society. Infatuation, for example, elicits positive emotions such as euphoria [25], and romantic relationships enhance happiness and life satisfaction [36]. It is often overlooked, however, that love has many negative effects on people and society as well.

First, love can elicit several negative emotions. For example, infatuation is stressful [37], love can be accompanied by jealousy [38], the death of a romantic partner may elicit intense grief [39], and unreciprocated love and romantic breakups elicit sadness and shame [26]. Second, love may reduce general well-being. For example, romantic breakups are a main risk factor for major depressive disorder in adolescents [40] and dysfunctional romantic relationships and romantic breakups are associated with decreased happiness and life satisfaction [41,42]. Third, people who are in love may be distracted from their duties (e.g., work or homework) because they think about their beloved all the time [43,44]. Even though this may not bother the infatuated individual, it may result in a loss of productivity. Fourth, love plays a role in several mental disorders, including sexual dysfunctions, paraphilic disorders, and erotomanic and jealous delusional disorders [45], as well as in suicide behavior [46]. Finally, love is associated with various forms of criminal behavior including stalking [47], domestic violence [48,49], and homicide [50].

It may be clear that love has both positive and negative effects. Taken together, the negative effects of love cause substantial individual, social, and economic burden, and underscore the great need to study romantic love. It is my hope that thorough research on romantic love can both increase the positive effects of love and decrease its negative effects on individuals and society.

5. Romantic Love Is Not Uncontrollable

The fourth misconception is that love should not and/or cannot be controlled. An anonymous reviewer for one of my grant proposals on love regulation asked: "Do we want to be able to control our love feelings?"

Indeed, it is not uncommon for people to think that love should not be controlled because it is a natural process [28]. Nevertheless, there are many situations in which it might be beneficial to regulate love feelings. For example, love feelings may be stronger than desired, such as when people are still in love with their ex-partner after a breakup, when the love is forbidden, and when people are in love with someone who treats them poorly. In situations like those, people may want to decrease how in love they are. Successful down-regulation of love feelings could ameliorate heartbreak. It could also help people to stop pursuing an inappropriate partner or to put an end to a dysfunctional (e.g., abusive) relationship. At other times, love feelings may be weaker than desired, such as when they decline in long-term relationships [9,30]. Successful up-regulation of love may stabilize long-term relationships.

In addition, some people think that love regulation is difficult or even impossible [25,28]. People think that other people are better at love regulation than they are, that who they are in love with is less controllable than love intensity, and that infatuation is even less controllable than attachment and sexual desire [10,28,51,52]. Nevertheless, a series of studies have shown that people *can* control different types of love using behavioral and cognitive strategies. Specifically, looking at pictures of the beloved increases infatuation and attachment [16], positive reappraisal of the beloved, the relationship, and/or the future increases attachment [28,53], and sexual imagery increases sexual desire and infatuation [53]. Conversely, negative reappraisal of the beloved, the relationship, and/or the future decreases infatuation and attachment [10,28].

In short, misconceptions that love regulation is undesirable and/or difficult exist. Given that love regulation is possible and can be adaptive, these misconceptions have negative consequences for well-being. Therefore, lay people need to be educated about the feasibility and benefits of love regulation, and scientists should not let their own misconceptions keep them and others from studying this important topic.

6. There Is No Dedicated Love Brain Region, Love Neurotransmitter, or Love Hormone

The fifth misconception is that there is a dedicated love brain region, love neurotransmitter, and/or love hormone. This misconception is more prevalent in lay people than in scientists (the #1 question that I am asked in interviews for popular media is which brain region is involved in love) and reflects a lack of knowledge of how the brain and body work more than a misconception about love specifically.

Generally, there is no one-to-one mapping between anatomy and function. Each brain region, neurotransmitter, and hormone has multiple functions, and each function requires multiple brain regions, neurotransmitters, and/or hormones. Love affects behaviors, feelings, cognition, and physiology in many different ways [25]. Each of these 'components' of romantic love depends on a different network of brain regions, and multiple neurotransmitters and/or hormones. Take, for example, the enhanced memory for information that is related to the beloved, which is related to the arousal that this information elicits [54]. We know that enhanced memory for arousing information depends on the amygdala and hippocampus, the neurotransmitter noradrenaline, and the hormones adrenaline and cortisol [55,56]. Therefore, it can be expected that those brain regions, neurotransmitters, and hormones are involved in the memory bias for the beloved. And, take the increased skin conductance response to the beloved [57]. We know that skin conductance responses result from the release of the neurotransmitter acetylcholine in the sympathetic nervous system, which, in turn, is innervated by the paraventricular nucleus of the hypothalamus [58]. Therefore, that brain region and neurotransmitter likely play a role in the skin conductance response to the beloved. I hope that these two examples clarify how different brain networks, neurotransmitters, and hormones are involved in the different components of romantic love. This component process model reflects an approach that aims to understand romantic love as an emergent process that consists of numerous components, each with its own neurobiological basis.

Even though scientists typically understand that there is no dedicated love brain region, love neurotransmitter, or love hormone, they could improve the focus of their research questions and designs according to the component process model. Many neuroimaging studies on romantic love (including some of my own) use a passive viewing design, which makes it difficult to interpret the findings without resorting to reverse inference, which is the inference of mental states from neuroimaging data [59]. By having participants complete specific tasks during neuroimaging (e.g., a memory, attention, or regulation task) instead, the findings become more interpretable in terms of mental states, which will then allow us to learn that brain network/neurotransmitter/hormone X plays a role in component Y of romantic love.

7. Pharmacological Manipulation of Romantic Love Is Not Near

The final misconception is that our recent knowledge of the biological basis of romantic love will soon lead to a pharmacological route to control romantic love [60–63], which is something that people have pursued for ages. Even nowadays, people across the world wishfully use aphrodisiac substances and love philters [64]. However, although evidence-based pharmacological manipulation of love feelings may be feasible at some point in the future, several issues prevent the development of an effective and safe 'love pill' in the short term.

First, the scientific community has only just begun to unravel the psychopharmacology of love. We are only starting to learn which neurotransmitters and hormones might play a role in the different types of love. For example, several functional Magnetic Resonance Imaging (fMRI) studies have shown that brain regions such as the caudate, putamen, ventral tegmental area, insula, cingulate cortex, and inferior frontal gyrus are more active when people view pictures of their beloved than when they view pictures of other people [65–72]. Some of those regions (especially the caudate, putamen, and ventral tegmental area) are dopaminergic brain regions, and their activation in response to the beloved has been interpreted as evidence for the notion that romantic love is associated with increased levels of the neurotransmitter dopamine. However, it is important to note that fMRI studies cannot reveal whether dopamine is released in response to the beloved. To my knowledge, there is only one study that has actually measured dopamine levels when people view pictures of their beloved (compared to when they view pictures of friends), using positron emission tomography (PET). That study showed more dopamine release in response to the beloved pictures than the friend pictures in the medial orbitofrontal and prefrontal cortices, but surprisingly not in the more typical dopaminergic regions [73]. So, more research is needed on whether and where dopamine is released when people see their beloved. As another example, it has been hypothesized that romantic love is associated with reduced levels of serotonin because of its resemblance with obsessive–compulsive disorder [25]. In one study, however, women who were in love had higher blood serotonin levels than women who were not in love, and obsessive thinking about the beloved in women was associated with an increased serotonin level in serum [43]. So we cannot conclude at this time that romantic love is associated with reduced serotonin levels. In addition, we are still far from understanding any *causal* relationships between psychopharmacology and love feelings. For example, many studies compare people who are in love when they view stimuli that are related to their beloved with when they view other stimuli. It would be informative, but more difficult, to compare participants who are in love with participants who are not in love or even to compare people before and after they fall in love. Crucially, in order to develop a 'love pill' we would have to prove that alteration of neurotransmitter or hormone levels actually results in a change in the intensity of love.

Second, it would be challenging to design a drug that targets love feelings for one person specifically, which would be desirable in at least some situations. For example, someone who is married might want to decrease their love feelings for a crush without changing (or while increasing) their love for their spouse. Third, because the neurotransmitters and hormones involved in love have many different functions, any love drug that affects the levels of these neurotransmitters or hormones may have side effects that could be adverse. Finally, pharmacological manipulation of love feelings is associated with ethical issues such as who decides whether and when someone takes a love drug to increase or decrease their love feelings [60,61]. Compared to pharmacological manipulation of love feelings, behavioral and cognitive strategies to regulate love feelings like the ones mentioned before (i.e., looking at pictures of the beloved, positive or negative reappraisal of the beloved, the relationship, and/or the future, and sexual imagery) are associated with fewer physical and ethical risks and can be implemented right away.

In addition, I hope that the examples about dopamine and serotonin show that we need to be careful when citing previous work. That is, we should be specific when describing previous research findings (e.g., dopaminergic regions becoming more active vs. dopamine levels being elevated). Additionally, when citing researchers' suggestions and hypotheses (e.g., love being associated with high dopamine and low serotonin levels), we need to label them as such so that they are not taken as empirical evidence by the reader.

8. Conclusions

Science is making great strides in understanding romantic love. In this article, I have refuted six common misconceptions that exist in lay people and/or scientists, in the hopes that this will allow us to make even greater progress. Alongside the social science of romantic relationships, the cognitive and affective neuroscience of romantic love could mature into its own important field of research that focuses on the intrapersonal aspects of romantic love, including the intensity of love. Different types of love and the various emotions have some similarities, so we can be inspired by our knowledge of emotions, but because love is not an emotion we cannot assume that anything we know about emotions also applies to romantic love. We need to realize that love has multiple negative effects, which underscores the importance of research on this topic. And despite what people may think, it is possible and may be beneficial to control love feelings. Future research can explore what strategies are effective and adaptive in which situations. I also recommend focusing our research questions and designs using a component process model of romantic love. Finally, more work needs to be done to understand the (causal) role that various brain networks, neurotransmitters, and hormones play in romantic love. When citing previous work, we need to distinguish suggestions from empirical findings and recognize the limits of information that a certain research method provides.

To conclude, research on romantic love is extremely important because it pertains to almost everyone and because it affects people to a great extent, both good and bad. I recommend that we do not let our misconceptions guide what we study and that we cite previous work precisely, so that the science of romantic love can be an even more fruitful field of research that will benefit individuals and societies.

Funding: This research received no external funding.

Data Availability Statement: No new data were created or analyzed in this study. Data sharing is not applicable to this article.

Conflicts of Interest: The author declares no conflicts of interest.

References

1. Carver, K.; Joyner, K.; Udry, J.R. *National Estimates of Adolescent Romantic Relationships, in Adolescent Romantic Relations and Sexual Behavior: Theory, Research, and Practical Implications*; Florsheim, P., Ed.; Lawrence Erlbaum Associates Publishers: Mahwah, NJ, USA, 2003; pp. 23–56.
2. Jankowiak, W.R.; Fischer, E.F. A cross-cultural perspective on romantic love. *Ethnology* **1992**, *31*, 149–155. [CrossRef]
3. Aron, E.N.; Aron, A. Extremities of love: The sudden sacrifice of career, family, dignity. *J. Soc. Clin. Psychol.* **1997**, *16*, 200–212. [CrossRef]
4. Berscheid, E. Love in the fourth dimension. *Annu. Rev. Psychol.* **2010**, *61*, 1–25. [CrossRef] [PubMed]
5. Fisher, H.E. Lust, attraction, and attachment in mammalian reproduction. *Hum. Nat.* **1998**, *9*, 23–52. [CrossRef]
6. Hatfield, E. Passionate and companionate love. In *The Psychology of Love*; Sternberg, R.J., Barnes, M.L., Eds.; Yale University Press: New Haven, CT, USA, 1988; pp. 191–217.
7. Sternberg, R.J. A triangular theory of love. *Psychol. Rev.* **1986**, *93*, 119–135. [CrossRef]
8. Thoits, P.A. The sociology of emotions. *Annu. Rev. Sociol.* **1989**, *15*, 317–342. [CrossRef]
9. Langeslag, S.J.E.; Muris, P.; Franken, I.H. Measuring romantic love: Psychometric properties of the infatuation and attachment scales. *J. Sex Res.* **2013**, *50*, 739–747. [CrossRef]
10. Langeslag, S.J.E.; Sanchez, M.E. Down-regulation of love feelings after a romantic break-up: Self-report and electrophysiological data. *J. Exp. Psychol. Gen.* **2018**, *147*, 720–733. [CrossRef] [PubMed]
11. Zsok, F.; Haucke, M.; De Wit, C.Y.; Barelds, D.P. What kind of love is love at first sight? An empirical investigation. *Pers. Relatsh.* **2017**, *24*, 869–885. [CrossRef]
12. Erickson, S.E. Romantic parasocial attachments and the developments of romantic scripts, schemas and beliefs among adolescents. *Media Psychol.* **2018**, *21*, 111–136. [CrossRef]
13. Tuchakinsky, R.H. Para-romantic love and para-friendships: Development and assessment of a multiple-parasocial relationships scale. *Am. J. Media Psychol.* **2011**, *3*, 73–94.
14. Karhulahti, V.; Välisalo, T. Fictosexuality, fictoromance, and fictophilia: A qualitative study of love and desire for fictional characters. *Front. Psychol.* **2021**, *11*, 575427. [CrossRef] [PubMed]
15. Finkel, E.J.; Cheung, E.O.; Emery, L.F.; Carswell, K.L.; Larson, G.M. The suffocation model: Why marriage in America is becoming and all-or-nothing institution. *Curr. Dir. Psychol. Sci.* **2015**, *24*, 238–244. [CrossRef]
16. Langeslag, S.J.E.; Surti, K. Increasing love feelings, marital satisfaction, and motivated attention to the spouse. *J. Psychophysiol.* **2022**, *36*, 199–214. [CrossRef]
17. Acevedo, B.P.; Aron, A. Does a long-term relationship kill romantic love? *Rev. Gen. Psychol.* **2009**, *13*, 59–65. [CrossRef]
18. Funk, J.L.; Rogge, R.D. Testing the Ruler with Item Response Theory: Increasing Precision of Measurement for Relationship Satisfaction with the Couples Satisfaction Index. *J. Fam. Psychol.* **2007**, *21*, 572–583. [CrossRef] [PubMed]
19. Busby, D.M.; Christensen, C.; Crane, D.R.; Larson, J.H. A revision of the Dyadic Adjustment Scale for use for distressed and nondistressed couples: Construct hierarchy and multidimensional scales. *J. Marital. Fam. Ther.* **1995**, *21*, 289–308. [CrossRef]
20. Fehr, B.; Russell, J.A. Concept of emotion viewed from a prototype perspective. *J. Exp. Psychol. Gen.* **1984**, *113*, 464–486. [CrossRef]
21. Shaver, P.; Schwartz, J.; Kirson, D.; O'connor, C. Emotion knowledge: Further exploration of a prototype approach. *J. Personal. Soc. Psychol.* **1987**, *52*, 1061–1086. [CrossRef]
22. Shaver, P.R.; Morgan, H.J.; Wu, S. Is love a "basic" emotion? *Pers. Relatsh.* **1996**, *3*, 81–96. [CrossRef]
23. Cowen, A.S.; Keltner, D. Sematic space theory: A computational approach to emotion. *Trends Cogn. Sci.* **2021**, *25*, 124–136. [CrossRef] [PubMed]
24. Langeslag, S.J.E. Liefde is een motivatie, niet een emotie: Een neurobiologische benadering [Love is a motivation, not an emotion: A neurobiological approach]. *De Psycholoog* **2006**, *41*, 260–265.
25. Fisher, H.E.; Aron, A.; Mashek, D.; Li, H.; Brown, L.L. Defining the brain systems of lust, romantic attraction, and attachment. *Arch. Sex. Behav.* **2002**, *31*, 413–419. [CrossRef]
26. Leary, M.R.; Koch, E.J.; Hechenbleikner, N.R. Emotional responses to interpersonal rejection. In *Interpersonal Rejection*; Leary, M., Ed.; Oxford University Press: Oxford, UK, 2001; pp. 145–166.

27. Miceli, M.; Castelfranchi, C. Meta-emotions and the complexity of human emotional experience. *New Ideas Psychol.* **2019**, *55*, 43–49. [CrossRef]
28. Langeslag, S.J.E.; Van Strien, J.W. Regulation of romantic love feelings: Preconceptions, strategies and feasibility. *PLoS ONE* **2016**, *11*, e0161087. [CrossRef] [PubMed]
29. Verduyn, P.; Lavrijsen, S. Which emotions last longest and why: The role of event importance and rumination. *Motiv. Emot.* **2015**, *39*, 119–127. [CrossRef]
30. Hatfield, E.C.; Pillemer, J.T.; O'Brien, M.U.; Le, Y.C. The endurance of love: Passionate and companionate love in newlywed and long-term marriages. *Interpersona* **2008**, *2*, 35–64. [CrossRef]
31. Rubin, Z. Measurement of romantic love. *J. Personal. Soc. Psychol.* **1970**, *16*, 265–273. [CrossRef] [PubMed]
32. Skolnick, A. *The Intimate Environment: Exploring Marriage and the Family*, 2nd ed.; Little, Brown: Boston, MA, USA, 1987.
33. Lamy, L. Beyond emotion: Love as an encounter of myth and drive. *Emot. Rev.* **2016**, *8*, 97–107. [CrossRef]
34. Aron, A.; Aron, E.N. Comment: An inspiration for expanding the self-expansion model of love. *Emot. Rev.* **2016**, *8*, 112–113. [CrossRef]
35. Fisher, H.; Aron, A.; Brown, L.L. Romantic love: An fMRI study of a neural mechanism for mate choice. *J. Comp. Neurol.* **2005**, *493*, 58–62. [CrossRef] [PubMed]
36. Kim, H.K.; McKenry, P.C. The relationship between marriage and psychological well-being. *J. Fam. Issues* **2002**, *23*, 885–911. [CrossRef]
37. Marazziti, D.; Canale, D. Hormonal changes when falling in love. *Psychoneuroendocrinology* **2004**, *29*, 931–936. [CrossRef] [PubMed]
38. De Silva, P. Jealousy in couple relationships: Nature, assessment, and therapy. *Behav. Res. Ther.* **1997**, *35*, 973–985. [CrossRef] [PubMed]
39. Rosenzweig, A.; Prigerson, H.; Miller, M.D.; Reynolds, C.F., III. Breavement and late-life depression: Grief and its complications in the elderly. *Annu. Rev. Med.* **1997**, *48*, 421–428. [CrossRef] [PubMed]
40. Monroe, S.M.; Rohde, P.; Seeley, J.R.; Lewinsohn, P.M. Life events and depression in adolescence: Relationship loss as a prospective risk factor for first onset of major depressive disorder. *J. Abnorm. Psychol.* **1999**, *108*, 606–614. [CrossRef] [PubMed]
41. Amato, P.R. The consequences of divorce for adults and children. *J. Marriage Fam.* **2004**, *62*, 1269–1287. [CrossRef]
42. Proulx, C.M.; Helms, H.M.; Buehler, C. Marital quality and personal well-being: A meta-analysis. *J. Marriage Fam.* **2007**, *69*, 576–593. [CrossRef]
43. Langeslag, S.J.E.; Van der Veen, F.M.; Fekkes, D. Blood levels of serotonin are differentially affected by romantic love in men and women. *J. Psychophysiol.* **2012**, *26*, 92–98. [CrossRef]
44. Van Steenbergen, H.; Langeslag, S.J.; Band, G.P.; Hommel, B. Reduced cognitive control in passionate lovers. *Motiv. Emot.* **2014**, *38*, 444–450. [CrossRef]
45. American Psychiatric Association. *Diagnostic and Statistical Manual of Mental Disorders*, 5th ed.; DSM-5; American Psychiatric Association: Arlington, VA, USA, 2013.
46. Canetto, S.S.; Lester, D. Love and achievement motives in women's and men's suicide notes. *J. Psychol. Interdiscip. Appl.* **2002**, *136*, 573–576. [CrossRef] [PubMed]
47. Meloy, J.R.; Fisher, H. Some thoughts on the neurobiology of stalking. *J. Forensic Sci.* **2005**, *50*, 1472–1480. [CrossRef] [PubMed]
48. Garcia-Moreno, C.; Jansen, H.A.; Ellsberg, M.; Heise, L.; Watts, C.H. Prevalence of intimate partner violence: Findings from the WHO multi-country study on women's health and domestic violence. *Lancet* **2006**, *368*, 1260–1269. [CrossRef] [PubMed]
49. Wilt, S.; Olson, S. Prevalence of domestic violence in the United States. *J. Am. Women's Assoc.* **1996**, *51*, 77–82.
50. Wilson, M.; Daly, M. Spousal homicide risk and estrangement. *Violence Vict.* **1993**, *8*, 3–16. [CrossRef] [PubMed]
51. Horner, S.B.; Langeslag, S.J.E. Negative and positive reappraisal after a romantic break-up. *J. Stud. Res.* **2019**, *8*, 9–17. [CrossRef]
52. Surti, K.; Langeslag, S.J.E. Perceived ability to regulate love. *PLoS ONE* **2019**, *14*, e0216523. [CrossRef]
53. Langeslag, S.J.E.; Davis, L.L. A preliminary study on up-regulation of sexual desire for a long-term partner. *J. Sex. Med.* **2022**, *19*, 872–878. [CrossRef] [PubMed]
54. Langeslag, S.J.; Olivier, J.R.; Köhlen, M.E.; Nijs, I.M.; Van Strien, J.W. Increased attention and memory for beloved-related information during infatuation: Behavioral and electrophysiological data. *Soc. Cogn. Affect. Neurosci.* **2015**, *10*, 136–144. [CrossRef]
55. Roozendaal, B.; McEwen, B.S.; Chattarji, S. Stress, memory, and the amygdala. *Nat. Rev. Neurosci.* **2009**, *10*, 423–433. [CrossRef]
56. Phelps, E.A. Human emotion and memory: Interactions of the amygdala and hippocampal complex. *Curr. Opin. Neurobiol.* **2004**, *14*, 198–202. [CrossRef] [PubMed]
57. Guerra, P.; Campagnoli, R.R.; Vico, C.; Volchan, E.; Anllo-Vento, L.; Vila, J. Filial versus romantic love: Contributions from peripheral and central electrophysiology. *Biol. Psychol.* **2011**, *88*, 196–203. [CrossRef] [PubMed]
58. Iversen, S.; Iversen, L.; Saper, C. The autonomic nervous system and the hypothalamus. In *Principles of Neuroscience*; Kandel, E.R., Schwartz, J.H., Jessell, T.M., Eds.; McGraw Hill: New York, NY, USA, 2000; pp. 960–981.
59. Poldrak, R.A. Inferring mental states from neuroimaging data: From reverse inference to large-scale decoding. *Neuron* **2011**, *72*, 692–697. [CrossRef] [PubMed]
60. Earp, B.D.; Wudarczyk, O.A.; Sandberg, A.; Savulescu, J. If I could just stop loving you: Anti-love biotechnology and the ethics of a chemical breakup. *Am. J. Bioeth.* **2013**, *13*, 3–17. [CrossRef] [PubMed]

61. Wudarczyk, O.A.; Earp, B.D.; Guastella, A.; Savulescu, J. Could intranasal oxytocin be used to enhance relationships? Research imperatives, clinical policy, and ethical considerations. *Curr. Opin. Psychiatry* **2013**, *26*, 474–484. [CrossRef] [PubMed]
62. Earp, B.D.; Savulescu, J. What is love? Can it be chemically modified? Should it be? reply to commentaries. *Philos. Public Issues (New Ser.)* **2020**, *10*, 93–151.
63. Garasic, M.D. Love in the posthuman world: How neurointerventions could impact on our societal values. *Philos. Public Issues (New Ser.)* **2020**, *10*, 29–43.
64. Wedeck, H.E. *Love Potions through the Ages: A Study of Amatory Devices and Mores*; Open Road Media: New York, NY, USA, 2021.
65. Acevedo, B.P.; Aron, A.; Fisher, H.E.; Brown, L.L. Neural correlates of long-term intense romantic love. *Soc. Cogn. Affect. Neurosci.* **2012**, *7*, 145–159. [CrossRef]
66. Aron, A.; Fisher, H.; Mashek, D.J.; Strong, G.; Li, H.; Brown, L.L. Reward, motivation, and emotion systems associated with early-stage intense romantic love. *J. Neurophysiol.* **2005**, *94*, 327–337. [CrossRef]
67. Bartels, A.; Zeki, S. The neural basis of romantic love. *Neuroreport* **2000**, *11*, 3829–3834. [CrossRef]
68. Fisher, H.E.; Brown, L.L.; Aron, A.; Strong, G.; Mashek, D. Reward, addiction, and emotion regulation systems associated with rejection in love. *J. Neurophysiol.* **2010**, *104*, 51–60. [CrossRef] [PubMed]
69. Stoessel, C.; Stiller, J.; Bleich, S.; Boensch, D.; Doerfler, A.; Garcia, M.; Richter-Schmidinger, T.; Kornhuber, J.; Forster, C. Differences and similarities on neuronal activities of people being happily and unhappily in love: A functional magnetic resonance imaging study. *Neuropsychobiology* **2011**, *64*, 52–60. [CrossRef] [PubMed]
70. Xu, X.; Aron, A.; Brown, L.; Cao, G.; Feng, T.; Weng, X. Reward and motivation systems: A brain mapping study of early-stage intense romantic love in Chinese participants. *Hum. Brain Mapp.* **2011**, *32*, 249–257. [CrossRef] [PubMed]
71. Younger, J.; Aron, A.; Parke, S.; Chatterjee, N.; Mackey, S. Viewing pictures of a romantic partner reduces experimental pain: Involvement of neural reward systems. *PLoS ONE* **2010**, *5*, e13309. [CrossRef] [PubMed]
72. Langeslag, S.J.E.; Van der Veen, F.M.; Röder, C.H. Attention modulates the dorsal striatum response to love stimuli. *Hum. Brain Mapp.* **2014**, *35*, 503–512. [CrossRef]
73. Takahashi, K.; Mizuno, K.; Sasaki, A.T.; Wada, Y.; Tanaka, M.; Ishii, A.; Tajima, K.; Tsuyuguchi, N.; Watanabe, K.; Zeki, S.; et al. Imaging the passionate stage of romantic love by dopamine dynamics. *Front. Hum. Neurosci.* **2015**, *9*, 191. [CrossRef]

Disclaimer/Publisher's Note: The statements, opinions and data contained in all publications are solely those of the individual author(s) and contributor(s) and not of MDPI and/or the editor(s). MDPI and/or the editor(s) disclaim responsibility for any injury to people or property resulting from any ideas, methods, instructions or products referred to in the content.

MDPI AG
Grosspeteranlage 5
4052 Basel
Switzerland
Tel.: +41 61 683 77 34

Behavioral Sciences Editorial Office
E-mail: behavsci@mdpi.com
www.mdpi.com/journal/behavsci

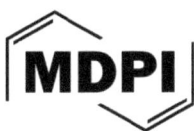

Disclaimer/Publisher's Note: The title and front matter of this reprint are at the discretion of the Guest Editors. The publisher is not responsible for their content or any associated concerns. The statements, opinions and data contained in all individual articles are solely those of the individual Editors and contributors and not of MDPI. MDPI disclaims responsibility for any injury to people or property resulting from any ideas, methods, instructions or products referred to in the content.

www.ingramcontent.com/pod-product-compliance
Lightning Source LLC
LaVergne TN
LVHW072333090526
838202LV00019B/2414